EVIDENCE-BASED PRACTICE
ACROSS THE **HEALTH PROFESSIONS**

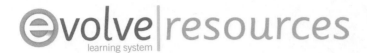

Evolve – the Latest Evolution in Learning

Evolve provides online access to free learning resources and activities designed specifically to enhance the textbook you are using in your class.

Visit this website and start your learning Evolution today!
Login: http://evolve.elsevier.com/AU/Hoffmann/evidence/

This website contains additional activities not covered in the book for most chapters. These materials are designed to encourage and consolidate learning and should be used by readers to further examine and explore the content of the relevant chapters.

Evolve online courseware for **Evidence-based Practice across the Health Professions** offers:

- Multiple-choice questions and answers
- True/false questions and answers
- Short answer questions and answers
- Classification questions and answers
- Completion questions and answers.

Think outside the book…evolve.

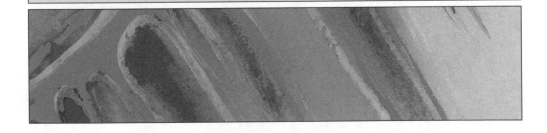

EVIDENCE-BASED PRACTICE
ACROSS THE **HEALTH PROFESSIONS**

Tammy Hoffmann
Sally Bennett
Chris Del Mar

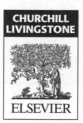

CHURCHILL
LIVINGSTONE

ELSEVIER

Sydney Edinburgh London New York Philadelphia St Louis Toronto

BS

Churchill Livingstone
is an imprint of Elsevier

Elsevier Australia. ACN 001 002 357
(a division of Reed International Books Australia Pty Ltd)
Tower 1, 475 Victoria Avenue, Chatswood, NSW 2067

ELSEVIER

National Library of Australia Cataloguing-in-Publication Data

Hoffmann, Tammy.

Evidence based practice across the health professions /
Tammy Hoffmann, Sally Bennett, Chris Del Mar.

ISBN: 978 0 7295 3902 9 (pbk.)

Includes index.
Bibliography.

Clinical medicine--Decision making.
Evidence-based medicine.

Bennett, Sally.
Del Mar, Chris.

616

Publishing Editor: Sunalie Silva
Developmental Editor: Meg O'Hanlon
Publishing Services Manager: Helena Klijn
Editorial Coordinator: Eleanor Cant
Edited by Linda Littlemore
Proofread by Tim Learner
Cover and internal design by Avril Makula
Index by Michael Ferreira
Typeset by TNQ Books and Journals
Printed by Ligare

PEFC
PEFC/21-31-17

This book has been printed on paper certified
by the Programme for the Endorsement of
Forest Certification (PEFC). PEFC is
committed to sustainable forest management
through third party forest certification
of responsibly managed forests.

10/7/10

Contents

Foreword

Clinicians have talked for decades, concentrating on the meaning of words without worrying too much about the clarity of their propositions. The concept of evidence-based decision making has smashed into the pack ice like a small but well-designed icebreaker, and it is now clear that the propositions made by clinicians can be divided into those assertions that can be substantiated by evidence and those which are made on the basis of experience or beliefs. Propositions based on evidence are not morally superior to other types of propositions but they do provide a stronger base for decision making, hence the term 'evidence-based decision making'.

Evidence-based decision making, like most paradigms, was fiercely resisted by the clinical professions when it was first raised, but Iain Chalmers, who counselled me when going to speak at one of the debates that were once common along the lines of 'This House deplores the concept of evidence-based medicine', said that I should take heart and simply tell the clinicians that when patients were campaigning against evidence-based medicine then we would be worried.

Evidence-based medicine does not do away with the need for human skills or clinical judgement; in fact, it makes their role clearer and more accountable. Evidence-based clinical practice is just what it says on the tin—evidence-based. To the evidence has to be brought the needs of the particular patient (their other diagnoses and risk factors, for example), and the third factor is their values. Evidence, particular needs and values—these three things must come together; the evidence helps make the decision but the decision has to be taken by the clinician and the patient.

If evidence-based decision making was the paradigm of the 1990s, what is the paradigm of the 21st century? The answer is clear. The 20th century was the century of the clinician; the 21st century is the century of the patient, and all patients should have full and equal access to all evidence; that is the next move.

This book provides an excellent foundation for evidence-based decision making, covering a wide range of topics and skills. It provides worked examples from multiple health professions and discusses the importance of clinical reasoning and communication with patients in detail.

Health care is still delivered by professions whose shape has remained largely unchanged since the 19th century. There are two approaches to dealing with this problem. The first is to try to reshape the boundaries of the professions as we know them; that does not seem a very profitable line to take. Another approach is to focus on the tasks and functions that all need to be involved in, and worry less about who does what and more about what needs to be done. Evidence-based decision making is common to all professions and provides an ideal platform for multidisciplinary work. Different professions bring different perspectives to bear on the evidence, on relating the evidence to the individual and on helping the individual reflect on their values as they consider how the evidence affects the options presented to them. With this in mind, this book provides examples of the use of evidence from many different health professions. Importantly, the evidence-based approach offers the opportunity for professionals to work more closely together without agonising over their roles.

Sir Muir Gray, CBE
Director, National Knowledge Service
Chief Knowledge Officer to the National Health Service (NHS)

Preface

This book aims to provide enough basic knowledge to enable any health professional to develop skills for evidence-based practice. We hope that this book will be useful regardless of whether the reader is a practising health professional or an undergraduate, graduate-entry or post-graduate student, either with or without clinical experience. Little, if any, previous exposure to the concepts of evidence-based practice is needed.

So why do we think that another book about evidence-based practice is needed? This book deliberately targets a wide range of health professions (medicine, occupational therapy, physiotherapy, speech pathology, podiatry, nursing, nutrition therapy, complementary and alternative medicine, medical imaging and radiation therapy). Other health professions that are not specifically mentioned, such as social work or psychology, are also likely to find it relevant and useful to clinical practice.

We have led classes in evidence-based practice for students from a range of health professions. We noted how worked examples from their own health profession were preferred by students as they were more quickly understood, relevant and helped contextualise learning. One of the unique features of this book is that it includes examples written by, and for, a wide range of health professions to facilitate learning and to make it easier to provide training in evidence-based practice to interdisciplinary groups.

This book also contains content that we consider to be very important to the process of evidence-based practice, but that most books about evidence-based practice do not explicitly address. Specifically, we have included a chapter about how to talk with clients about evidence. It includes a range of practical strategies to facilitate shared decision making and effective communication with clients. There is also a chapter about clinical reasoning and its interface with evidence-based practice, as an understanding of clinical reasoning can clarify, and hopefully improve, clinical decision making.

Special thanks go to all of the contributors who wrote this book with us and to the people who also reviewed chapters (John Bennett, Annie McCluskey, Denise O'Connor, Leigh Tooth). Any errors are ours. Please send us information about errors or improvements. If you send them to us (feedback@elsevier.com.au) and we incorporate them in future editions, we will acknowledge your contribution. We hope that the skills learnt through reading this book will help make sense of some of the complexity of clinical decision making and contribute to better outcomes for clients.

Tammy Hoffmann, Sally Bennett and Chris Del Mar
30th January 2009

Contributors

Marilyn Baird BA, DCR, PhD **Associate Professor and Foundation Head, Department of Medical Imaging and Radiation Sciences, Monash University, Melbourne, Victoria, Australia;** Marilyn created the curriculum for the four-year Bachelor of Radiography and Medical Imaging which commenced in 1998. Subsequently she has successfully supervised the introduction of an articulated masters degree in medical ultrasound and graduate entry masters programs in radiation therapy and nuclear medicine. Her research interests are primarily directed towards improving clinical teaching and learning. In June 2008 she was re-appointed by the Minister of Health (Victoria) as President of the Medical Radiation Practitioners Board of Victoria for 2008–2011.

John W Bennett BMedSc, MBBS, BA(Hons), PhD, FRACGP, FACHI **Discipline of General Practice, School of Medicine, and The University of Queensland Health Service, The University of Queensland, Brisbane, Australia;** John is a practice principal at the University Health Service, The University of Queensland, and regularly uses evidence-based medicine in his clinical practice. He has taught evidence-based medicine in Brisbane and Oxford (at the Centre for Evidence-Based Medicine) and has co-authored a number of articles relevant to evidence-based practice. He is on the Royal Australian College of General Practitioners' Quality Care committee that uses evidence in the production of resources for general practitioners.

Sally Bennett BOccThy(Hons), PhD **Lecturer, Division of Occupational Therapy, School of Health and Rehabilitation Sciences, The University of Queensland, Brisbane, Australia;** Sally is an occupational therapist with both clinical and research experience. She has designed an evidence-based practice curriculum and taught evidence-based practice to occupational therapy, physiotherapy and speech pathology students for eight years. She has undertaken research in evidence-based practice, including her PhD, and is contributing to multiple Cochrane reviews. She helped establish the OTseeker database (which she currently manages) that contains citations of systematic reviews and randomised controlled trials relevant to occupational therapy. She is active in both national and international professional committees as an advisor on evidence-based practice and is also a member of the Critically Appraised Papers Advisory Board for the Australian Occupational Therapy Journal.

Jeff Coombes BEd(Hons), BAppSc, MEd, PhD **Associate Professor in Exercise Science, The University of Queensland, Brisbane, Australia;** Jeff Coombes is also the President of the Australian Association for Exercise and Sports Science and is an accredited exercise physiologist and lectures to students on exercise prescription and programming and interprofessional education. He directs a research program that attempts to improve the evidence base about the effects of exercise training on conditions such as cardiovascular disease, diabetes and kidney disease.

Chris Del Mar BSc, MA, MB BChir, MD, FRACGP, FAFPHM **Dean of Health Sciences and Medicine and PVC (Research), Bond University, Gold Coast, Queensland, Australia;** Chris was educated in science and medicine and worked as a general practitioner until 1988 when he took up an academic position at the University of Queensland, where he was Professor of General Practice from 1995 to 2004. He has undertaken research into health services and also clinical areas, including evidence-based practice. He has published over 250 research articles, reviews, book chapters and books. He was Editor of the research section of the *Australian Family Physician*; Chair of the Royal Australian College of General Practitioners (RACGP) National Research Committee; President of the Australian Association for Academic General Practice and Chair of the editorial committee of the Australian Government's health web portal, HealthInsite. He is a Coordinating Editor of the International Cochrane Collaboration and is a Visiting Professor of General Practice at Oxford University.

Jenny Doust BA, BEcons, BMBS, Grad Dip Clin Epi, PhD, FRACGP **Professor of Public Health, Faculty of Health Sciences and Medicine, Bond University, Gold Coast, Queensland, Australia;** Jenny has worked and trained as a general practitioner, clinical epidemiologist and economist. Since graduating in medicine, she has worked in positions that combine her interests in these three areas. Her main research areas of interest are diagnosis, screening and evidence-based practice in clinical practice. She is a member of the Cochrane Systematic Reviews of Diagnostic Accuracy Methods Working Group.

Mark R Elkins BPhty, BA, MHSc, PhD **Senior Research Physiotherapist, Royal Prince Alfred Hospital, Sydney, New South Wales, Australia;** As part of his research position Mark conducts original research and performs systematic reviews, primarily in the areas of physiotherapy and respiratory disease. He is a co-director of the Centre for Evidence-Based Physiotherapy, which maintains the Physiotherapy Evidence Database (PEDro). He is also a Clinical Senior Lecturer at the Central Clinical School of Medicine at the University of Sydney and has published and presented workshops in the area of evidence-based physiotherapy.

Joy Higgs AM, BSc, Grad Dip Phty, MHPEd, PhD **Strategic Research Professor in Professional Practice in The Research Institute for Professional Practice, Learning and Education and Director of The Education for Practice Institute, Charles Sturt University, North Paramatta, New South Wales, Australia ;** Joy has worked in health sciences research and education for over 25 years. She has published widely, including 14 books, in her fields of expertise in professional practice, practice knowledge, clinical reasoning, qualitative research and professional education. In 2008 she published the third edition of *Clinical Reasoning in the Health Professions* with Mark Jones and colleagues. Joy is an experienced research supervisor and many of her students have researched clinical reasoning and professional practice.

Tammy Hoffmann BOccThy(Hons), PhD **Lecturer, Division of Occupational Therapy, School of Health and Rehabilitation Sciences, The University of Queensland, Brisbane, Australia;** Tammy is an occupational therapist with clinical, academic and research experience. One of her teaching interests is evidence-based practice and she coordinates and lectures in evidence-based practice courses to undergraduate, graduate entry and postgraduate students from a number of health professions. Evidence-based practice is also one of her research interests and she has published a number of articles in this area. Tammy has also researched and published widely in the area of client education. She has delivered numerous workshops on evidence-based practice to interdisciplinary groups of health professionals. Tammy is a member of the team that developed and maintains the occupational therapy evidence database, OTseeker (www.otseeker.com) and is a member of the Critically Appraised Papers Advisory Board for the *Australian Occupational Therapy Journal*.

Jonathon Kruger BPhysio, MPH **Manager, Policy and Communication, The Australian Physiotherapy Association;** Jonathon was previously a senior physiotherapist at a major teaching hospital in Melbourne, Australia. During this time he was responsible for the successful strategic restructure of the service to improve customer focus through establishment of a sustainable evidence-based framework for clinical practice in physiotherapy. In recent years he has moved into the field of health policy and has undertaken senior advisory roles for a number of organisations. This work has involved analysing and developing evidence-based public health policy and programs in areas such as developmental health and wellbeing, environmental health, men's health, chronic disease and the health workforce.

Susan Leicht Doyle MS, OTR/L **Lead Therapist and Occupational Therapist, Inpatient Rehabilitation Unit, Southwest Washington Medical Center, Vancouver, USA;** Sue has worked as an occupational therapist for almost three decades in Australia and the USA. She was Assistant Professor, Occupational Therapy, at Ithaca College NY from 1999 to 2004 where she was involved with incorporating evidence-based practice into the curriculum. Sue is also a Cochrane Review author for the stroke group. Her post-professional masters degree research was in clinical reasoning and her current PhD research includes exploring how therapists define and incorporate evidence into their reasoning process when working with people who have had a stroke.

Craig Lockwood RN, BN, GradDip, MNsc **Associate Director—Evidence Review and Innovation, The Joanna Briggs Institute, Adelaide, South Australia, Australia;** Craig Lockwood is the Associate Director for Evidence Review and Innovation at the Joanna Briggs Institute (JBI) and coordinates the JBI Evidence Review team which maintains and develops the JBI COnNECT nodes and content. His interests are in methods and outcomes of qualitative synthesis; the conduct of systematic reviews of healthcare interventions, practices and experiences; and in methods to promote the implementation and evaluation of evidence-based practice. Craig is a registered general nurse with a clinical background in renal and dermatological nursing.

Annie McCluskey DipCOT, MA, PhD **Senior Lecturer (Occupational Therapy) and NHMRC-NICS-HCF Foundation Fellow (2007–2009), Faculty of Health Sciences, The University of Sydney, New South Wales, Australia;** Annie is an occupational therapist, health services researcher, NHMRC-NICS-HCF Foundation Fellow, and co-developer of the freely available OTseeker evidence database (www.otseeker.com) and OT CATs website (www.otcats.com). Her research has investigated the effect of teaching health professionals how to search for and appraise evidence, the process of becoming an evidence-based practitioner and evidence indexed on OTseeker. Annie is currently investigating the implementation of evidence by community rehabilitation teams in Sydney, to help improve outcomes for people with stroke. NICS is an institute of the National Health and Medical Research Council (NHMRC), Australia's peak body for supporting health and medical research. The NHMRC-NICS fellowships aim to identify and support future leaders in evidence-based practice and to build a community of practitioners with the expertise to support other health professionals to overcome the barriers to applying evidence.

Ann McKibbon MLS, PhD **Associate Professor, Health Information Research Unit, Department of Clinical Epidemiology and Biostatistics, McMaster University, Hamilton, Ontario, Canada;** Ann's background is information sciences and her PhD is in informatics. She teaches in the Health Research Methodology program although most of her recent effort has been to develop a new MSc in eHealth and an affiliated eHealth Research Network. Her research focuses on the use of information resources by health professionals, information retrieval and knowledge translation.

Angela Morgan BSpAud (Hons), PhD **Postdoctoral Research Fellow, Murdoch Children's Research Institute, Melbourne, Victoria, Australia; Speech Pathology Department, Royal Children's Hospital, Melbourne, Victoria, Australia; Department of Paediatrics,**

University of Melbourne, Victoria, Australia; Angela has over 10 years of clinical and research experience in paediatric rehabilitation in Australia and the United Kingdom (UK). She gained an international view of evidence-based practice in paediatric rehabilitation through her experience as a Research Lecturer in the UK from 2004 to 2006 (at the Institute of Child Health, University College London, conjointly with The Children's Trust Rehabilitation Centre). She returned to Australia in 2006 to develop an NHMRC-funded research program focused on paediatric speech and swallowing problems associated with acquired brain injury.

Denise O'Connor BAppScOT(Hons), PhD **Senior Research Fellow, Monash Institute of Health Services Research, Monash University, Melbourne, Victoria, Australia;** Denise currently project manages a cluster randomised controlled trial concerned with knowledge transfer and exchange (KTE) in allied health. She is also an investigator on other KTE research projects, an active Cochrane systematic review author and editor with the Cochrane Neuromuscular Disease Group. Previously she worked as a Lecturer with the Australasian Cochrane Centre where she coordinated training and support for Australasian Cochrane authors.

Alan Pearson RN, ONC, DipNEd, MSc, PhD, FCN, FRCNA, FAAG, FRCN **Executive Director, The Joanna Briggs Institute, Adelaide, South Australia, Australia; Professor of Evidence-Based Health Care, The University of Adelaide, South Australia, Australia;** Alan has extensive experience in clinical practice in the UK, the USA, Papua New Guinea and Australia. He is the Editor of the *International Journal of Nursing Practice* and is Expert Adviser to the World Health Organisation's World Alliance on Patient Safety; Expert Adviser to Guidelines International Network; Co-Convenor of the Cochrane Qualitative Research Methods Group; and is the foundation Executive Director of the Joanna Briggs Institute. He has been involved in advancing evidence-based practice in China, Taiwan, Korea, Hong Kong, Singapore, Thailand, Myanmar (Burma), Spain, fourteen African countries, the USA, Canada, Romania, the UK and Australia.

Sheena Reilly BAppSc, PhD **Professor of Paediatric Speech Pathology, Department of Paediatrics, The University of Melbourne, Victoria, Australia; Professor–Director of Speech Pathology, The Royal Children's Hospital, Melbourne, Victoria, Australia; Director, Healthy Development Research, Murdoch Children's Research Institute, Melbourne, Victoria, Australia;** Sheena holds a National Health and Medical Research Council (NHMRC) practitioner fellowship and her research focuses on speech and language development, and the prevalence and predictors of communication and swallowing difficulties in children. Sheena has a strong interest in evidence-based practice, particularly the application of evidence-based practice to speech pathology. She is co-editor of the book *Evidence-Based Practice in Speech Pathology* and is on the editorial board of Evidence-Based Communication Assessment and Intervention.

Sharon Sanders BSc(Pod), MPH **Discipline of General Practice, The University of Queensland, Brisbane, Australia;** While working as a podiatrist in the public health service Sharon completed a Masters of Public Health and, for the last 10 years, she has been working at The University of Queensland researching and teaching the skills of evidence-based practice to students and health professionals from a range of disciplines.

Michal Schneider-Kolsky Sc, DipEd, MRepSc, GradCertHealthProfEdu, PhD **Senior Lecturer, Department of Medical Imaging and Radiation Sciences, Monash University, Melbourne, Victoria, Australia;** Michal trained as a scientist with a PhD in Obstetrics and Gynaecology and a Masters in Reproductive Physiology. She conducts lectures and workshops on evidence-based practice and research methodology to undergraduate and postgraduate students.

Jemma Skeat BSpPath(Hons), PhD **Postdoctoral Research Fellow, Murdoch Children's Research Institute, Melbourne, Victoria, Australia; Speech Pathology Department, Royal Children's Hospital, Melbourne, Victoria, Australia; Department of Paediatrics, University of Melbourne, Victoria, Australia;** Jemma is a clinical speech pathologist and researcher, with a background in both qualitative and quantitative research. Jemma has an interest in evaluating qualitative evidence and speech pathologists' use of evidence in practice.

Alan Spencer MPH, Grad Dip Diet, BSc(Hons) **Director of Nutrition Services, Gold Coast Health Service District, Queensland, Australia;** Alan is a clinical dietitian for the Intensive Care Unit and parenteral nutrition services at the Gold Coast Hospital. He is also a teaching fellow for the School of Health Science at Bond University. He has a long-standing interest in evidence-based practice and is a member of the Gold Coast District evidence-based practice committee and is an active contributor to Bond University's evidence-based practice workshops.

Leigh Tooth BOccThy(Hons) PhD **Senior Research Fellow, Australian Longitudinal Study on Women's Health, School of Population Health, The University of Queensland, Brisbane, Australia;** Leigh is a graduate in occupational therapy and has had both a clinical and research career. She was previously an NHMRC Fellow with the Longitudinal Studies Unit in the School of Population Health researching statistical methodology and teaching in the epidemiology program. Her current research interests include women's health, outcome evaluation, longitudinal methods, quality of life, comorbidity and epidemiology. Leigh is one of the founding chief investigators of the OTseeker database.

Merrill Turpin BOccThy, Grad Dip Counsel, PhD **Lecturer, Division of Occupational Therapy, School of Health and Rehabilitation Sciences, The University of Queensland, Brisbane, Australia;** Merrill's professional areas of expertise include occupational therapy philosophy and professional issues and clinical/professional reasoning and evidence-based practice. She uses a range of qualitative research methods to understand diverse aspects of people's experiences as well as organisational culture and service development processes.

Luis Vitetta GradDip IntegrMed, GradDip Nutr/EnvironMed, PhD **Associate Professor and Principal Research Fellow, Unit of Health Integration, School of Medicine, The University of Queensland, Brisbane, Australia; Director, The University of Queensland National Institute of Complementary Medicine Collaborative Centre;** From 2000 to 2005, Luis was the Deputy Head and Director of Research of the Graduate School of Integrative Medicine at Swinburne University, where he was involved in developing and delivering evidence-based complementary medicine modules for postgraduate programs to medical practitioners and allied health professionals.

Nancy L Wilczynski MSc, PhD **Assistant Professor and Research Manager, Health Information Research Unit (HIRU), Department of Clinical Epidemiology and Biostatistics, McMaster University, Hamilton, Ontario, Canada;** Nancy teaches in the Health Research Methodology Program in the Faculty of Sciences which provides training at the MSc and PhD levels. She oversees the research conducted in the HIRU which is focused on the field of health information science and is dedicated to the generation of new knowledge about the nature of health and clinical information problems, the development of new information resources to support evidence-based health care and the evaluation of various innovations in overcoming healthcare information problems.

Caroline Wright Msc, PGCE, BSC (Hons), DCR (T) **Senior Lecturer in Radiation Therapy, Department of Medical Imaging and Radiation Sciences, Monash University, Melbourne, Victoria, Australia;** Caroline's current role is convening the graduate entry Masters of Radiation Therapy at Monash University. Her research interests include the assessment and regulation of fitness to practice in students and professionals, clinical assessment and advancing practice in the profession. She is a member of the Editorial Review Board for the *Journal of Radiotherapy in Practice* and a member of the Medical Radiations Practitioner Board of the Victoria Education Committee.

Rachel Yates BTEC (UK), BSc(Hons) **Director of Policy, The Australian General Practice Network;** Prior to Rachel's current position, she was a Research Manager in an academic general practice unit with a research focus on asthma and obesity. The Australian General Practice Network is the peak Australian body for the general practice network and supports the delivery of quality primary care to Australian communities through general practice and the broader multidisciplinary team. This includes a focus on promoting the uptake of evidence-based practice.

Reviewers

Jenny Wilkinson BSc, PhD, GradDipFET, MHEd
Associate Professor in Anatomy and Physiology, Course Coordinator BHlthSc(ComplMed), School of Biomedical Sciences, Charles Sturt University, New South Wales, Australia

Megan Davidson BAppSci(Physio), PhD
Head of School, School of Physiotherapy, La Trobe University, Victoria, Australia

CHAPTER 1

Introduction to evidence-based practice

Tammy Hoffmann, Sally Bennett and Chris Del Mar

LEARNING OBJECTIVES

After reading this chapter, you should be able to:

- Explain what is meant by the term evidence-based practice
- Understand the origins of evidence-based practice
- Explain why evidence-based practice is important
- Describe the scope of evidence-based health care
- List and briefly explain each of the five steps that make up the evidence-based practice process

What is evidence-based practice?

There is a famous definition by Professor David Sackett and some of his colleagues which declares evidence-based medicine to be explicit and conscientious attempts to find the best available research evidence to assist health professionals to make the best decisions for their clients.[1] Even though this definition was originally given with respect to evidence-based medicine, it is often extended beyond the medical profession and used to define evidence-based practice as well. The definition may sound rather ambiguous, so let us pick its elements apart so that you can fully appreciate what is meant by the term evidence-based practice.

The purpose of evidence-based practice is to assist in clinical decision making. To make informed clinical decisions, we need to integrate lots of pieces of information. As health professionals, we are typically very good at seeking information from our clients and their families and from the settings in which we work but, traditionally, have not been as aware of the information that we can gain from research. When Sackett and his colleagues refer to 'evidence', they clarify it by specifying 'evidence from research'. So, although we need information from many sources, evidence-based practice shows how research can also play a role in informing clinical decisions. Let us sidetrack for a moment to look briefly at what research can offer us to enhance our clinical decision making.

We are familiar with the importance of research for testing theories and for providing us with the background information that forms part of our clinical knowledge. Knowledge about subjects such as anatomy, pathology, psychology and social structures that is essential to our work has been refined over many years through research. Our science-based training gives us models on which to base our clinical management of clients. Of course, having an understanding of the mechanisms is important—for example, we could never have made sense of heart failure or diabetes without understanding the basic mechanisms of these illnesses. Yet, focussing only on the mechanisms of illness can be misleading. Evidence-based practice encourages us to concentrate instead on testing the information directly. This is actually difficult for health professionals to do because we have been trained to consider primarily the underlying mechanisms. Table 1.1 gives some clinical examples to illustrate how the two approaches differ.

Returning to exploring the elements of the definition of evidence-based practice, the definition very deliberately states that attempts to find evidence should be 'explicit' and 'conscientious'. There is a good reason for this. Prior to the advent of evidence-based practice, the way in which many health professionals accessed research was somewhat haphazard and their understanding of how to accurately interpret research results was often superficial. In other words, we may not have been making the best use of research to inform our clinical decision making. For example, simply using whatever research evidence you happen to obtain from reading the few journals that you subscribe to is not going to sufficiently meet your clinical information needs. Hence, the definition of evidence-based practice encourages us to be 'explicit' and 'conscientious' in our attempts at locating the best evidence from research.

That leads us to explore what is meant by the term *best* evidence from research. Understanding what the different study designs can and cannot help you with and, if you like, what their pros and cons are is important. Part of the skill of evidence-based practice is being able to locate the type of study design that is best suited to the particular type of information that you need in order to make a clinical decision. Further, as we will explain in more detail later in this chapter, some studies have not been designed very well

Previous recommendation (based on a mechanism approach)	Rationale based on a mechanism approach	The empirical research that showed it was wrong
Put babies onto their fronts when they go to sleep	If they should vomit in their sleep, they might swallow the vomit into their lungs and develop pneumonia (Dr Spock in the 1950s)[2]	Observational data have shown that babies are more likely to die of sudden infant death syndrome (SIDS) if they lie on their fronts, rather than on their backs, when sleeping[3]
Bed rest after a heart attack (myocardial infarct)	The heart needs resting after an insult in which some of the heart muscle dies	Randomised controlled trials showed that bed rest makes thromboembolism (a dangerous condition in which a clot blocks the flow of blood through a blood vessel) much more likely[4]
Covering skin wounds after removal of skin cancer	To prevent bacteria gaining access and therefore causing infection	A randomised controlled trial showed that leaving the skin wounds open does not increase the infection rate[5]

TABLE 1.1 Examples of how focussing only on the mechanisms of illness can be misleading

and this reduces the confidence that we have in their conclusions. We therefore need to attempt to find the best quality research that is available.

The beginning of the definition of evidence-based medicine according to Sackett and colleagues (1996), introduced at the beginning of this chapter, is well known and often quoted. However, the section that follows is also important. It reads:

The practice of evidence-based medicine means integrating individual clinical expertise with the best available external clinical evidence from systematic research. By individual clinical expertise we mean the proficiency and judgement that individual clinicians acquire through clinical experiences and clinical practice. Increased expertise is reflected in many ways, but especially in more effective and efficient diagnosis and in the more thoughtful identification and compassionate use of individual patients' predicaments, rights, and preferences in making clinical decisions about their care.[1]

This definition makes it clear that evidence-based practice also requires clinical expertise, which includes thoughtfulness and compassion as well as knowledge of effectiveness and efficiency. As this is a key aspect of evidence-based practice, we will consider the concept of clinical expertise in more depth in Chapter 15.

A simple definition of evidence-based practice

Over time, the definition of evidence-based practice has been expanded upon and refined. Nowadays one of the most frequently used and widely known definitions of evidence-based practice acknowledges that it involves the integration of the best research evidence with clinical expertise and the client's values and circumstances.[6] It also requires the health professional to take into account characteristics of the practice context in which

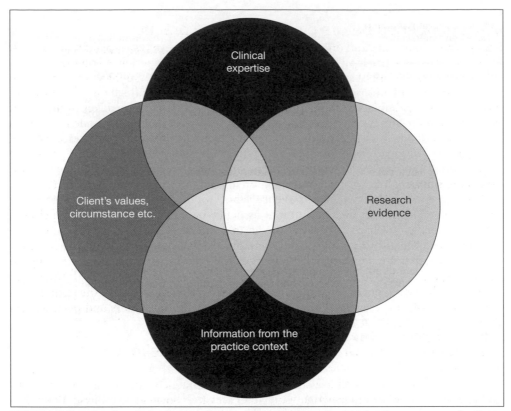

FIGURE 1.1 Evidence-based practice involves using clinical reasoning to integrate information from four sources: research evidence, clinical expertise, the client's values and circumstances and the practice context

they work. This is illustrated in Figure 1.1. As you read this book, keep this definition in mind. Evidence-based practice is *not* just about using research evidence as some critics of it may suggest. It is also about valuing and using the education, skills and experience that you have as a health professional. Furthermore, it is also about considering the client's situation and values when making a decision, as well as considering characteristics of the practice context in which you are interacting with your client. This requires judgement and artistry, as well as science and logic. The process that health professionals use to integrate all of this information is clinical reasoning. When you take these four elements and combine them in a way that enables you to make decisions about the care of a client, then you are engaging in evidence-based practice.

Where did evidence-based practice come from?

It came from a new medical school that started in the 1970s at McMaster University in Canada. The new medical program was unusual in several respects. One difference was that it was very short (only three years). This meant that its teachers realised that the notion of teaching medical students everything that they needed to know was clearly impossible. All they could hope for was to teach them how to find for themselves what they needed to know. How could they do that? The answer was the birth of evidence-based medicine, and hence evidence-based practice.

What happened before evidence-based practice?

This is a good question, and one that clients often ask whenever we explain to them what evidence-based practice is all about. We often relied just on 'experience', on the expertise of colleagues who were older and 'better' and on what we were taught as students. Each of these sources of information can be flawed and there is good data to show this.[7] Experience is very subject to flaws of bias. We overemphasise the mistakes of the recent past, and underestimate the rare mistakes. What we were taught as students is often woefully out of date.[8] The health professions are, by their nature, very conservative, and so relying on colleagues who are older and better (so-called 'eminence-based practice'[9]) as an information source will often provide us with information that is out of date, biased and, quite simply, often wrong.

This is not to say that clinical experience is not important. In fact, it is so important that it is a key feature in the definition of evidence-based practice. Clinical experience (discussed further in Chapter 15) is knowledge that is generated from practical experience and involves thoughtfulness and compassion as well as knowledge about the practices and activities that are specific to a discipline. However, rather than simply relying on clinical experience alone for decision making, we need to use our clinical experience together with other types of information. To help us make sense of all of the information that we have—from research, from clinical settings, from our clients and from clinical experience—we use clinical reasoning processes.

Is evidence-based practice the same as 'guidelines'?

No. As you will see in Chapter 13, guidelines are one way that evidence-based practice can help to get the best available evidence into clinical practice, but they are by no means the only way. To make matters worse, guidelines are often not evidence-based. When this is the case, they are worse than any evidence-based practice alternatives.

Is evidence-based practice the same as randomised controlled trials?

No. As you will see in Chapter 4, it is certainly true that randomised controlled trials are the cornerstone of research investigating whether *interventions* ('treatments') work. However, questions about interventions are not the only type of question that health professionals need good research information about. For example, health professionals also need good information about questions of: *aetiology* (what causes disease or makes it more likely); *frequency* (how common it is); *diagnosis* (how we know if the client has the disease or condition of interest); *prognosis* (what happens to the condition over time); and what the *client's experiences and concerns* are in particular situations. In this book, we will primarily focus on how to answer four main types of questions—concerning the effects of interventions, diagnosis, prognosis and clients' experiences and concerns—as these questions are relevant to a range of health professionals and are asked commonly by them. Each question type requires a different type of research design (of which randomised controlled trials are just one example) to address it. Other research designs include *qualitative research, case-control studies, cross-sectional studies* and *cohort studies*. There are many others. They can all be examples of the best evidence for some research questions. This is explored in more depth in Chapter 2.

Can anyone practise evidence-based practice?

Yes. With the right training, practice and experience, any of us can learn how to do evidence-based practice competently. You do not have to be an expert in anything. Having access to the internet and databases (such as PubMed and the Cochrane Library) is good. And having some trustworthy colleagues to check your more surprising findings is also good.

Do health professionals have time for an activity like evidence-based practice?

Health professionals do not have to commit more time to evidence-based practice than they are comfortable with. Actually, if you are a practising health professional, you will probably find that you can replace a lot of what you currently do (for example, reading journals, attending in-services or other continuing professional development activities) with evidence-based practice.

Why is evidence-based practice important?

Put simply, the main reason why evidence-based practice is important is because it aims to provide the most effective care that is available, with the aim of improving client outcomes. However, there are many other reasons why it is important. When you seek health care for yourself from a health professional, do you expect that you will receive care that is based on the best available evidence? Of course you do. Likewise, our clients expect that we will provide them with the most effective care and the most accurate healthcare information that is available. As the internet plays such a large role in today's society, clients are now more aware of and educated about health conditions and issues such as intervention options and available tests. For example, it is not uncommon for clients to show their health professional information about a new intervention that they read about on the internet and ask to receive that intervention. As their treating health professional, we need to be able to assess the accuracy of this information, determine the suitability of the intervention for our client and work with them to decide if this intervention is an appropriate and effective option for them.

Evidence-based practice promotes an attitude of inquiry in health professionals and gets us thinking about questions such as: Why am I doing this in this way? Is there evidence that can guide me to do this in a more effective way? As such, evidence-based practice has an important role in facilitating our professional accountability. By definition, we are *professionals* whose job is to provide health care to people who need it (hence the term, health professionals). As part of providing a professional service it is our responsibility, when it is possible, to ensure that our practice is informed by the best available evidence. When we integrate the best available evidence with information from our clinical knowledge, clients and practice context, the reasoning behind our clinical decisions becomes more apparent and this serves to reinforce both our professional accountability and our claim of being a health professional.

Evidence-based practice also has an important role to play in ensuring that health resources are used wisely and that relevant evidence is considered when decisions are made about funding health services. There are finite resources available to provide health care to people. As such, we need to be responsible in our use of healthcare resources. For example, if there is good quality evidence that a particular intervention is harmful or not effective and will not produce clinically meaningful improvement in our clients, we should not waste precious resources providing this intervention— even if it is an intervention that has been provided for years. That is not to say, however, that if no research exists that clearly supports what we do, the interventions that we provide should not be funded. As discussed later in this book, absence of evidence and evidence of ineffectiveness (or evidence of harm) are quite different things.

Scope of evidence-based health care

As you will have gathered by now, evidence-based practice is a concept that has emerged out of evidence-based medicine. Although this book will concentrate largely on the use of evidence-based practice in clinical settings, evidence-based concepts now permeate all of health care (and beyond). That is why you will hear, from time to time, terms such as 'evidence-based purchasing' (where purchasers are informed by research to make purchases of health and social care services and resources that are useful and safe), 'evidence-based policy' (where policy makers integrate research evidence into the formation of policy documents and decisions to address the needs of the population) or 'evidence-based management' (where managers integrate research findings into a range of management tasks). Evidence-based practice has had a significant impact in more than just the clinical domain and its influence can be seen in many of the major health systems and government health policies across the world. In fact, if you are interested, you might like to do a quick internet search that will show that 'evidence-based' principles are now being applied in social care, criminology, education, conservation, engineering, sport and many other disciplines.

Common criticisms of evidence-based practice

Once you start reading widely in this area you will notice that many have criticised evidence-based practice. Criticisms that have been raised are often due to lack of knowledge or misinformation, so let us have a look at some of them here. Some authors criticise evidence-based practice for relying too heavily on quantitative methods. However, qualitative research is very important in helping us to understand more about how individuals and communities perceive health, manage their own health and make decisions related to health service usage.

Authors from a range of health professions have also highlighted the limitations of relying on research to provide the evidence upon which to base practice. They point to limited available research, particularly in allied health. Similarly, questions have been raised as to whether it is possible to develop sufficient and appropriate research to support the complexity and rapidly changing nature of professional practice.[10] While we agree that there will never be enough research to provide answers to every possible clinical question, evidence-based practice emphasises using the best research evidence *available* and acknowledges the need to draw on expert opinion where research does not exist. Further, clinical experience, which is one of the key components of evidence-based practice, must be relied on even more where there is a lack of evidence or uncertainty.

Many authors have debated the nature of 'evidence', arguing that evidence comes from many sources other than research. While it is vital to incorporate information from many different sources, the term 'evidence' in evidence-based practice serves a specific purpose. Its purpose is to highlight the value of information from research which has so often been ignored. In fact, some have suggested that, instead of the term evidence-based practice, 'knowledge-based practice' or 'information-based practice' should be used. While these alternatives avoid the contentiousness about what evidence is and what it is not, it would be impossible to find a health professional who does not base their practice on knowledge or information. In other words, use of the term 'evidence' (where evidence is taken to mean evidence from research) helps to highlight a source of information that has been under utilised. Use of the term 'evidence' to highlight the role of research in clinical decision making by no means discounts the importance of information and knowledge from clients and health professionals themselves, and this is something we hope to demonstrate throughout this book.

The process of evidence-based practice

Rather than just being a vague concept that is difficult to incorporate into everyday clinical practice, the process of evidence-based practice is actually quite structured. The process can be viewed as a number of steps that health professionals need to perform when an information need (that can be answered by research evidence) arises:[6]

1. Convert your information needs into an answerable clinical question.
2. Find the best evidence to answer your clinical question.
3. Critically appraise the evidence for its validity, impact and applicability.
4. Integrate the evidence with clinical expertise, the client's values and circumstances, and information from the practice context.
5. Evaluate the effectiveness and efficiency with which steps 1–4 were carried out and think about ways to improve your performance of them next time.

Some people may prefer to remember these steps as the five **A**s:[11]

- **A**sk a question
- **A**ccess the information
- **A**ppraise the articles found
- **A**pply the information
- **A**udit

Regardless of which list you prefer to use to remember the process of evidence-based practice, the basic steps are the same and they are explained in more detail below.

Step 1: Convert your information needs into an answerable clinical question

The process of evidence-based practice begins with the recognition that you, as a health professional, have a clinical information need. Some types of clinical information needs can be answered with the assistance of research evidence. Chapter 2 describes the different types of clinical information needs and which ones research evidence can help you to answer. An important step in the evidence-based practice process is turning this information need into an answerable clinical question and there are some easy ways to do this which are demonstrated in Chapter 2.

You may have a question about:

- **intervention** (that is, treatment)—for example, in adults with rheumatoid arthritis, is education about joint protection techniques effective in reducing hand pain and improving function?
- **diagnosis**—for example, in adults admitted to a chest pain unit, which elements of serial diagnostic testing are the most sensitive and specific predictors of cardiac involvement?
- **prognosis**—for example, in people undergoing total knee replacement for osteoarthritis, what improvement in walking ability is expected after six weeks?
- **clients' experiences and concerns**—for example, what does the lived experience of older adults transitioning to residential aged care facilities mean for their ability to integrate and find a sense of identity?

The type of question will determine the type of research that you need to look for in order to answer your question. All of this is explained further in Chapter 2.

Step 2: Find the best evidence to answer your clinical question

Once you have structured your clinical question appropriately and know what type of question you are asking and, therefore, what sort of research you need to look for, the next step is to find the research evidence to answer your question. It is important that you are aware of the many online evidence-based resources and which will be most appropriate for you to use to search for the evidence to answer your question. Being able to *efficiently* search the online evidence-based resources is a crucial skill to have for anyone who practises evidence-based practice. Chapter 3 contains information about the key online evidence-based resources and how to efficiently look for evidence.

Step 3: Critically appraise the evidence for its validity, impact and applicability

Upon finding the evidence, you will need to critically appraise it. That is, you need to examine the evidence closely to determine whether it is worthy of being used to inform your clinical practice.

Why do I need to critically appraise the evidence? Is not all published research of good quality?

Unfortunately not all published research is of good quality. In fact, there are a number of studies that suggest that much of it is of poor quality (see, for example, references 12–18). There are a range of reasons why this is the case. Conducting a well-designed research study is hard work—there are many issues to consider during the design phase. Sometimes, even when researchers have designed a great study, things that they have no control over can happen—such as losing many of the participants to follow-up (despite their best attempts to avoid this happening) or an unexpected change in the type or number of clients who are eligible for recruitment into the study. There are many practical and ethical considerations that can also make it difficult to conduct a study that uses methods to avoid introducing bias into a trial. For example, in the overwhelming majority of randomised controlled trials that evaluate an allied health intervention, it is not possible to blind either the participants or the therapists who are providing the intervention as to whether the participants are in the intervention group or the control group. As you will see in Chapters 2 and 4, lack of blinding can introduce bias in a study but, for most of these studies, it is not possible to blind the participants or therapists. Too often, research is conducted by people who do not have a full awareness of the issues surrounding research design and, as a result, the studies that they conduct are flawed. The way in which some researchers report their studies also can be incomplete and, as readers, we are often left wondering about the details of some aspects of the study and unsure if they did or did not consider particular aspects of study design. Sadly, the people who peer-review the studies for journals are sometimes no more informed about all of the latest issues in study design than the researchers who conducted the studies.

Fortunately, it appears that this situation is changing, with some emerging data showing that the quality of studies is improving over time as researchers increase their use of methods to minimise the risk of bias.[17,19,20] This is most likely because there is now a growing awareness of the importance of strong study design (thanks in part to the proliferation of evidence-based practice) on the part of authors of studies, reviewers of studies and journal editors. As you will see in Chapter 4, guides for how certain types of studies (such as randomised controlled trials) should be reported have been developed and a growing number of journals now require authors of studies to carefully follow these guides if they wish their article to be considered for publication. All of this is good news for us, as it has the potential to make interpreting research reports easier, but there is still a very long way to go.

Because of this, before you can use the results of a research study to assist you in making a clinical decision, you need to determine whether the study methods are sound enough to provide you with potentially useful information or, alternatively, whether the methods are so flawed that they might potentially provide misleading results. Studies that are poorly designed may produce results that are distorted by bias (and often more than one type of bias). Some of the common types of bias are introduced in Chapter 2. The main types of bias that are relevant to each of the question types are explained in detail in the corresponding chapter that discusses how to appraise the evidence for each question type.

What is involved in critically appraising evidence?

There are three main aspects of the evidence (that is, each study) that you need to appraise (in the following order):

1. **Internal validity.** This refers to whether the evidence is trustworthy. That is, can you believe the results of the study? You evaluate the validity of the study by determining whether the study was carried out in a way that was methodologically sound. In this step, we are concerned with the study's *internal validity*—this is explained more fully in Chapter 2.
2. **Impact.** If you decide that the validity of the study is sufficient that you can believe the results, you then need to look closely at the results of the study. The main thing that you need to determine is the impact (that is, the clinical importance) of the evidence. For example, in a study that compared the effectiveness of a new intervention with an existing intervention, did the new intervention have a *large enough effect* on the clinical outcome(s) of interest that you would consider altering your practice and using the new intervention with your client?
3. **Applicability.** If you have decided that the validity of the study is adequate and that the results are clinically important, the final step of critical appraisal is to evaluate whether you can apply the results of the study to your client. Essentially you need to assess whether your client is so different from the participants in the study that you cannot apply the results of the study to your client. This step is concerned with assessing the *external validity* (or the 'generalisability' or 'applicability') of the study— this is explained more fully in Chapter 2.

Many of the chapters of this book (Chapters 4–12) are devoted to helping you learn how to critically appraise various types of evidence. There are plenty of appraisal checklists that you can use to help you to critically appraise the evidence. Many of the checklists are freely available on the internet. Most of them contain more or less the same key items. The checklists that we have used in this book as a general guide for the appraisal of quantitative research are based on those that were developed by the UK National Health Service Public Health Resource Unit as part of the Critical Appraisal Skills Programme (CASP). In turn, these checklists were derived from the well-known *Journal of the American Medical Association (JAMA)* Users' Guides.[21] The CASP checklists are freely available at http://www.phru.nhs.uk/Pages/PHD/resources.htm. For the appraisal of qualitative research, we have used the Qualitative Assessment and Review Instrument (QARI), which was developed by the Joanna Briggs Institute. The QARI can be accessed as part of a software package which you can download for free (once you have registered) at http://www.joannabriggs.edu.au/services/sumari.php.

Each of the CASP checklists begins by asking two screening questions. These questions are designed to filter out studies of low methodological quality, so that you do not waste your time proceeding to appraise the validity, impact and applicability of a study that is going to be of too poor quality for you to use in clinical decision making. In the worked examples in Chapters 5, 7 and 9, you will notice that these screening questions are not included in the examples. This is because, prior to appraising their chosen article, the authors of each of the worked examples had already conducted a screening process when they decided which article was the best available evidence to use to answer their clinical question. When you are critically appraising research articles, keep in mind that no research is perfect and that it is important to not be overly critical of research articles. It just needs to be *good enough* to assist you in making a clinical decision.

Step 4: Integrate the evidence with clinical expertise, the client's values and circumstances, and information from the practice context

The fourth step in the evidence-based practice process involves integrating the findings from the critical appraisal step with your clinical expertise, your client's needs and the practice (clinical) context. As discussed earlier in this chapter and illustrated in Figure 1.1, these four elements form the definition of evidence-based practice. Clinical expertise refers to a health professional's cumulated experience, education and clinical skills. As evidence-based practice is a problem-solving approach that initially stems from a client's needs, any clinical decision that is made in relation to the client should involve consideration of the unique needs, values, preferences, concerns and experiences that each client brings to the situation. Many of the chapters of this book discuss the need for and process of integrating research evidence with clinical expertise and the client's needs, with appropriate consideration also given to the practice context.

Step 5: Evaluate the effectiveness and efficiency with which steps 1–4 were carried out and think about ways to improve your performance of them next time

As evidence-based practice is a process that is intended to be incorporated into the clinical practice of health professionals, it is important that you learn to do it as efficiently as possible so that it does not become a time-consuming onerous task. Asking yourself self-reflection questions after you have completed the previous four steps of the evidence-based practice process can be a useful way to identify which steps you are doing well and areas where you could improve. Box 1.1 contains some examples of self-reflection questions that you could ask when evaluating how well you performed steps 1 to 4 of the evidence-based practice process.

BOX 1.1 **EXAMPLES OF SELF-REFLECTION QUESTIONS WHEN EVALUATING YOUR PERFORMANCE OF STEPS 1 TO 4 OF THE EVIDENCE-BASED PRACTICE PROCESS**

- Am I asking well-formulated clinical questions? (See Chapter 2.)
- Am I aware of the best sources of evidence for the different types of clinical questions? (See Chapter 3.)
- Am I searching the databases efficiently? (See Chapter 3.)
- Am I using the hierarchy of evidence for each type of clinical question as my guide for the type of evidence that I should be searching for? (See Chapter 2.)
- Where possible, am I searching for and using information that is higher up in the pyramid of levels of organisation of evidence (for example, syntheses, synopses, summaries and pre-appraised original studies)? (See Chapter 3.)
- Am I integrating the critical appraisal into my clinical practice? (See Chapters 4–12.)
- Am I proactively monitoring for newly emerging evidence in my field of practice? (See Chapter 3.)

How this book is structured

The process of evidence-based practice that was just described has been used as a structure for this book. In addition to the key steps that form the evidence-based practice process, other topics that are important for health professionals who wish to practise evidence-based practice to know about (such as how to implement evidence into practice and how to communicate with clients about evidence) are also addressed in chapters of this book.

Chapter 1: Introduction to evidence-based practice	This chapter addresses some of the background information about evidence-based practice, such as what it is, why it was developed, why it is important and the five key steps that underlie the process of evidence-based practice.
Chapter 2: Information needs, asking questions and some basics of research studies	Chapter 2 provides you with details about clinical information needs, how to convert them into an answerable question and how the type of research that you should look for differs according to the type of question that you are asking. This chapter also contains some of the background statistical information that you need to understand before being able to critically appraise the research evidence.
Chapter 3: Finding the evidence	Chapter 3 contains information about how to undertake the second step of the evidence-based practice process, which is searching for the evidence to answer your clinical question.
Chapter 4: Evidence about effects of interventions	This chapter explains what to do when you have a clinical question about the effects of an intervention, with the focus on how to perform the third and fourth steps of the evidence-based practice process. It gives details about how to assess the validity of the evidence, understand the results and use the evidence to inform clinical practice.
Chapter 5: Questions about the effects of interventions: examples of appraisals from different health professions	As the steps of evidence-based practice become easier with practice, this chapter provides you with a number of worked examples of questions about interventions so that you can see, step-by-step, for various clinical scenarios how questions are formulated and evidence is found, appraised and applied. In keeping with the multidisciplinary nature of this book, examples from a range of health professions are provided.
Chapter 6: Evidence about diagnosis	This chapter follows the same structure as Chapter 4, but the content is focussed on how to appraise the evidence when your clinical question is about diagnosis.
Chapter 7: Questions about diagnosis: examples of appraisals from different health professions	Chapter 7 contains a number of worked examples of questions about diagnosis from a range of health professions that commonly have diagnostic/assessment informational needs.

Chapter 8: Evidence about prognosis	This chapter follows the same structure as Chapters 4 and 6, but the content is focussed on how to appraise the evidence when your clinical question is about prognosis.
Chapter 9: Questions about prognosis: examples of appraisals from different health professions	Chapter 9 contains a number of worked examples of questions about prognosis from a range of health professions that commonly consider prognostic issues.
Chapter 10: Evidence about clients' experiences and concerns	This chapter follows the same structure as Chapters 4, 6 and 8, but the content is focussed on how to appraise the evidence when your question is about clients' experiences and concerns and you are using qualitative research to answer the question.
Chapter 11: Questions about clients' experiences and concerns: examples of appraisals from different health professions	Chapter 11 contains a number of worked examples of questions about clients' experiences and concerns from a range of health professions.
Chapter 12: Appraising and understanding systematic reviews and meta-analyses	As you will see in Chapter 2, systematic reviews and meta-analyses are a very important research study type in evidence-based practice. They are so important that we have devoted an entire chapter to explaining how to appraise and make sense of them.
Chapter 13: Clinical guidelines	Clinical practice guidelines can be a useful tool in evidence-based practice. Chapter 13 provides you with information about what they are, how they are developed, where to find them and how to assess their quality to determine if you should use them in your clinical practice.
Chapter 14: Talking with clients about evidence	Knowing how to talk with clients about the evidence that you have found and appraised and how to explain to them what it all means in a way that they can understand is an important skill for health professionals to have. Chapter 14 describes how to do this as well as how to involve your clients in the decision-making process.
Chapter 15: Clinical reasoning and evidence-based practice	Clinical reasoning is the process by which health professionals integrate information from many different sources. Having an understanding of clinical reasoning can clarify, and hopefully improve, our clinical decision making.

Chapter 16:
Implementing
evidence into practice

After finding and appraising the evidence, client outcomes will only be altered if the evidence is then implemented into clinical practice. Chapter 16 describes the process for doing this, along with some of the barriers that may be encountered during the process, and strategies for overcoming them.

Summary points of this chapter

- Evidence-based practice is a problem-based approach where research evidence is used to inform clinical decision making. It involves the integration of the best available research evidence with clinical expertise, our client's values and circumstances, and consideration of the clinical (practice) context.
- Evidence-based practice is important because it aims to improve client outcomes and it is what our clients expect. However, it also has a role in facilitating professional accountability and guiding decisions about the funding of health services.
- Evidence-based practice has extended to all areas of health care and is now used in areas such as policy formulation and implementation, purchasing and management.
- There are five main steps in the evidence-based practice process: 1) asking a question; 2) searching for evidence to answer it; 3) critically appraising the evidence; 4) integrating the evidence with your clinical expertise, the client's values and information from the practice context; and 5) evaluating how well you performed steps 1–4 and how you can improve your performance the next time you complete this process.
- Not all research evidence is of sufficient quality that you can confidently use it to inform your clinical decision making. Therefore you need to critically appraise it before deciding whether to use it. The three main aspects of the evidence that you need to critically appraise are its: 1) validity (can you trust it?), 2) impact (are the results clinically important?) and 3) applicability (can you apply it to your client?).

References

1. Sackett D, Rosenberg W, Gray J et al. Evidence based medicine: what it is and what it isn't: it's about integrating individual clinical expertise and the best external evidence. BMJ 1996; 312: 71–72.
2. Spock B. Baby and child care. London: The Bodley Head; 1958.
3. Gilbert R, Salanti G, Harden M et al. Infant sleeping position and the sudden infant death syndrome: systematic review of observational studies and historical review of recommendations from 1940 to 2002. Int J Epidemiol 2005; 34:874–887.
4. Allen C, Glasziou P, Del Mar C. Bed rest: a potentially harmful treatment needing more careful evaluation. Lancet 1999; 354:1229–1233.
5. Heal C, Buettner P, Raasch B et al. Can sutures get wet? Prospective randomised controlled trial of wound management in general practice. BMJ 2006; 332:1053–1056.
6. Straus S, Richardson W, Glasziou P et al. Evidence-based medicine: how to practice and teach EBM. 3rd edn. Edinburgh: Elsevier Churchill Livingstone; 2005.
7. Oxman A, Guyatt G. The science of reviewing research. Ann NY Acad Sci 1993;703:125–133 discussion 133–134.
8. Sibley J, Sackett D, Neufeld V et al. A randomised trial of continuing medical education. N Engl J Med 1982; 306:511–515.
9. Isaacs D, Fitzgerald D. Seven alternatives to evidence based medicine. BMJ 1999; 319:1618.
10. Higgs J, Titchen A, eds. Practice knowledge and expertise in the health professions. Oxford: Butterworth–Heinemann; 2001.
11. Jackson R, Ameratunga S, Broad J et al. The GATE frame: critical appraisal with pictures. ACP J Club 2006; 144:2.

12. Anyanwu C, Treasure T. Surgical research revisited: clinical trials in the cardiothoracic surgical literature. Eur J Cardiothorac Surg 2004; 25:299–303.
13. Kjaergard L, Frederiksen S, Gludd C. Validity of randomised clinical trials in gastroenterology from 1964–2000. Gastroenterology 2002; 122:1157–1160.
14. Dickinson K, Bunn F, Wentz R et al. Size and quality of randomised controlled trials in head injury: review of published studies. BMJ 2000; 320:1308–1311.
15. Chan S, Bhandari M. The quality of reporting of orthopaedic randomised trials with use of a checklist for nonpharmacological therapies. J Bone Joint Surg Am 2007; 89:1970–1980.
16. Hoffmann T, McKenna K, Hadi T et al. Quality and quantity of paediatric research: an analysis of the OTseeker database. Aust Occup Ther J 2007; 54:113–123.
17. Hoffmann T, Bennett S, McKenna K et al. Interventions for stroke rehabilitation: analysis of the research contained in the OTseeker evidence database. Top Stroke Rehabil 2008; 15:341–350.
18. Bennett S, McKenna K, McCluskey A et al. Evidence for occupational therapy interventions: effectiveness research indexed in the OTseeker database. Br J Occup Ther 2007; 70:426–430.
19. Moseley A, Herbert R, Sherrington C et al. Evidence for physiotherapy practice: a survey of the physiotherapy evidence based database (PEDro). Aust J Physiother 2002; 48:43–49.
20. McCluskey A, Lovarini M, Bennett S et al. What evidence exists for work-related injury prevention and management? Analysis of an occupational therapy evidence database (OTseeker). Br J Occup Ther 2005; 68:447–456.
21. Guyatt G, Rennie D. Users' guides to the medical literature. JAMA 1993; 270:2096–2097.
22. Keister D, Tilson J. Proactively monitoring for newly emerging evidence: the lost step in EBP? Evid Based Med 2008; 13:69.

CHAPTER 2

Information needs, asking questions and some basics of research studies

Chris Del Mar and Tammy Hoffmann

LEARNING OBJECTIVES

After reading this chapter, you should be able to:
- Describe the types of clinical information needs that can be answered using evidence-based practice
- Differentiate between just-in-case information and just-in-time information
- Convert your informational needs into answerable, well-structured clinical questions, using the PICO format
- Describe the basic design of some of the common study types that are used in evidence-based practice
- Explain the hierarchy of evidence for questions about the effects of interventions, the hierarchy for diagnostic questions and the hierarchy for prognostic questions
- Explain what is meant by internal validity and external validity
- Describe some of the main types of bias that can occur in studies
- Differentiate between statistical significance and clinical significance and briefly explain how each of them is determined

This chapter will provide background information that you need to know in order to understand the details of the evidence-based practice process that follow in the subsequent chapters of this book. In that sense, this chapter is a somewhat diverse but important collection of topics. We start by describing the types of clinical information needs health professionals commonly have and discuss some of the methods that health professionals use to obtain information to answer their needs. As we saw in Chapter 1, converting informational needs into an answerable, well-structured question is the first step in the process of evidence-based practice and, in this chapter, we will explain how to do this. We then explain the importance of matching the type of information you need with the type of study design that is most appropriate to answer your question. As part of this, we will introduce and explain the concept of 'hierarchies of evidence' for each type of question. In the last sections of this chapter, we will explain some concepts that are fundamental to the critical appraisal of research evidence, which is the third step in the evidence-based practice process. The concepts that we will discuss include internal validity, chance, bias, confounding, statistical significance, clinical significance and power.

Clinical information needs

Health professionals need information all the time to make decisions, to reassure clients, to make practical arrangements and so on. Some of the information that we need can be usefully assembled from research and some of it cannot. Table 2.1 provides examples of some of the obvious types of information that can or cannot be gathered from research. This book will help you to learn how to deal with information needs that can be answered to some extent by research. Along the way we will also discuss the types of information that come from clients and the types of information that come from clinical experience. When we consider these together—information from research, clients and experience— we are working in an evidence-based practice framework.

Dealing effectively with information needs

Having established that health professionals have many information needs, this section explains how you can effectively deal with these information needs. A simple overview of one way of doing this is as follows:
- Recognise when we have a question.
- Record the question—do not lose that moment!
- Attempt to find the answer.
- Record the answer.
- Stop and reflect on what you have been looking up and dealing with. Is it helping you to answer your question?

The size of the problem

The clinical literature is big. Just how big is staggering. There are thousands of new studies published hourly. For example, randomised controlled trials are published at the rate of 20,000 per year. That is roughly 50–60 per day, or one every 20–30 minutes. Worse than that, randomised controlled trials represent a small proportion (less than 5%) of the research that is indexed in Medline and, as you will see in Chapter 3, it is just one of the databases that are available for you to search in to find evidence. This means that the accumulated literature is a massive haystack in which are embedded some important needles we have to find. One of those needles of information might be the difference

	Information		Examples
These questions typically *cannot* be answered by research	Local	Background information	• Is this client eligible for treatment subsidy? • What are the regulations for the use of a type of treatment? • Who can be referred to this service? • What are the opening hours of the hospital outpatients' administration? • Is there an organisation that runs a chronic disease self-management program in this community? • What is a Colles 'fracture'?
These questions *can* usually be informed by research	General	Aetiology/ frequency	• Is this risk factor associated with that disease? • How many people with those symptoms have this disease?
		Prognosis	• What happens to this illness without treatment?
		Diagnosis	• If I elicit this sign among people with these symptoms, how many have that disease? • If this test is negative how sure can I be that the client does *not* have the disease?
		Treatment/ intervention	• How much improvement can I expect from this intervention? • How much harm is likely from the intervention? • Is this intervention more effective than that intervention?
		Clients' experiences and concerns	• What is the experience of clients concerning their condition or intervention? • What is happening here and why is it happening?

TABLE 2.1 Clinical information needs—examples of those that can and those that cannot be answered by evidence-based practice

between effective or ineffective (or even harmful) care for your client. One of the purposes of this book, then, is to help you find needles in haystacks.

Noting it down

It is important that we keep track of the questions that we ask. It is very easy to lose track of them and then the opportunity evaporates. If you cannot remember what you wanted to know when in the midst of managing a client, chances are you will also forget later.

How should we do this? One way is to keep a little book in which to write them down in your pocket or handbag. Date and scribble. A more modern way is electronically, of course, using a personal digital assistant (PDA) or computer (if simultaneously making client records). Some of us tell the client what we are doing:

I am just making a note of this to myself to look it up when I have a moment.

or

Let us get online and look that up right now, because I want to make sure that I am using the latest research for you …

In Chapter 1, we discussed the general process of looking up, appraising and applying the evidence that we find. But also remember to keep track (in other words, write it down!) of the information that you found and how you evaluated and applied it. In the end, the information that is found might result in you changing (hopefully improving) your clinical practice. The way it does this is often uncoupled from the processes you undertook, so it takes some time to realise what led you to make the changes—often systematic—to the way you do things. Sometimes the research information just reassures us that we are on the right track but this is important also.

Different ways of obtaining information: Push or pull? Just-in-case or just-in-time?

Push: just-in-case information

In advertising jargon, the term 'push' is used, meaning that the information is pushed out. This is the traditional means by which information is disseminated. This is basically the function of journals. Research is undertaken and either sent directly to you, or pre-digested in some way (perhaps as an editorial, review article, systematic review or guideline). 'Just-in-case' information is made available when it is generated, or when it is thought (by someone other than you, the health professional) that health professionals ought to hear about it.

Figure 2.1 shows some examples of information that can be *pushed*. Other sources of 'push' information include conferences, professional newsletters, textbooks and informal chats to colleagues and other people from other professional groups.

As can be seen, there are many ways that a piece of research can percolate through to you as a health professional. The picture is actually more complex than this: what

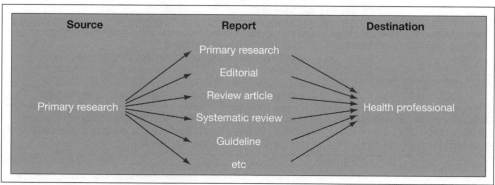

FIGURE 2.1 How does research data get to you?

is picked up for review, systematic review and so on is determined by a number of different factors, including which journal the primary data were first published in, how relevant readers think it is and how well it fits into the policy being formulated or already in existence. There are, in fact, different sorts of information that we might consider accessing and this is explained in detail in Chapter 3 (see Figure 3.1). But this is only the start. All these methods rely on the information arriving at your place of work (or home, post box, email inbox etc). Then it has to be managed before it is actually put into practice. How does this happen? There are a number of different stages that can be considered and these are explained in Table 2.2.

Clearly this is not an easy process. There are many steps where the flow can be interrupted. All the steps have to happen for the research to run the gauntlet through to the client. One solution is to use one of the abstracting services. One of these is the *Evidence Based* journal series (see http://ebm.bmj.com/). This type of service is described in depth in Chapter 3 but, in a nutshell, these journals only provide reports of previous research (that is, they contain no primary research). Papers are reported only if they

Task	Explanation
Read the title	Decide whether something is worth reading at all.
Read the abstract	
Read the full paper	We have obviously not tossed this paper aside (that means we have turned the page).
Decide if it is …	
a. relevant	A lot of research is not aimed at us (as health professionals looking for better information to manage our clients). Much of it is researcher-to-researcher information. Just some of it is information that we think might be useful to us, either now or in the future when this might become part of everyday practice.
b. believable	Methodologically sound. That means the information is not biased to the extent that we cannot believe the result. This is explained further later in this chapter and in Chapters 4–12.
Wonder if the technique is available	A lot of research does not spell out the treatment, diagnostic procedure or definitional terms adequately so that we can simply put the research into practice—even if we believe it!
Store the paper so we can recall it when the right client comes along	Different health professionals do this in different ways: • tear out the paper and file it • meticulously make out references cards or electronic databases • just try to remember it. Most health professionals do the last. And then forget!
Ensure we have the necessary resources to incorporate the research into our practice	There may be prerequisites, such as availability of resources and skills to carry it out or perhaps some policy needs to be instituted before this can happen.
Persuade the client	… that this is the best management …

TABLE 2.2 The processes involved in making sure that *just-in-case* information is used properly to help clients

survive a rigorous selection process that begins with a careful methodological appraisal, and then, if the paper is found to be sufficiently free of bias, it is sent for appraisal by a worldwide net of health professionals who decide if the research is relevant. The resultant number of papers that is reported in each discipline is surprisingly small. In other words, only a few papers are not too biased *and* also relevant! Happily for health professionals, there is another option.

Pull: just-in-time information

Pull is advertising jargon for the way potential customers go looking for information, rather than simply waiting for it to be *pushed* to them. In this context, it is information that the health professional seeks in relation to a specific question arising from their clinical work. This gives it certain characteristics. This is illustrated in Table 2.3 using the five As that were introduced in Chapter 1 as a way of simply describing the steps in the evidence-based practice process.

If this looks familiar to you, well, this is the essential core of evidence-based practice. How feasible is it to incorporate this way of finding information 'just-in-time'? Again, there are a number of steps that have to be undertaken. These are not easy either—they all need mastering and practice (like almost everything in clinical care). For example, asking questions is difficult. It requires us to be open to not knowing everything. This is more difficult for some people than others (doctors were notorious for having trouble with this—perhaps because society bestowed some god-like attributes on them that made it potentially too disappointing if they admitted not knowing stuff). The truth is, most people in modern times welcome the honesty that goes with questioning the best management. It makes the health professional appear to be taking infinite and meticulous care.

How often do we ask questions? Is this something that we can aspire to realistically? Most health professionals are worried that they do not ask questions enough. Relax. You do. Studies have been undertaken in a number of settings (all to do with doctors, sadly) to show that they ask questions much more than they thought they did. For example, a study undertaken in Iowa, USA, examined what questions family doctors working in the community asked during the course of their work. Just over 100 doctors asked >1100 questions over 2.5 days, which is approximately 10 each.[1] A similar Spanish study found

Task	Explanation
Ask a question: re-format the question into an answerable one	This ensures relevance—by definition!
Access the information: searching	Decide whether to look now (in front of the client) or later. Searching is a special skill, which is described in Chapter 3.
Appraise the papers found	We talk about this (in fact, we talk about this a lot!) in Chapters 4–12.
Apply the information	This means with the client who is in front of you.
Audit	Check whether the evidence-based practice processes that you are engaged in are working well.

TABLE 2.3 Processes involved in *just-in-time* information: the five As

that doctors had a good chance (nearly 100%) of finding an answer if it took less than 2 minutes, but were much less likely to do so (<40%) if it took 30 minutes.[2] A study of doctors found that they are more likely to chase an answer if they estimate that an answer exists, or if the information need is urgent.[3] Nurses working in a similar setting were more likely to ask someone or look in a book in order to answer their questions.[4] Despite advances in electronic access, health professionals do not seem to be doing well at effectively seeking answers to clinical questions.[5] If we are not able in the hurly burly of daily clinical practice to look up questions immediately, it is important (as we mentioned earlier in the chapter) to write them down.

How to convert your information needs into an answerable clinical question

Let us look at how we can take our clinical information needs and convert them into answerable clinical questions which we can then effectively search to find the answers to. You may remember from Chapter 1 that forming an answerable clinical question is the first step of the evidence-based practice process. Asking a good question is central to successful evidence-based practice. A focussed, well-constructed question typically has four components,[6] which can be easily remembered using the PICO mnemonic:

- **P**atient or **p**roblem or **p**opulation
- **I**ntervention, diagnostic test or prognostic factor
- **C**omparison
- **O**utcome(s)

Patient or problem

In this component, you are stating who or what the question is about. This may include the primary problem, disease or coexisting conditions—for example, '*In children with autism …*' Sometimes you may also wish to specify the sex and age of a client if that is going to be relevant to the diagnosis, prognosis or intervention—for example, '*In elderly women who have osteoporosis …*'

Intervention or issue

The term intervention is used here in its broadest sense. It may refer to the intervention (that is, treatment) that you wish to use with your client—for example, '*In people who have had a stroke, is home-based rehabilitation as effective as hospital-based rehabilitation in improving ability to perform self-care activities?*' In this case, home-based rehabilitation is the intervention that we are interested in. Or, if you have a diagnostic question, this component of the question may refer to which diagnostic test you are considering using with your clients—for example, '*Does the Mini-Mental State Examination accurately detect the presence of cognitive impairment in older community-living people?*' In this example, the Mini-Mental State Examination is the diagnostic test that we are interested in. Or, if you have a question about prognosis, you may sometimes wish to specify a particular factor or issue that may influence the prognosis of your client—for example, in the question '*What is the likelihood of hip fracture in women who have a family history of hip fracture?*', the family history of hip fracture is the particular factor that we are interested in. If you want to understand more about clients' perspectives you may want to focus on a particular *issue*. For example, in the question '*How do adolescents who are being treated with chemotherapy feel about hospital environments?'*, the issue of interest is adolescent perceptions of hospital environments.

Comparison

Your questions may not always include this component. It is mainly questions about the effects of intervention (and sometimes diagnosis) that use this component. Add a comparison element to your question if you are interested in comparing the intervention component of your question to another intervention and wish to know if one intervention is more effective than another. In the example that we used above, *'In people who have had a stroke, is home-based rehabilitation as effective as hospital-based rehabilitation in improving ability to perform self-care activities'*, the comparison is hospital-based rehabilitation. Sometimes, the comparison that you are interested in may be usual (or standard) care and, sometimes, you may not wish to have any comparison.

Outcome(s)

This component of the question should clearly specify what outcome (or outcomes) you are interested in. For some outcomes you may also need to specify whether you are interested in increasing the amount of the outcome (such as the score on a functional assessment) or decreasing it (such as the reduction of pain). In the stroke question example above, the outcome of interest was an improvement in the ability to perform self-care activities. As you will see in Chapter 14, shared decision making is an important component of evidence-based practice and it is important, where possible, to involve your client in choosing the goals of intervention that are most important to them. As such, there will be many circumstances where the outcome component of your question will be guided by your client's preferences.

The exact way that you should structure your clinical question varies a little depending on the type of question that you have. This is explained more in the relevant chapter—Chapter 4 for questions about the effects of intervention, Chapter 6 for diagnostic questions, Chapter 8 for prognostic questions and Chapter 10 for qualitative questions.

Now that I have my question formulated, what types of information should I look for?

Not all types of information are equally useful—some are much more useful than others. This is because useful pieces of information are …
1. more relevant or
2. more truthful …
… than others.

Relevant information

One of the problems is that there is so much information that deciding what to download and use can be distorted by finding something that *nearly* answers what you asked, *but not quite*. Deciding how relevant information is can be partly met by using the PICO mnemonic that was explained above. This can help you decide in advance what you need to ask, and then ensure that you are not distracted by interesting looking (but sadly, not directly relevant) information.

Truthful information

Some information only purports to answer your question but either does not or, worse, cannot. In fact much of the information published as research is actually unhelpful to us health professionals. There are many reasons for this:

1. The information is published as *researcher-to-researcher* communication. For example, research into the best instrument to use for measuring outputs is unlikely to be directly useful to any question you need answered as a practising health professional.
2. The research (even though it does attempt to answer the question that you need an answer for) was undertaken using a method that cannot answer the question. As we shall see shortly, this is often because the wrong study type was used. There are many different study types, and the right one must be used to answer the question at hand.
3. The research (even though it does attempt to answer the question that you need an answer for) was undertaken insufficiently well to answer the question. For example, the research may have failed in a large number of different ways so that we are unsure that the apparent 'result' is true.

We will now look at the last two reasons in the list above in detail.

What are the different study types?

First we need to understand some of the different study types that exist. They are given and briefly explained in Table 2.4.

There are some important things to notice about the study types that are listed in Table 2.4:

1. Only one study type is particularly good at addressing intervention questions—randomised controlled trials. This means that the best evidence about intervention questions will come from them, or possibly their meta-analysis. A meta-analysis is a part of a systematic review where the results from individual studies are combined. Systematic reviews and meta-analyses are discussed in detail in Chapter 12.
2. All the other study types are observational studies. They are not the best at answering questions about the effect of interventions, but they are good at answering *other* types of questions, including questions about prognosis, diagnosis, frequency and aetiology.
3. Different questions require different study designs and this is explained more fully in the next section. Although randomised controlled trials can answer questions about prognosis (for example), by examining just the control group (who did not receive any intervention) of a randomised controlled trial, this can be inefficient.
4. This means that there is no universal 'hierarchy of evidence', as is sometimes claimed. Hierarchies of evidence only exist for each question type.

Hierarchies of evidence for each question type

Hierarchies of evidence exist for each question type and are useful as they tell you what type of study you should look for first when searching for evidence to answer your question. If there are no relevant studies of the type that are at the top of the hierarchy (for example, systematic reviews of randomised controlled trials if an intervention question), you then proceed to search for the type of study that is next down the list (for example, randomised controlled trials). This way, you are searching for the best available evidence. The higher up the hierarchy that a study is, the more likely it is that the study can minimise the impact of bias on the results of the study. We can also think of the hierarchy as representing a continuum of certainty (with higher levels of

Study type	How it works	The type of questions that it is good at answering
Randomised controlled trial	This is an experiment. Participants are randomised into two (or more) different groups and each group receives a different intervention. At the end of the trial, the effects of the different interventions are measured.	Questions about interventions, such as: Is the intervention effective? Is one intervention more effective than another?
Cohort	This is an observational study. It is a type of longitudinal study where participants are followed over time. Participants with specific characteristics are identified as a 'cohort', differences between them are measured and they are followed over time. Finally, differences in outcome are observed and related to the initial differences.	Several questions: Risks—what risk factors predict disease? Aetiology—what factors cause these outcomes? Prognosis—what happens with this disease over time? Diagnosis—if the test is positive, what happens to the client?
Case-control	Observational study. Participants who have experienced an outcome already (such as developing a disease) are identified. They are then 'matched' with other participants who are similar— except they do *not* have the outcome (for example, the disease being studied). Differences in risk factors between the two groups of participants are then analysed.	Several questions: Risks—what risk factors predict disease? Prognosis—what happens with this disease over time?
Cross-sectional	Sample a population at a particular point in time and measure them to see who has the outcome. Often, associations between risk factors and a certain outcome are analysed.	Observational: Frequency—how common is the outcome (disease, risk factor etc)? Aetiology—what risk factors are associated with these outcomes?
Qualitative	• Interviews (asking people) • Focus groups (representative people are encouraged to talk) • Participant observation (the researcher joins the group to understand what is going on)	Observational: Why do people …? What are the possible reasons for …? How do people feel about …?

TABLE 2.4 Some of the main study types that you need to know about for evidence-based practice

certainty at the top of the hierarchy). Consider, for example, the hierarchy of evidence for intervention questions—the continuum of certainty represents how certain we are that the effects found in the study are actually due to the intervention and not something else. This introduces two very important concepts in evidence-based practice, bias and confounding, which are explained in the next section of this chapter.

Be aware that there are a number of published hierarchies of evidence which have been put together by various organisations. On the whole, they are fairly similar, but there are subtle differences between them. So, if you are a reading a document and it refers to a particular study as being (for example) level III-1 evidence, it is a good idea to check which hierarchy of evidence the document followed when making that classification because what level III-1 evidence means in one hierarchy scheme may differ slightly from what it means according to another hierarchy scheme. The hierarchies of evidence for the various types of questions that are shown in Table 2.5 are a simplified version of the hierarchies of evidence that have been developed by the National Health and Medical Research Council (NHMRC) of Australia.[7] Note that, at the time of writing this chapter, these NHMRC hierarchies of evidence were considered a draft document and were undergoing a stage of public consultation as they were recently modified from the hierarchies that appeared in a previously published document.

Level	Intervention	Diagnosis	Prognosis
I	A systematic review of level II studies	A systematic review of level II studies	A systematic review of level II studies
II	Randomised controlled trial	A study of test accuracy with an independent, blinded comparison with a valid reference standard, among consecutive persons with a defined clinical presentation	Prospective cohort study
III-1	Pseudo-randomised controlled trial (that is, alternate allocation or some other method was used rather than true randomisation—see Chapter 4 for details about this)	As for level II, but a study that used *non-consecutive* participants	
III-2	Comparative study *with* concurrent controls: • non-randomised experimental trial • cohort study • case-control study • interrupted time series with a control group	A comparison with a reference standard that does not meet the criteria required for level II or/and III-1 evidence	Analysis of the prognostic factors among the participants in one group of a randomised controlled trial
III-3	Comparative study *without* concurrent controls: • historical control study • two or more single arm study • interrupted time series without a parallel control group	Diagnostic case-control study	Retrospective cohort study
IV	Case series	Study of diagnostic yield (no reference standard)	• Case series *or* • Cohort study where participants are at different stages of the disease/condition

TABLE 2.5 **Hierarchies and levels of evidence for questions about intervention, diagnosis and prognosis**

As such, the final NHRMC hierarchies of evidence may differ slightly to those that are shown in Table 2.5. We suggest that you check the NHMRC website (http://www.nhmrc.gov.au) for the final hierarchies of evidence once they are published.

Most of the study types that are included in Table 2.5 have been explained already in this chapter. The intricate details of the main study types will be explained in the relevant chapter that deals with how to appraise evidence for each of the question types. However, we will now briefly consider the study types[7] shown in Table 2.5 but not yet explained:

- A **non-randomised experimental trial** is essentially the same as a randomised controlled study, but there is no randomisation (hence it is lower down the hierarchy as this opens it up to all kinds of bias). Participants are allocated to either an intervention or control group and the outcomes from each group are compared.

- The basic premise of a **case-control study** was explained in Table 2.4, but not in relation to how it can be used to answer questions about the effects of intervention. When a case-control study has been used to answer a question about the effect of an intervention, 'cases' are participants who have been exposed to an intervention and 'controls' are participants who have not.

- In an **interrupted time series study** (with a control group), trends in an outcome are measured over multiple time points *before* and *after* the intervention is provided to a group of participants, and then compared to the outcomes at the same time points for a group of participants who did not receive the same intervention. This type of study can also be conducted without a parallel control group being involved. When this occurs, the before and after data for just the one group is compared. As there is no control group, this variation of this study design is lower down the hierarchy of evidence.

- In a **historical control study,** the key word is historical as the control group does not participate in the study at the same time as the intervention group. There are two main forms that this type of study can take. Data about outcomes are prospectively collected for a group of participants who received the intervention of interest. This data is compared with either: 1) data about outcomes from a group of people who were treated at the same institution before the intervention of interest was introduced—this group is, in a sense, considered to be a control group who received standard care—or 2) data about outcomes from a group of people who received the control (or an alternative) intervention but the data comes from a previously published document.

- A **two or more single arm study** gathers the data from two or more studies and compares the outcomes of a single series of participants (in each study) who received the intervention of interest.

- A **case series** is simply a report on a series of clients (that is, 'cases') who have an outcome of interest (or received the intervention that is being studied). There is no control group involved.

- In a **diagnostic (test) accuracy study**, the outcomes from the test that is being evaluated (known as the *index test*) are compared with outcomes from a *reference standard test* to see how much agreement there is between the two tests. The outcomes are measured in people who are suspected of having the condition of interest. A reference standard test (often called the 'gold standard' test) is the test that is considered to be the best available method for establishing the presence or absence of the target condition of interest.

- In a **diagnostic case-control study**, the results from a reference standard test are used to create two groups of people—those who are known to have the condition of interest (the 'cases') and those who do not have it (the 'controls'). The index test results for the cases are then compared with the index test results for the controls.
- In a **study of diagnostic yield**, the index test is used to identify people who have the condition of interest. A reference standard test is not used to confirm the accuracy of the diagnosis and, therefore, this study design is at the bottom of the hierarchy of evidence for diagnostic questions.
- The basic idea of a **cohort** study was explained in Table 2.4, but there are two broad types of cohort studies that can be conducted and, as you can see in the prognosis column of Table 2.5, they sit at very different levels in the hierarchy of evidence for prognostic questions. The reasons for this are explained in Chapter 8, but for now we will just explain the main difference between them. In a **prospective cohort study,** groups of participants are identified as a 'cohort' (based on whether they have or have not been exposed to a certain intervention or situation) and then followed prospectively over time to see what happens to them. In a **retrospective cohort study,** the cohorts are defined from a previous point in time and the information is collected (for example, from past records) about the outcome(s) of interest. Participants are not followed up in the future to see what happens to them, as happens in a prospective cohort study.

Hierarchy of evidence for questions about clients' experiences and concerns

Questions about clients' experiences and concerns are answered using qualitative evidence. The various qualitative research methodologies will be explained in depth in Chapter 10. There is currently no universally agreed upon hierarchy of evidence for study types that seek to answer questions about clients' experiences and concerns.

Internal validity: What have bias and confounding got to do with evidence-based practice?

Internal validity and external validity

As we saw in Chapter 1 when the process of evidence-based practice was explained, when reading a research study you need to know if you can believe the results of the study. Internal validity refers to whether the evidence is trustworthy. That is, are the conclusions that the authors have stated for that particular study valid? Can we be sure that the association or effect found is not really due to some other factor? Three common alternative explanations that must be considered for the association or effect that is found in a study are: 1) chance, 2) bias and 3) confounding. We will now look at each of these in turn. But before we do, let us briefly explain what external validity is so that you do not confuse it with internal validity. External validity is something entirely different and refers to the generalisability of the results of a study. That is, to what extent can we apply the results of the study to people other than the participants of the study?

Chance

One possible explanation for the results that are found in a study is the possibility that the findings might be due to random variation. The measurements that are made during research with a *sample* of participants are nearly always subject to random variation. As we will explain later in this chapter, determining whether findings are due to chance is a key feature of statistical analysis (hypothesis testing). The best way to avoid error due to random variation is to ensure that the sample size (that is, the number of participants) of the study is adequate. This will be discussed in more detail later in the chapter.

Bias

To understand why some studies might be more trusted sources of evidence than others, it is important that you understand the concept of bias. Bias can be visualised as the characteristic of lawn bowls which enables them to roll in a curve. Although this characteristic of lawn bowls to 'not run true' (that is, in a straight line) is useful in the game of bowls, it is a problem in study design, and therefore we use the term bias for any effect that prevents a study from running true. Whereas chance is caused by *random* variation, bias is caused by *systematic* variation. Bias is a systematic error in the way that participants are selected for a study, outcomes are measured or data are analysed which, in turn, leads to inaccurate results.

Biases can operate in either direction. That is, they can lead to the underestimation or overestimation of the effect that is reported in a study. Let us consider an example of a randomised controlled trial of the effectiveness of a new intervention for back pain. If the participants allocated to the new intervention had less severe symptoms (that is, had less back pain) at the start of the trial than the participants who were allocated to the 'comparison' intervention group, any differences at the end of the study might be the result of that initial difference and not the new intervention that was provided. This bias would be called 'allocation bias'. This means that the way in which the participants were allocated to the two different intervention groups was biased and therefore we cannot know what caused the effect. But there are dozens of other kinds of bias, and we need to be able to recognise them. Table 2.6 briefly describes some of the common kinds of bias that can occur. Some are relevant to non-randomised studies and some to randomised studies. Chapter 4 discusses the biases that can occur in randomised controlled trials in more detail.

Assessing whether bias has occurred in a study is the main focus of the first step (is the evidence valid?) in the three-step critical appraisal process that was described in Chapter 1. Being able to assess whether the evidence is valid is a key skill that is needed for those who wish to practise evidence-based practice. As such, this topic is given a lot of attention in this book, primarily in Chapters 4, 6, 8, 10 and 12.

Confounding

'Confound' comes from the Latin *confundere*—*com-* (together) + *fundere* (to pour)—meaning to confuse. Add another liquid to the pure initial one and they become mixed. So it is with confounding factors. The confounding factor (the 'confounder') becomes confused with the factor of interest, and we lose its purity. In other words, confounding variables are generally variables that are causally associated with the outcome variable under investigation and non-causally associated with the explanatory variable of interest. Whereas bias might arise from error in the measurement of a variable, confounding involves error in the *interpretation* of what may be an accurate measurement.

In research study design, we want to minimise confounders. In randomised controlled trials, the easiest way of doing this is to randomly allocate participants to groups. This ensures that confounders are spread throughout the groups fairly, and not stacked up

Type	How it operates	How study design can prevent it	What to look for when critically appraising an article
Selection or sampling bias	Systematic differences between those who are selected for study and those who are not selected. This means that the results of the study may not be generalisable to the population from which the sample is drawn.	Good sampling ensures that the people who are participating are representative of the population you want to generalise to.	Check how the sampling was done. Look for any data that compares this sample with the population's characteristics.
Allocation bias	In experimental studies, allocation or selection bias can refer to intervention and control groups being systematically different.	Randomisation attempts to evenly distribute both known and unknown confounders. Assess differences between groups at baseline. Statistically control for differences in analysis.	Check the article for a comparison of the groups before an intervention to see if they look sufficiently similar (also known as baseline similarity).
Maturation bias	The effect might be due to changes that have occurred naturally over time, not because of any intervention.	Use a control group and random allocation to intervention or control group.	Check to see if a control group and random allocation were used.
Attrition bias	Participants who withdraw from studies may differ systematically from those who remain. Alternatively, there may be more participants lost from one group in the study than the other group.	Minimise loss to follow-up. Analyse the results by intention-to-treat.	Reject articles with a loss to follow-up of >15%. Check if results were analysed by intention-to-treat.
Measurement bias in experimental studies	Errors in measuring exposure or outcome can lead to differential accuracy of information between groups. In other words, if the way that data are measured differs systematically between groups, this introduces bias. In experimental studies, this can be due to bias in the expectations of study participants, health professionals or researchers.	'Blinding' participants, health professionals or researchers will reduce this bias. Blinding is discussed further in Chapter 4.	Look to see if the study used methods to reduce the participants', health professionals' and/or researchers' awareness of a participant's group allocation (blinding).

TABLE 2.6 Some common kinds of bias

(Continued)

Type	How it operates	How study design can prevent it	What to look for when critically appraising an article
Placebo effect	An improvement in the participants' condition may occur because they expect or believe that the intervention they are receiving will cause an improvement.	Have a control group of participants that receive approximately the same intervention (that is, raise no different expectations). 'Blinding' participants, health professionals or researchers will reduce this bias.	Check if there is a suitable control group and look to see if the study used methods to reduce the participants', health professionals' and/or researchers' awareness of a participant's group allocation (blinding).
Hawthorne effect	Participants may experience changes because of the attention that they are receiving from being a part of the research process.	Have a control group that is studied in the same way (except for the intervention)— that is, a randomised controlled trial.	Check if there is a suitable control group to control for attention and if the randomised controlled trial is designed properly.

TABLE 2.6 Some common kinds of bias —(Cont'd)

in one group unfairly. Another way of addressing this is to make a list of confounders and ensure that they are evenly distributed across the groups. In fact, this is the method employed for observational studies (since there is no other option).

However the problem is *unknown* confounders—factors that we either cannot measure, or do not even know about—that could influence the results. For example, participants' level of motivation to participate fully in an intervention (consider one that required people to perform certain exercises daily) is very difficult to measure accurately and could be a potential unknown confounder for a study that was examining the effectiveness of this intervention. Randomisation is the key, because the act of randomisation distributes all confounders both known and unknown fairly. A problem remains, though. What about the chance of an unequal distribution of confounders between groups? The answer to that is to do with two things: numbers and statistics.

Statistical significance, clinical significance and power

Statistical significance

The concern that we identified above is that a randomised controlled trial could be biased because of a chance uneven distribution of confounders across the groups. The chance of this happening is reduced if the number of participants in the trial is increased (as the numbers get larger, the chance of unevenness decreases). The problem is that, however large the trial is designed to be, the chance of unevenness never decreases to zero, meaning that there is always a chance of bias from confounders. This means that we have to tolerate some uncertainty, less as the trial size gets larger, until the trial is sufficiently large that we can relax. The question is: how large? The answer is assisted by statistics, which is the science of dealing with this uncertainty and quantifying it. There are two main ways of deciding whether a difference in the summaries of two groups of participants is due to chance or to a real difference between them.

1. The **p value**

P is short for 'probability'. The test is based on one of the cornerstones of scientific philosophy: that we cannot ever prove anything, but rather can only disprove it.[8] This means that we have to invert the test from the intuitive which is

  •   'Are the measurements between the two groups different enough to assume that it is because of some factor other than chance?'

  to

  •   'Are the measurements between the two groups *similar* enough to assume that it is because of chance alone?'

If we can show that the latter statement is unlikely, then we can say that there must be some *other* factor responsible for the difference. In other words the *p* value is estimated to establish 'how likely it is that the difference is because of chance alone'. Statisticians estimate a value of *p* that will be somewhere between 1.0 (absolutely sure that the difference is because of chance alone) and 0.0 (absolutely sure that the difference is *not* because of chance alone). Traditionally we set the arbitrary value of *p* as <0.05, at which point we assume that chance was so unlikely that we can rule it out as the cause of the difference. A value of 0.05 (5/100) is the same as 5% or 1:20. What we say when we use this cut-off point for the *p* value is: 'We would have to repeat the study an average of 20 times for the result to happen once by chance alone'. When a study produces a result where the *p* value is <0.05, that result is considered to be 'statistically significant'.

2. **Confidence intervals**

Confidence intervals take a different approach and instead estimate what range of values the true value lies within. True value refers to the population value, not just the estimate of a value that has come from the sample of one study (such as an estimate about how effective an intervention is)—this is explained in more depth in Chapter 4. The range of values is called the confidence interval, and is most commonly set at the same arbitrary level as *p* values (0.95, or 20:1), which is also called the 95% confidence interval. Another way to think of the value is graphically, as shown in Figure 2.2.

Figures 2.2A and 2.2B show the range of possible values for an estimated measurement for two different studies. In each figure the two vertical lines indicate the two limits (or boundaries) of the confidence interval. The values in between these lines indicate the range of values within which we are 95% certain (or confident, hence the term confidence intervals) that the true value is likely to lie. The probability that the true value lies outside of this confidence interval is 0.05 (or 5%), with half of this value (2.5%) in each tail of the curve. The most likely value is central and, in most cases, the distribution of possible values forms a normal distribution (that is, a bell-shaped curve). The spread of values will form a different shape according to different influences on the 95% confidence interval. For example, in the study that is represented by Figure 2.2B, the sample size is larger. This has the effect of narrowing the 95% confidence interval because the normal curve is more peaked. The same effect is achieved by samples that yield greater uniformity of the participants (that is, decreased variance of the sample). This is summarised in Table 2.7.

Confidence intervals are an important concept to understand if you wish to practise evidence-based practice as they help you with the second step (what is the impact of the

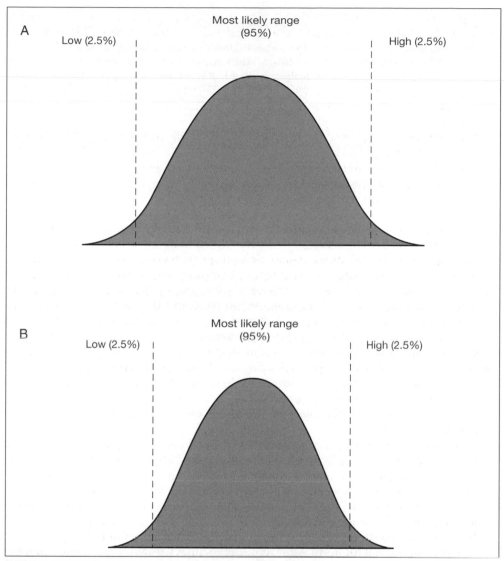

FIGURE 2.2 For two different studies, the range of possible values for an estimated measurement (with the 95% confidence interval) is shown. In 2.2B, the 95% confidence interval is smaller (narrower) than the one in 2.2A. A smaller confidence interval can occur when the sample size of a study is larger.

evidence?) of the three-step critical appraisal process that was described in Chapter 1. The role that confidence intervals play in helping you to determine the impact of the evidence is explained in more detail in Chapter 4.

Clinical significance

There is one more essential consideration: how big a difference is worthwhile? Once we have established a difference that is unlikely to be attributable to chance (that is, it is statistically significant), how can we decide whether the difference is important? Clinical significance is defined as just that: the minimum difference that would be important. (Because of this, some people use the term 'clinical importance' rather than 'clinical

Factor	Effect on the confidence interval
Sample size (that is, the number of participants in the study)	The confidence interval narrows as the sample size increases—there is more certainty about the effect estimate. This is one of the reasons why it is important that studies have an adequate sample size. The importance of a smaller (narrower) confidence interval is explained in Chapter 4.
Variance (the amount of 'noise' or differences in values between participants in the sample)	The confidence interval widens as the variance increases— there is less certainty about the effect estimate.

TABLE 2.7   Effect of sample size and variance on a study's confidence interval

significance' to refer to this concept.) We cannot use statistics to measure it because it is a judgement: we have to decide what difference would be important (meaning, would change clinical practice). This means choosing some difference based on what is clinically important. Such differences are called 'clinically significant'. For example, consider an intervention study where the outcome being measured was pain, using a visual analogue scale (a straight line with one end meaning 'no pain' and the other end meaning 'the most pain imaginable'). If the intervention had the effect of reducing participants' pain (on average) by 4 points on a 10-point visual analogue scale (where 1 = 'no pain' and 10 = 'the most pain imaginable'), we would probably judge a difference of this size to be clinically significant, whereas a reduction of 0.5 would probably not be considered clinically significant. Chapter 4 discusses in further detail the various approaches that can be used to help determine clinical significance.

Hopefully it is now clear that there are three main categories that the results of a study can fall into:
- a result that is not statistically significant—when this is the case, you do not need to bother deciding whether the result is clinically significant as you cannot even be very sure that the result was not due to chance
- a result that is statistically significant but *not* clinically significant—this is unfortunately a common scenario, and regrettably means that you cannot use a result such as this to inform your clinical decision making
- a result that is statistically significant *and* clinically significant—this is the type of result that we hope for as it means that this result is potentially useful in our clinical practice and we can proceed to the third step in the three-step critical appraisal process— deciding whether you can apply the evidence to your client.

Outcome measures—what you need to know about them
The issue of clinical significance raises another issue that is important when it comes to appraising articles—you need to know about the outcome measure that a study used as this helps you to make a judgement about clinical significance. In our pain study example, if the visual analogue scale that was used to measure pain was a 0–100 scale, then we would probably no longer consider a reduction in pain of 4 points (on a 100-point scale) to be clinically significant (although on a 10-point scale, we felt that it was). If you are lucky, the study that you are reading will include the scale range of the continuous outcome measures used in the study somewhere in the article (usually in the methods section or in a results table). If they do not, then you will need to find this information out for yourself. If it is an outcome measure that you are familiar with, great! If not,

perhaps searching for it on the internet (even Google can be useful in this instance) may help you to find out more about it.

In addition to knowing about the actual measures that a study used to measure the outcomes, it is important that you consider whether the outcomes themselves are relevant, useful and important to your client. When referring to intervention studies, put simply, a good intervention is one that improves outcomes that matter to clients. For example, you may have a client who has had a stroke and, as a result, has difficulty using their arm to perform functional activities such as eating and getting dressed. The client's goal is to return to doing these activities independently. You are considering using a physical rehabilitation technique on them to improve their ability to carry out these activities, primarily by working on the quality of the movement that they have in their affected arm. Let us suppose that when evaluating the evidence for the effectiveness of this intervention, there are two studies that you can use to inform your practice (for the sake of simplicity, we will assume that they both have a similar level of internal validity): the outcomes measured in one study (study A) are arm function and the ability to perform self-care activities, whereas the outcome measured in the other study (study B) is quality of arm movement. In this (very simplified!) example, if you choose study A to inform your clinical practice you will be able to communicate the results of the study to the client and explain to them the estimated effect that the intervention may have on their ability to perform these activities. Remember that this is what your client primarily wants to know about. Although study B may provide you with information that is useful to you as a health professional, the effect that the intervention may have on the quality of arm movement may be of less interest to your client than knowing how it may improve the function of their arm. Considering whether the outcomes measured by a study are useful to your client is one way of considering the client-centredness of the study. In Chapter 14, the concept of client-centred care is explained and the importance of encouraging clients' involvement in decisions about their health care is discussed.

Putting it all together: thinking about power

As we mentioned earlier, we can have results that are statistically significant but not clinically significant. But statistical significance can be made more likely by increasing the size of the sample (or reducing the 'noise', more properly called 'variance'). If a study is large enough, its results will become statistically significant even though the differences are not important clinically—which is why we call on clinical significance to decide what is worthwhile. This means we can decide on the minimum size a study's sample has to be to give a definitive answer. This is important because it helps decide what would be wasteful (above the minimum is wasteful of research resources). Estimating the minimum is called a 'power calculation'. A study has enough power (meaning there is a large enough sample) if a statistically significant difference is found.

In other words, the power of a study is the degree to which we are certain that, if we conclude that a difference does *not* exist, that it in fact does *not* exist. The accepted level of power is generally set at the arbitrary level of 80% (or 0.80).

But what happens if the minimum sample size is not reached? Such a study is called 'underpowered', meaning that if a non-significant difference was found, it might nevertheless correspond to a truly clinically significant difference, but this was something that was not detected because the sample was too small. In other words, a non-significant result might mean either that there is truly no difference or that the sample was too small to detect one. This state of affairs, where a study has incorrectly concluded that a difference does not exist, is also called a type-2 error. Because of the risk of this type of error occurring, when evaluating a study, you need to decide whether the study had adequate power (that is, a large enough sample size). This can be determined by checking an article to see if the researchers did a power calculation. When researchers do a power analysis prior to conducting the study, it enables them to estimate how many participants they will need to recruit to be reasonably sure (to a given level of uncertainty) that they will detect an important difference if it really exists. You can then check if they actually did recruit at least as many participants as they estimated would be needed.

Can a study be too large? Surprisingly, the answer is yes. If a study is too large, then effort and money have been wasted in undertaking research unnecessarily. A more subtle reason is that a difference that is statistically significant can be found, but the difference may be so small that we judge its significance to not be meaningful. This can mean having a situation that we discussed earlier in this chapter where a difference is *statistically* significant but *clinically* **not** significant.

Summary points of this chapter

- Questions about frequency, diagnosis, prognosis and the effects of interventions are among the types of clinical questions that can usually be answered using evidence-based practice.
- Converting your informational needs into answerable clinical questions is the first step of the evidence-based practice process. A well-structured question can be achieved by using the PICO (Patient/problem, Intervention, Comparison, Outcome[s]) format.
- Systematic reviews, randomised controlled trials, cohort studies, cross-sectional studies and case-control studies are some of the common study types that are used in evidence-based practice.
- For each type of question, there is a different hierarchy of evidence. The higher up the hierarchy that a study is, the more likely it is that the study can minimise the impact of bias on the results of the study. You should use the hierarchy of evidence that is appropriate to your question to guide your search for and selection of evidence to answer your question.
- For all question types, a systematic review of level II evidence is at the top of the hierarchy and you should always search for this type of evidence first. The study type that is level II evidence is different for each question type. For intervention questions, level II evidence is a randomised controlled trial; for prognostic questions it is a prospective cohort study; and for diagnostic studies it is a study of test accuracy that involved an independent, blinded comparison with a valid reference standard, among consecutive persons with a defined clinical presentation.
- Being able to recognise if bias and/or confounding have occurred in a study is a crucial part of the critical appraisal process as it enables you to determine the internal validity of the evidence. There are many types of bias and you need to be able to recognise them. Internal validity refers to how much we can trust the results of a study and is a reflection of the degree to which chance, bias and/or confounding are operating in a study.
- If the result of a study is statistically significant, it means that we are reasonably sure that the result (such as a difference in outcomes between two groups in a study) did not occur because of chance. Statistical significance can be indicated by *p* values or confidence intervals. In evidence-based practice, confidence intervals are much more useful than *p* values. If a result is statistically significant, you then need to consider if it is also clinically significant—that is, is the result important enough that you will use it in your clinical practice? Clinical significance is determined by judgement.

References

1. Ely J, Osheroff J, Ebell M et al. Analysis of questions asked by family doctors regarding patient care. BMJ 1999; 319:358–361.
2. Gonzalez-Gonzalez A, Dawes M, Sanchez-Mateos J et al. Information needs and information-seeking behaviour of primary care physicians. Ann Fam Med 2007; 5:345–352.
3. Gorman PN, Helfand M. Information seeking in primary care: how physicians choose which clinical questions to pursue and which to leave unanswered. Med Decis Making 1995; 15:113–119.
4. Cogdill KW. Information needs and information seeking in primary care: a study of nurse practitioners. J Med Libr Assoc 2003; 91:203–215.
5. Coumou HC, Meijman FJ. How do primary care physicians seek answers to clinical questions? A literature review. JAMA 2006; 94:55–60.
6. Straus S, Richardson W, Glasziou P et al. Evidence-based medicine: how to practice and teach EBM. 3rd edn. Edinburgh: Elsevier; 2005.
7. National Health and Medical Research Council (NHMRC). NHMRC additional levels of evidence and grades for recommendations for developers of guidelines. 2008. Online. Available: http://www.nhmrc.gov.au (23 Aug 2008).
8. Hacking I. An introduction to probability and inductive logic. 1st edn. New York: Cambridge University Press; 2001.

CHAPTER 3

Finding the evidence

Nancy Wilczynski and Ann McKibbon

LEARNING OBJECTIVES

After reading this chapter, you should be able to:
- Describe the basics of searching
- Understand how literature services are organised
- Be aware of the major online evidence-based resources and how they fit into the organisation of literature services
- Be aware of the discipline-specific online evidence-based resources
- Know which databases will likely have an answer when searching for evidence for each type of question (that is, intervention, diagnosis, prognosis and qualitative)
- Know how to search for evidence for each type of question

One of the most important and challenging aspects of implementing evidence-based practice can be finding the current best evidence relevant to your clinical question. The internet provides ready and free access to information but the information explosion and the ever-increasing availability of online resources makes finding the current best evidence difficult. Many online resources falsely claim to be 'evidence-based', making it difficult for health professionals to navigate internet sites. In addition to discerning if the information provided on the internet site is based on sound evidence, research shows that some of the obstacles that are most frequently encountered when attempting to find the answer to a clinical question are:
- the excessive amount of time required to find information
- difficulty in selecting an optimal strategy to search for information
- failure of the selected resource to provide an answer.[1]

These barriers can be reduced by approaching the search for the current best evidence in a systematic way that harnesses the organisation of the literature to your advantage. In this chapter, we will show you some of the main ways that you can do this. We will begin by describing the basics of searching, followed by a description of a model that outlines a categorisation of evidence-based information services and how this evidence is processed and presented. Within each category of this model, we will describe the types of evidence that are included and the resources that are available to find that type of evidence. We will concentrate on the resources which have the strongest evidence base as these resources are the ones that are likely to be of most use to you in your clinical practice and are also typically the resources that are easier and faster to use. The chapter concludes with a number of clinical questions and examples of how you can find an answer to these questions using the model and the information resources that are described in the chapter.

The basics of searching

So that your search for evidence is as efficient as possible, it is a good idea to understand some of the basic principles of effective searching, which are:
1. Carefully define your clinical question.
2. Choose your key search terms.
3. Broaden your search if necessary, with synonyms, truncation and/or wildcards.
4. Use Boolean operators.

Carefully define your clinical question

Information about how to construct a well-formulated clinical question, using the PICO format, was provided in Chapter 2.

Choose your key search terms

Using the PICO format to structure your clinical question makes choosing key search terms relatively easy. Typically you would start your search using the 'P' (patients [or population]) and 'I' (intervention) terms or phrases from your question. For example, if your question was 'In people with chronic low back pain, is an operant-behavioural graded activity program more effective than physical training in improving functional ability?' you would start your search with the phrases "chronic low back pain" ('P' terms) and "operant-behavioural graded activity" ('I' terms).

Broaden your search if necessary

Once you have identified key terms or phrases you should consider broadening your search, particularly if your initial search yields no relevant articles.

- The first way to broaden your search is to consider using **synonyms and related terms**. For example, if you are searching for articles on clients with "rheumatoid arthritis" you can broaden your search by also searching with the terms "RA" and "rheumatologic disease". Several online resources list synonyms and related terms for many diseases and conditions, for example, eMedicine from WebMD (http://www.emedicine.com/; choose a condition), eMedicineHealth from WebMD (http://www.emedicinehealth.com/script/main/hp.asp) and Genetics Home Reference from the U.S. National Library of Medicine (http://ghr.nlm.nih.gov/glossary).
- Another way to widen your search is to use **truncation and wildcards**. When using truncation in a search you enter the first part of a keyword, insert a symbol (usually an asterisk symbol*) and accept any variant spellings or word endings, from the occurrence of the symbol onward. For example, "disease*" would retrieve records with the word disease, as well as the words diseases, diseased etc. When using wildcards in a search you enter a wild card character (usually "?") within or at the end of a keyword to substitute for only one character. Wildcards are particularly useful when searching for some plural forms, such as "wom?n", which would retrieve records with the words woman and women. Wildcards are also very useful when searching for terms where there is a variation between the American and Australian spelling of the words, such as orthopaedic and paediatric. Searching with the term "orthop?edic" will find articles that use orthopaedic as well as orthopedic. Truncation symbols and wildcard characters vary between databases and database providers; for example, in PubMed the truncation symbol is an asterisk (*) whereas when searching MEDLINE in Ovid it is a colon (:) or dollar sign ($). Consult each database's online help section to determine which symbols or characters to use.

Use Boolean operators

Once you have determined the terms or phrases that you will include in your search you should consider combining your search terms using the Boolean logical operators. The Boolean AND command is used when you want all search terms to be present in each article that is retrieved. For example, when searching using 'P' terms and 'I' terms you would combine these using the Boolean AND command as you would want to retrieve articles that have both your patient/population of interest *and* the intervention of interest. Using our example above, your search strategy would be "(chronic low back pain) AND (operant-behavioural graded activity)", thus narrowing your search.

The Boolean OR command is used when you want *any* of the specified search terms to be present in the articles. When incorporating synonyms and related terms you would search using the Boolean OR command, for example, "rheumatoid arthritis OR RA OR rheumatologic disease", thus broadening your search. When using this search you will retrieve articles that have any one of 'rheumatoid arthritis' OR 'RA' OR 'rheumatologic disease'. How search terms should be grouped together, that is, whether "double inverted commas" or brackets () should be used, varies between different databases, so it is useful to check this in the database's help section.

Basics of searching—an example

To illustrate these basics of searching further we will work through a step-by-step example.

Clinical scenario

You are a rehabilitation consultant who has recently seen a number of individuals with work-related neck muscle pain, especially pain from the descending part of the trapezius muscle. You know that physical exercise is generally recommended but you do not know which type of training is more effective in relieving muscle pain—strength training of the painful muscle or general fitness training without direct involvement of the painful muscle.

Step 1: Identify the components of your question in PICO format

P Patient population	I Intervention (therapy, diagnostic test, prognostic factor)	C Comparison	O Outcomes
Work-related neck muscle pain	Strength training of the painful muscle	General fitness training	Pain relief

Step 2: Compose your clinical question

Clients with work-related neck muscle pain	Patients
Strength training of the painful muscle	Intervention
General fitness training without direct involvement of the painful muscle	Comparison
Greater pain relief	Outcomes

Step 3: Construct the final clinical question

For clients with work-related neck muscle pain, does strength training of the painful muscle versus general fitness training without direct involvement of the painful muscle result in greater pain relief?

Step 4: Record keywords and phrases

Keyword 1:	Keyword 2:	Keyword 3:	Keyword 4:
Neck muscle pain	Muscular strength training	General fitness	Pain relief

Step 5: Identify synonyms and variant words

Keyword 1:	Keyword 2:	Keyword 3:	Keyword 4:
Neck strain Neck strains Neck strain injury Neck strain injuries Neck sprain Neck sprains Stiff neck Trapezius muscle pain	Strength training Muscle strengthening	Exercise	Pain

Step 6: Use truncation and wildcards where appropriate and Boolean operators to combine terms

(Neck muscle pain OR Neck strain* OR Neck strain injur* OR Neck sprain* OR Stiff neck OR Trapezius muscle pain) AND (Strength training OR Muscle strengthening) AND (General fitness OR Exercise) AND (Pain*)

Note: The truncation symbol used in this example is for conducting a search in PubMed.

Step 7: Decide which online resource(s) to search

The online resource that you decide to search in will depend on the type of question that you are asking (for example, intervention, diagnostic, prognostic or qualitative question). As was explained in Chapter 2, for each type of question there is a hierarchy of evidence. This hierarchy should be used to guide your search so that you know what type of study design you are hoping to find when searching. The type of study design that you are looking for will, in turn, influence which online resource(s) you should search in. For example, if your clinical question is a prognostic one related to rehabilitation, then you will be looking for a cohort study (or systematic review of cohort studies). Therefore, there is no point in searching the Cochrane Library, PEDro or OTseeker as these resources do not contain cohort studies. The best resource for you to start your search in would probably be PubMed, using the Clinical Queries feature. All of these resources, and many others, are described in the following section and in the examples at the end of this chapter.

A model of evidence-based information services

In this chapter, we will use a five-level pyramid to discuss the organisation of evidence-based information services.[2] This '5S' model (see Figure 3.1) is hierarchical in nature and has:

- **original studies** (what was done in one study) at the base
- **syntheses** (what the evidence is across several studies on the same topic)—that is, systematic reviews of the literature
- **synopses** (what the evidence is across several studies, along with an expert telling you its strengths and potential practice changes)—that is, succinct descriptions of original studies and reviews, often accompanied by expert commentaries such as those found in evidence-based secondary journals like *ACP Journal Club*, *Evidence-Based Medicine* and *Evidence-Based Nursing*

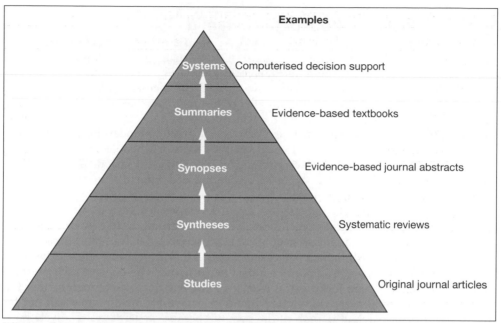

FIGURE 3.1 The 5S pyramid showing levels of organisation of evidence from healthcare research
Reproduced with permission from Haynes RB, Of studies, syntheses, synopses, summaries, and systems: the "5S" evolution of information services for evidence-based healthcare decisions; American College of Physicians; 2006[2]

- **summaries**—that is, management options for diseases or conditions arranged by clinical topics such as those that appear in the Physician's Information and Education Resource (PIER) and Clinical Evidence (quite like a textbook chapter with a broad-based summary of a content area)
- **systems**—that is, integrated decision support services which provide evidence plus 'actions' that should be taken in relation to a specific client or situation.

As you are seeking the current best evidence, begin your search as high up in the pyramid as possible. The higher you go in the pyramid, the more the evidence has been collected, sifted and synthesised. As the synthesis and evaluation work has already been done by others, using evidence from the higher levels will save you time and labour and assist you to apply the best quality evidence that is currently available.

Deciding where to start on the pyramid depends largely on the question being asked and what resources are available to you. As explained earlier, you should be guided by the hierarchy of evidence for the type of question that you are asking. Additionally, you will also find that much of the content that is available at the higher levels of the pyramid is aimed at the medical profession and that most of the evidence for nursing and the allied health questions are found in the bottom two levels of the pyramid and, at times, level three. At each level of the '5S' pyramid, users of the evidence must appraise the quality of the evidence presented ensuring that the methods used to generate this evidence were sound. Detailed information about how to critically appraise evidence, once you have found it, is presented in Chapters 4–12 of this book. Each level of the pyramid will now be discussed further, starting at the top of the pyramid, where the best and most highly synthesised evidence can be found.

Systems—first layer (top) of the pyramid

Systems are found at the top of the '5S' pyramid. A system is an integrated clinical decision support service designed to improve clinical decision making. Such a system may be integrated into an electronic client health record system or hospital clinical information system. Alternatively, the system may allow for entry of client-specific characteristics, such as age, gender, renal function and allergy history. These computerised decision support systems reliably link client characteristics with the current evidence-based guidelines for care. The system generates client-specific recommendations (for example, lower the dose of insulin because of hypoglycaemic events or schedule a mammography because it is due next month). A key component of a clinical decision support service that differentiates it from other types of evidence-based information services is the integration of client-specific variables.

Clinical decision support systems have been developed for various clinical issues, including the diagnosis of chest pain, the management of chronic disease (such as diabetes care) and the timely administration of preventive services (such as immunisations). A systematic review of the effects of computerised clinical decision support systems showed that many improve health professionals' performance.[3] If you have such a system in your workplace, you are lucky as it is likely that you will not need to look further for the best evidence to answer your clinical question. However, most people will not be able to begin their search at the top of the pyramid because systems are relatively rare, existing for only a few diseases or conditions, and usually have a medical focus. Not all health professions have electronic client medical records and, even if they do, many are not integrated with a decision support system that has an evidence-based guideline summarising the current best evidence on a topic of interest. Therefore, if you do not have access to a system that addresses your information needs, you will need to start your search for the current best evidence at the next level down in the pyramid.

Summaries—second layer of the pyramid

Summaries are information resources that provide regularly updated evidence, which is usually arranged by clinical topics. They are considered to be similar to traditional textbook chapters in form and content. Evidence-based clinical guidelines are also located at this level of the pyramid. Summaries provide guidance and/or recommendations for client management and often provide links to other aspects of the disease or condition. Summaries can be found in disease-specific textbooks such as *Evidence-based Endo-crinology*[4] but, unless the textbook is accompanied by a website where the content can be regularly updated, the content in a print textbook becomes quickly outdated. Online textbooks that are regularly updated are becoming more common. Medicine has the most of these online textbooks and some of these contain information which may be of interest to allied health professionals or nurses. All of the online textbooks listed below are available on a subscription basis but many workplaces, particularly academic and healthcare institutions, may have institutional subscriptions. Examples of these online textbooks are:

• *Clinical Evidence* (http://clinicalevidence.bmj.com/ceweb/index.jsp) is provided by the BMJ Publishing Group and summarises evidence on the benefits and harms of healthcare interventions for selected medical conditions. The evidence is drawn from systematic reviews and original studies. The content is presented in question format (for example, what are the effects of interventions aimed at reducing relapse rates and disability in people with multiple sclerosis?), with the levels of evidence used to answer the question and hyperlinks to the supporting evidence. A clinical guide (that is, a comment on how to use this information in clinical practice) is also presented.

- *Physician's Information and Education Resource (PIER)* (http://pier.acponline.org/index.html), from the American College of Physicians (ACP), is an integrated summary service that provides evidence-based guidance and practice recommendations for health professionals. It is organised into seven topic types (diseases, screening and prevention, complementary and alternative medicine, ethical and legal issues, procedures, quality measures and drug resources), with each topic containing several modules. *PIER*'s authors are supported by an explicit evidence-based process, where current best evidence is provided to the authors of the chapters after comprehensive literature searches are conducted.

  PIER is available online to ACP members but it can be accessed through *STAT!Ref* (http://www.statref.com/), an online healthcare reference that provides full text access to key medical reference sources and textbooks, some of which are evidence-based resources. *STAT!Ref* is a subscription-based resource that is usually available in academic or hospital environments where institutional subscriptions exist. *PIER* is more directive than *Clinical Evidence* as it contains recommendations rather than evidence summaries.

- *Up To Date* (http://www.uptodate.com/) is an online textbook that is very comprehensive in its topic coverage. It is currently organised into 16 medical specialties (for example, adult primary care and internal medicine, cardiovascular medicine, endocrinology and diabetes, family medicine). *UpToDate* provides specific recommendations (guidelines) for health professionals for client care and most, but not all, of these recommendations include an assessment of the quality of the evidence.

- *First Consult* (http://www.mdconsult.com/das/pdxmd/lookup/87695189-2?type=med) is part of *MD Consult*, from Elsevier, and is an evidence-based and continuously updated clinical information resource for primary care clinicians. Designed for use at point-of-care (for example, at the bedside, in the clinic), information is arranged around the components of medical topics, differential diagnosis and procedures. Recommendations are made but neither the levels of evidence nor links to supporting evidence accompany each recommendation.

- *EBM Guidelines: Evidence Based Medicine* (http://ebmg.wiley.com/ebmg/ltk.koti), from Wiley Interscience, is a collection of clinical guidelines for primary care combined with the best available evidence. There are approximately 1000 primary care practice guidelines, which are continuously updated and cover a wide range of medical conditions. Both diagnosis and treatment are included.

Synopses—third layer of the pyramid

If you do not find an answer to your clinical question in a summary, the next best place to search for an answer is in a synopsis. Synopses are structured abstracts or brief overviews of published individual studies and systematic reviews that have been screened for methodological rigour. This means you do not have to do this step yourself! Synopses can be found in the following online resources:

- *ACP Journal Club* (http://www.acpjc.org/), *Evidence-Based Medicine* (http://ebm.bmj.com/) and *Evidence-Based Nursing* (http://ebn.bmj.com/) are pre-appraised, secondary journals that are available online as well as in print. To produce the content for these journals, research staff hand-search over 130 core healthcare journals and critically appraise the articles in each issue to identify high quality primary studies and review articles that have potential for clinical application. From this pool of articles, practising health professionals rate the content for relevancy and newsworthiness. The studies and reviews that are considered to be the most clinically important are summarised in structured abstracts. A clinical expert comments on the methods and provides a clinical bottom line (that is, how to use the evidence in clinical practice).

The focus of the content in *ACP Journal Club* is internal medicine and it includes sections on therapy, diagnosis, prognosis, aetiology, quality improvement and continuing education, economics, clinical prediction guides and differential diagnosis. The focus of the content in *Evidence-Based Medicine* is general medical practice and includes the same sections as *ACP Journal Club* (for example, therapy, diagnosis etc). The focus of the content in *Evidence-Based Nursing* is nursing and includes the same sections as *ACP Journal Club* and *Evidence-Based Medicine* with an additional section that contains articles of a qualitative nature. These evidence-based journals are subscription-based resources. *ACP Journal Club* is also one of the databases available through Ovid (http://gateway.ovid.com/), a company that designs search engines and makes several evidence-based databases available on a subscription basis. Many institutions such as libraries, hospitals and universities use Ovid and therefore have institutional subscriptions.

- **Bandolier** (http://www.jr2.ox.ac.uk/bandolier/) provides a summary service that covers selected medical topics. Information comes from systematic reviews, meta-analyses, randomised trials and from high quality observational studies. The review of the clinical evidence is combined with a clinical commentary and a clinical bottom line. Bandolier's internet version is free of charge.
- **Several journals** also have sections where they highlight critically appraised papers. They generally use similar principles and format to *ACP Journal Club, Evidence-Based Medicine* and *Evidence-Based Nursing*. Examples in the allied health professions are the *Australian Journal of Physiotherapy, Australian Occupational Therapy Journal* and the Canadian Associations of Occupational Therapists *OT Now* publication.

A list of resources with hotlinks of pre-appraised resource journals (synopses) for various disciplines is maintained by The New York Academy of Medicine and is available at http://www.ebmny.org/journal.html.

Syntheses—fourth layer of the pyramid

When no synopses can be found, the next best place to look for an answer to your clinical question is a systematic review. Systematic reviews provide syntheses of the highest quality evidence available for a specific clinical question. Information about how to appraise systematic reviews is presented in Chapter 12 of this book. Systematic reviews can be found in the following resources:

- **Cochrane Database of Systematic Reviews** (http://www3.interscience.wiley.com/cgi-bin/mrwhome/106568753/HOME) is part of the Cochrane Library and is made up of several review groups that concentrate and synthesise the evidence in specific healthcare areas. For example, the focus of the Cochrane Musculoskeletal Group is synthesising the evidence from randomised controlled trials and controlled clinical trials of interventions that are concerned with the prevention, treatment and/or rehabilitation of musculoskeletal disorders.

Up until January 2008, the focus of the Cochrane Database of Systematic Reviews was solely on healthcare interventions. However, from Issue 1, 2008, reviews on diagnostic test accuracy were introduced. As of Issue 2, 2009, there were 5785 records available and most of these were completed reviews. Even with this many systematic reviews available, the Cochrane Collaboration contains less than half of the world's supply of systematic reviews.

The Cochrane Library, which houses the Cochrane Database of Systematic Reviews, is a subscription-based resource that is usually available in academic or hospital environments where institutional subscriptions exist. However, residents in a number of countries or regions can access The Cochrane Library online for free. A list of these countries and regions can be found at http://www3.interscience.wiley.com/cgi-bin/ mrwhome/106568753/AccessCochraneLibrary.html. Cochrane systematic reviews are indexed in several large biomedical electronic databases such as MEDLINE and are therefore also available through other vendors such as Ovid on a subscription basis and through PubMed (http://www.ncbi.nlm.nih.gov/sites/entrez?db=pubmed), which is free.

There are a number of ways to search in the Cochrane Database of Systematic Reviews, such as Quick Search, Advanced Search and MeSH search (see Box 3.1 for an explanation of MeSH). As the Cochrane Library is such an important evidence-based practice resource, it is important that you know how to search in it efficiently. We highly recommend that you read through the easy-to-read Cochrane Library User Guide, which is available for free at: http://www3.interscience.wiley.com/homepages/106568753/ CochraneLibraryUserGuide.pdf.

- **Database of Abstracts of Reviews of Effects (DARE)** (http://www.crd.york.ac.uk/ crdweb/) is produced by the Centre for Reviews and Dissemination at the University of York in the United Kingdom and contains abstracts of quality-assessed non-Cochrane systematic reviews. Each abstract includes a summary of the review together with a critical commentary about the overall quality of the review. DARE covers a broad range of health-related interventions. As of June 2009, it included over 15000 abstracts of systematic reviews. DARE is available free of charge. The Cochrane Library also includes DARE content.
- **Campbell Collaboration** (http://www.campbellcollaboration.org/) conducts and maintains systematic reviews about the effects of interventions in the social, behavioural and educational arenas (for example, social skills training). As of June 2009, the free searchable database contained 51 completed systematic reviews.
- **Various biomedical databases**—many systematic reviews are available in the large electronic biomedical databases such as MEDLINE and EMBASE. These databases are available through various providers such as Ovid (http://gateway.ovid.com/) on a subscription basis. MEDLINE is also available free of charge through PubMed.

It can be challenging to efficiently retrieve systematic reviews from these large databases because of the sheer volume of articles that they contain and because they also contain many other types of articles that are not useful for answering clinical questions. To assist with the retrieval of systematic reviews, researchers have developed search strategies for use in these large databases. The Clinical Queries screen in PubMed (http://www. ncbi.nih.gov/entrez/query/static/clinical.shtml; or accessed by a link on the PubMed homepage) offers some assistance to efficient searching by providing a ready-to-use search strategy for identifying systematic reviews. This feature is described in more detail later in this chapter when MEDLINE is discussed further.

- **Discipline-specific databases**—there are several discipline-specific databases which contain systematic reviews or index systematic reviews. For example:
  - **health-evidence.ca** (http://www.health-evidence.ca) is a free, searchable online registry of public health systematic reviews.
  - **OTseeker** (Occupational Therapy Systematic Evaluation of Evidence) is an occupational therapy evidence database and is freely available at http://www. otseeker.com/. OTseeker is described in more detail in the following section.
  - **PEDro** is the Physiotherapy Evidence Database, from the Centre for Evidence-based Physiotherapy in Australia, and is freely available at http://www.pedro.org. au. PEDro is described in more detail in the following section.
  - **PsycBITE** (the Psychological Database for Brain Impairment Treatment Efficacy) is freely available at http://www.psycbite.com/. PsycBITE is described in more detail in the following section.

- ◦ **speechBITE** (Speech Pathology Database for Best Interventions and Treatment Efficacy) is freely available at http://www.speechbite.com and is described in more detail in the following section.
- ◦ The **Joanna Briggs Institute** provides a library of systematic reviews that is available on a subscription basis (http://www.joannabriggs.edu.au/pubs/systematic_reviews.php). It contains reviews that are of relevance to nursing, physiotherapy, podiatry, occupational therapy, medical radiation and complementary therapy.

Studies—fifth layer (bottom) of the pyramid

When none of the upper layers of the pyramid provide an answer to your clinical question, you must look for individual studies. There are millions of individual studies, which can make it difficult for you to efficiently find the evidence that you need to answer your clinical question. When searching for individual studies, you should start your search using databases that have screened many sources for you, include only the most important clinical studies and have pre-appraised the studies for you. Examples are:

- **EvidenceUpdates** (http://plus.mcmaster.ca/EvidenceUpdates/) provides access to scientifically sound and clinically relevant studies that have been published in over 150 premier healthcare journals. The content found in these 150 journals is critically appraised by research staff, and those studies and reviews that are scientifically sound are then rated by practising health professionals for relevancy and newsworthiness. The content focuses on internal medicine and its subspecialties, general medical practice and nursing. Various types of articles are included such as those concerned with therapy, diagnosis, prognosis, aetiology, quality improvement and continuing education, economics, clinical prediction guides and differential diagnosis. A searchable database is available for use after registering for this free service.
- **OBESITY+** (http://plus.mcmaster.ca/obesity/Default.aspx) provides access to a subset of the content found in EvidenceUpdates. OBESITY+ provides access to the current best evidence about the causes, course, diagnosis, prevention, treatment and economics of obesity and its related metabolic and mechanical complications. A searchable database is available for use after registering for this free service.
- **REHAB+** (http://plus.mcmaster.ca/rehab/Default.aspx) provides access to the current best evidence about the causes, course, diagnosis, prevention, treatment and economics related to rehabilitation.
- **Cochrane Central Register of Controlled Trials** is part of the Cochrane Library and is the largest electronic registry of randomised controlled trials in existence (in June 2009, there were 575 595 records). It is available as part of a subscription to the Cochrane Library and is also available through Ovid's Evidence Based Medicine Review packages of databases (http://www.ovid.com/site/catalog/DataBase/904.jsp?top=2&mid=3&bottom=7&subsection=10) on a subscription basis, as well as through several other services such as Wiley Interscience.

  This registry of individual controlled trials is a companion database to the Cochrane Database of Systematic Reviews, which was described earlier in this chapter. The articles in this registry are sourced from large databases including MEDLINE and EMBASE, hand searches of major healthcare journals across many health disciplines and other sources that are utilised by the review groups within the Cochrane Collaboration.
- **OTseeker** (http://www.otseeker.com/) is a discipline-specific database that contains abstracts of systematic reviews and randomised controlled trials relevant to occupational therapy. The trials included in this database have been critically appraised and rated to help you interpret the results and assess the validity of the findings. OTseeker is available free of charge.

- **PEDro** (http://www.pedro.org.au/) is a discipline-specific database that contains abstracts of randomised controlled trials, systematic reviews and evidence-based clinical practice guidelines relevant to physiotherapy. As with the articles on OTseeker, most trials in the database have been critically appraised and this assessment helps you to discriminate between trials which are likely to be valid and interpretable and those which are not. PEDro is available free of charge.
- **PsycBITE** (http://www.psycbite.com/) catalogues studies (randomised and non-randomised controlled trials, case series and single subject design) and systematic reviews focusing on the cognitive, behavioural and other types of treatment for the psychological problems and issues that can occur as a result of acquired brain impairment. The methodological quality of most of the randomised trials, non-randomised controlled trials and case series has been rated.
- **speechBITE** (http://www.speechbite.com) is modelled on PsycBITE and contains treatment studies (systematic reviews, randomised and non-randomised controlled trials, case series and single subject design) across the scope of speech pathology practice. The randomised and non-randomised controlled trials have been critically appraised.

If you cannot find an answer to your clinical question using a pre-appraised service such as those outlined above, the next step is to use one or more of the large electronic bibliographic databases that are described in this section. When searching in the large electronic databases, it is often most effective if you search using a combination of **index terms** and **textwords**. These are explained further in Box 3.1.
- **MEDLINE** is the largest biomedical database and currently has over 16 million citations. MEDLINE is produced by the US National Library of Medicine and is available for free through PubMed (http://www.ncbi.nlm.nih.gov/sites/entrez?db=pubmed). Searching efficiently in MEDLINE is important because of the large size of the database and also because many of the articles that are included in the database are not appropriate for use in evidence-based practice (for example, literature reviews).
  MEDLINE is also available through providers, such as Ovid, on a subscription basis. When accessing MEDLINE via Ovid, content searches can also be limited by Clinical Queries for individual studies about therapy, diagnosis, prognosis, aetiology, clinical prediction guides, costs, economics and studies of a qualitative nature, as well as systematic reviews.
- As mentioned previously in this chapter, the **Clinical Queries** screen in PubMed can be a great tool to facilitate efficient clinical searching by listing ready-to-use search strategies. These search strategies filter the retrieval of appropriate study types for the **clinical categories of therapy, diagnosis, aetiology, prognosis and clinical prediction**. For example, when searching for an article about therapy, the search strategy attempts to restrict the retrieval to articles that report using a randomised controlled trial design.
- Search strategies that filter the retrieval of appropriate study types for the clinical categories of **healthcare costs** and **healthcare quality (and some qualitative topics)** can be found on the **Health Services Research Queries screen** (http://www.nlm.nih.gov/nichsr/hedges/search.html) after clicking on the Special Queries link in PubMed.

When using the Clinical Queries or Health Services Research Queries interfaces, you only need to:
1. Enter basic content information (such as the keywords from your clinical question—try starting with the 'P' and 'I' keywords and then broaden or narrow your search as needed).
2. Select the type of question that you are searching for an answer to (in Clinical Queries, you can choose from therapy, prognosis, diagnosis, aetiology or clinical prediction guides).

BOX 3.1   WHAT ARE INDEX TERMS AND TEXTWORDS?

INDEX TERMS

- These are somewhat like the index in a book. Index terms can be useful to search with as they are designed to overcome the problem of different authors using different terms to describe the same concept. Index terms (usually between 10 and 20) are assigned to each article by staff at the electronic databases using a database-specific thesaurus. Of course, to keep users on their toes, different databases use different index terms! For example, MEDLINE uses MeSH (Medical Subject Headings), CINAHL uses CINAHL subject headings and EMBASE uses Emtree.
- Index terms are organised hierarchically, using a tree structure, with broader terms higher up in the 'tree'. This structure provides an effective way for users to make their search broader and narrower as needed. For example, part of the MeSH tree structure for 'stroke' is as follows:

Nervous System Diseases
    Central Nervous System Diseases
        Brain Diseases
            Cerebrovascular Disorders
                Stroke
                    Brain Infarction
                        Brain Stem Infarction
                        Cerebral Infarction

- For some topics that you want to search on, there may be no corresponding index terms. Sadly, this is the case for many of the interventions that are used by allied health professionals. When this occurs, you need to search using textwords.
- How do you know what MeSH to use? You can search the MeSH browser online (http://www.nlm.nih.gov/mesh/MBrowser.html); when searching MEDLINE via Ovid, you can choose to have your search automatically mapped to relevant MeSH; or you can look at relevant articles to see what MeSH have been assigned to those articles.

TEXTWORDS

You can also search using textwords. These are free text words that are found in the title and abstract of the article and therefore are the words used by the authors of articles. The limitation of this method is that the authors may have used a different term (for example, 'cerebrovascular accident') to the search term that you are using (for example, 'stroke'). Although you are both describing the same thing, you may not retrieve their article in your search. The obvious way to overcome this is to use the relevant index term. However if there is no corresponding index term, using synonyms and related terms (combining them with OR) and truncation and wildcard symbols can help to broaden your search.

---

3. Decide if you want to conduct a sensitive (broad) or specific (narrow) search. A **sensitive search** increases the likelihood of retrieving every possible relevant study, which in PubMed can often result in an unmanageable number of search results. You may wish to begin by selecting a **specific search**, which will minimise the number of irrelevant studies that are returned. If you get very few, or no, search results, you can then repeat the search and change the emphasis to sensitive.

That is all you have to do. Everything else, such as the methodological refining of the search strategy, is done for you. A useful feature of Clinical Queries is that it also searches using the relevant MeSH terms (without you having to select them). Another handy feature of PubMed is the *Related Articles* feature—this is a list of related articles (as the name aptly

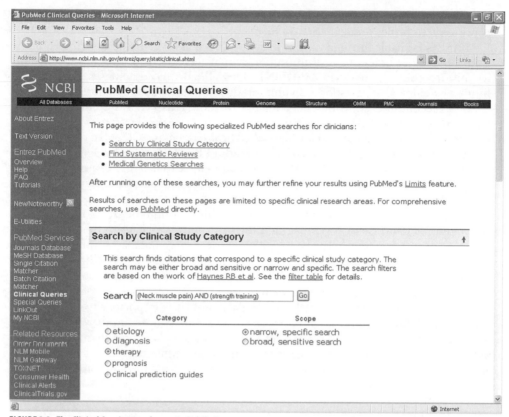

FIGURE 3.2   The Clinical Queries search page in PubMed

suggests!) that appears on the right-hand margin of the search results screen. This can be a quick and easy way to locate some additional articles that are relevant to your search.

Figure 3.2 shows the search page of Clinical Queries and a basic search related to the clinical scenario that was outlined earlier in this chapter. If you want to see what search Clinical Queries actually ran for you, click on the 'details' button on the search results page. In the example search that is shown in Figure 3.2, even though we only typed in (Neck muscle pain) AND (strength training), this is what was actually searched for:

(((("neck muscles"[MeSH Terms] OR ("neck"[All Fields] AND "muscles"[All Fields]) OR "neck muscles"[All Fields] OR ("neck"[All Fields] AND "muscle"[All Fields]) OR "neck muscle"[All Fields]) AND ("pain"[MeSH Terms] OR "pain"[All Fields])) AND ("resistance training" [MeSH Terms] OR ("resistance" [All Fields] AND "training" [All Fields]) OR "resistance training" [All Fields] OR ("strength" [All Fields] AND "training" [All Fields]) OR "strength training" [All Fields])) AND (randomized controlled trial[Publication Type] OR (randomized[Title/Abstract] AND controlled[Title/Abstract] AND trial[Title/Abstract])))

• **EMBASE**(http://www.elsevier.com/wps/find/bibliographicdatabasedescription.cws_home/523328/description#description) is a large European database with over 11 million citations. EMBASE is similar to MEDLINE in scope and content with an overlap in content between the two databases of about 30% to 50%. Compared to MEDLINE, EMBASE provides greater coverage of European and non-English-language publications and a broader coverage of topics concerned with pharmaceuticals, psychiatry, toxicology and alternative medicine.

EMBASE is available through various providers, such as Ovid, on a subscription basis. Your hospital or academic institution library may have an institutional subscription to this resource. As in Ovid MEDLINE, Ovid EMBASE content searches can be limited by Clinical Queries for individual studies about therapy, diagnosis, prognosis, aetiology, economics and studies of a qualitative nature, as well as systematic reviews.

- **CINAHL** (Cumulative Index to Nursing and Allied Health Literature http://www.cinahl.com/) is the premier nursing and allied health database. CINAHL contains over 800,000 records. CINAHL is offered by the vendor EBSCOHost. As in Ovid MEDLINE and Ovid EMBASE, EBSCO CINAHL offers content searches that can be limited by Clinical Queries for individual studies about therapy, prognosis, aetiology and studies of a qualitative nature, as well as systematic reviews.
- **PsycINFO** (http://www.apa.org/psycinfo/) is the comprehensive international bibliographic database of psychological literature from the 1800s to the present and contains over 2.4 million records. As with the other large databases, multiple access routes are available and all require a subscription. In Ovid PsycINFO, Clinical Queries can be used to limit retrieval to individual studies about therapy and those of a qualitative nature, as well as systematic reviews.

When searching using the large electronic databases, it is important to use the help function that is found within each database so that you become familiar with how to search the database efficiently. The features and interfaces of databases change from time to time and, as mentioned earlier, there are some subtle differences across databases in terms of refining search techniques, such as the symbols for truncation and the use of double quotation marks instead of parentheses for combining terms.

Some tips for locating qualitative research

Finding qualitative research can be very difficult. One of the reasons is that it is indexed in a number of different ways. Using the term 'qualitative' as a search term is often not useful, as sometimes qualitative research is indexed by the specific method that was used to collect data (for example, focus group or in-depth interview) and other times it is indexed according to the methodology that was used (for example, phenomenology or grounded theory). Table 3.1 shows some empirically derived[5-8] search strategies that can be used to locate qualitative studies in CINAHL, MEDLINE, EMBASE and PsycINFO. They are methodological search strategies meaning that they focus on the methods of qualitative research, not the content. Combine these methodological search strategies with your content terms, that is, the keywords from your clinical question. For example, to locate qualitative research about depression in women, you could try the following search string in Ovid MEDLINE: depression.tw. AND wom*n.tw. AND [interview:.tw. OR px.fs OR exp health services administration]. The search strategies shown in Table 3.1, except for the CINAHL strategy, are in Ovid syntax (that is, Ovid language) so they will need translation if you are searching using another interface. The CINAHL strategy provided is in EBSCO syntax as CINAHL will only be available through this provider as of 2009. The PubMed translation of the MEDLINE sensitive and specific search can be found on the Special Queries page of PubMed under Health Services Research Queries, which we described earlier in this chapter when MEDLINE was explained. As you can see in Table 3.1, there is a choice of three different search strategies—'sensitive', 'specific' or 'minimise the difference between sensitive and specific'. Use the sensitive search strategy when you want a very broad search and do not want to risk missing any relevant articles. Use the specific search strategy when you want to narrow your search and want to find

Hedge	MEDLINE (Ovid Syntax)	CINAHL (EBSCO Syntax)	EMBASE (Ovid Syntax)	PsycINFO (Ovid Syntax)
Sensitive	interview:.tw. OR px.fs. OR exp health services administration	((mh "study design+" not mm "study design+") or mh "attitude" or (mh "interviews+" not mm "interviews+"))	interview:.tw. OR qualitative. tw. OR health care organization	experience:.mp. OR interview:.tw. OR qualitative:. tw.
Specific	qualitative.tw. OR themes.tw.	((mh "grounded theory" not mm "grounded theory") or (ti thematic analysis or ab thematic analysis or mw thematic analysis))	qualitative.tw. OR qualitative study.tw.	qualitative:.tw. OR themes.tw.
Minimise difference between sensitive and specific	interview:.mp. OR experience:. mp. OR qualitative.tw.	((ti interview or ab interview) or (mh "audiorecording" not mm "audiorecording") or (ti qualitative stud* or ab qualitative stud*))	interview:.tw. OR exp health care organization OR experiences. tw.	experiences.tw. OR interview:.tw. OR qualitative.tw.

Colon = truncation; tw = textword; px = psychology; fs = floating subheading; exp = explosion; mp = multiple posting, term found in title, abstract or index terms; sh = subject heading; ti = title; ab = abstract; mh = subject heading; mm = exact major subject heading; mw = subject heading word; + = explode

TABLE 3.1 Search strategies (hedges) for locating qualitative research in MEDLINE, CINAHL, EMBASE and PsycINFO

just a few relevant articles, and use the 'minimise difference' search strategies for a search that is a balance between sensitivity and specificity.

Alerting or updating services

Although it is not on the '5S' pyramid specifically, electronic communication (i.e. email) can be a useful method of informing health professionals about newly published studies. Unlike all of the resources outlined above that require you to go and search for the evidence, alerting services bring the research literature to you in the form of email alerts or RSS (really simple syndication) feeds, which are simply a list of items that you sign up to receive. In Chapter 2, this was described as 'push' or 'just-in-case' information. Several alerting systems that target articles to individual health professionals have been developed. Some examples are:

• **EvidenceUpdates** (http://plus.mcmaster.ca/EvidenceUpdates/) is a free service that alerts health professionals to newly published studies and systematic reviews from over 150 premier healthcare journals that are published in their discipline. It is the same process that the *ACP Journal Club, Evidence-Based Medicine* and *Evidence-Based Nursing* use to select both clinically relevant and methodologically rigorous papers. If a paper is going to be clinically useful, it has a high probability of being selected in this database. Newly published studies and systematic reviews have been pre-appraised for methodological rigour and clinical relevancy and newsworthiness. Users choose the frequency at which they wish to receive email notifications or RSS feeds and the disciplines in which they are interested (for example, general medicine practice, endocrinology) and set the score level for clinical relevance and newsworthiness to a level that is acceptable to them.

- **OBESITY+** (http://plus.mcmaster.ca/obesity/Default.aspx) is a free alerting service that provides access to a subset of the content found in EvidenceUpdates. The content of OBESITY+ was described earlier in this chapter.
- **REHAB+** (http://plus.mcmaster.ca/rehab/Default.aspx) is a free alerting service that provides access to a subset of the content found in EvidenceUpdates that is relevant to rehabilitation.
- **MEDSCAPE** Best Evidence alerts (http://www.medscape.com/home) is a free alerting service of pre-appraised newly published studies about treatment, diagnosis, aetiology, prognosis and economics and also includes clinical prediction guides as well as systematic reviews. Topics covered by this service are the same as those included in the *ACP Journal Club, Evidence-Based Medicine* and *Evidence-Based Nursing.* After filling in an interest profile, users are sent email alerts about new evidence that contain links to the citation in PubMed plus clinical ratings and comments from practising health professionals.
- **My NCBI** (www.ncbi.nlm.nih.gov/books/bv.fcgi?rid=helppubmed.section.pubmedhelp. My_NCBI) is an alerting service within PubMed that will email users with new citations from MEDLINE in the clinical areas that they have specified. Users set up a search that will automatically email them citations of newly published articles based on content (for example, asthma in adolescents) or journal titles. My NCBI is offered free of charge through PubMed. However, the newly published articles are not filtered by methodological rigour and you will need to critically appraise the articles that are sent to you before considering their use in clinical practice.
- **Journals** may enable you to register to have the table of contents emailed to you as each new issue of the journal is published. You may wish to do this for journals that you frequently consult. As with My NCBI, the newly published articles are not filtered by methodological rigour and you will need to critically appraise the articles that are sent to you before considering their use in clinical practice.

Other resources

Again, although not specifically on the '5S' pyramid, many search engines are available for use on the internet. When using these search engines (for example, Google), you are not searching a defined database but are searching the internet in general. A major negative aspect of using these search engines is that evidence-based information may be difficult to find and a lot of high quality clinical research (such as that located in databases) cannot be located at all this way. On the other hand, positive aspects are that an internet search can be a quick way of tracking down a specific article and obtaining information about issues that keep changing such as listings of country-specific vaccination rules for travellers. Examples of internet search engines are:

- **Google** (http://www.google.com/), Yahoo (http://www.yahoo.com/), MSN (http://www.msn.com/) and Ask (formerly Ask Jeeves, http://www.ask.com/). All four internet search engines are commonly used and freely accessible. Search Engine Watch (http://searchenginewatch.com/links/article.php/2156221) maintains a list of major search engines on the web and rates the usefulness of each. Note that when searching using Google, truncations or wild cards for letters of the alphabet are not an option. In Google, the use of wild cards is for words rather than letters. For example, "personal * records" would retrieve items that include "personal health records", "personal medical records", "personal records" etc.

- Google Scholar (http://scholar.google.com/) is a free service provided by Google that provides searching of the scholarly literature. From one site, you are able to search across many disciplines and sources such as peer-reviewed papers, theses, books, abstracts and articles that are from academic publishers, professional societies, preprint repositories, universities and other scholarly organisations. Google Scholar sorts articles by weighting the full text of the article, the author, the publication in which the article appears and how often the article has been cited in other scholarly literature. This sorting results in the most relevant articles likely appearing on the first page.
- Search engines that retrieve and combine results from multiple search engines (meta-search engines) also exist. A list of these search engines can be found at http://searchenginewatch.com/links/article.php/2156241.

Finally, you may be faced with a clinical question and you do not know which of the evidence-based resources may be best for answering your particular clinical problem. In these situations 'federated search engines' provide a means to search many resources, with the retrieval of results organised according to the source of evidence.

- **SUMSearch** (http://sumsearch.uthscsa.edu/) is a free health-related meta-search engine that selects the best resources for your clinical question, formats your question for each resource and makes additional searches based on the results. You can focus (for example, intervention) and limit (for example, age) your search. By using SUMSearch, you can search multiple medical databases with one entry of search terms. For example, the entry of two words, "electrical stimulation" in SUMSearch provided links to 1285 entries in Wikipedia, 68 guidelines that are available through the US National Guidelines Clearinghouse, 29 guidelines in PubMed, 43 DARE or Cochrane systematic reviews, 245 other systematic reviews in PubMed and 295 original studies in PubMed. By contrast, when an internet search engine such as Google (http://www.google.com) was used to perform this search, it retrieved approximately 944,000 entries for "electrical stimulation" and the items were not grouped by source (for example, PubMed) or type of evidence (for example, systematic reviews).
- **TRIP** (Turning Research into Practice, http://www.tripdatabase.com/) is similar to SUMSearch in that it searches multiple databases and other evidence-based resources with just one entry of your search term(s). TRIP groups the search results into systematic reviews, evidence-based synopses, clinical practice guidelines (from North America, Europe and other locations), clinical questions, core primary research, e-textbooks and more. Any articles that are retrieved from MEDLINE are organised by purpose, that is, therapy, diagnosis, systematic review, prognosis and aetiology. You can filter your retrieval by choosing from one of 26 clinical specialties (for example, paediatrics). When searching MEDLINE, TRIP uses the PubMed Clinical Queries feature and multiple system-invoked synonyms. TRIP also searches EvidenceUpdates. TRIP was once a fee-based system but can now be accessed for free.

Search examples

In this section we will use some of the resources described in this chapter to answer several different clinical questions—one from each of the four major question types that are covered in this book (that is, effects of intervention, diagnosis, prognosis and questions about clients' experiences and concerns).

Clinical question about the effects of intervention

- You are a physiotherapist and currently have two clients who are pregnant and experiencing pelvic and back pain. You wonder:

  In pregnant women is acupuncture more effective than standard treatment in relieving pregnancy-related pelvic and back pain?

- Starting at the top of the pyramid, you confirm that there is nothing at the top three levels of the pyramid, which is often the case for allied health clinical questions. As your question is one about intervention effectiveness, you are ideally hoping to find a systematic review of randomised controlled trials. Therefore, your next step is to look for a systematic review (fourth level of the pyramid—syntheses) by searching in the Cochrane Database of Systematic Reviews, using the keywords from your clinical question (pregnan* AND acupuncture).
- Your search retrieves one review[9] that summaries interventions for preventing and treating pelvic and back pain in pregnancy. As all but one study included in the review had moderate to high potential for bias (as stated by the authors of the review), you decide to look for other systematic reviews, ideally ones where acupuncture was the only intervention of focus.
- Since PEDro contains systematic reviews and pre-appraised articles related to physiotherapy you decide to search there next. On the advanced search page, you type in the terms 'pregnancy acupuncture', and select the body part 'lumbar spine, sacro-iliac joint and pelvis'. Note that in PEDro you do not need to type in Boolean operators; just tick the box at the bottom of the advanced search page indicating whether you want the search terms to be combined with AND or OR. Your search retrieves eight records and two of these are systematic reviews. One was the Cochrane review that you had already found. The second review is a systematic review of acupuncture for pelvic and back pain in pregnancy[10] which appears to be exactly what you are after.
- Note that during this search you try the Cochrane Database of Systematic Reviews and the relevant discipline-specific database (PEDro in this case) before trying the large electronic databases such as MEDLINE, as it is typically much more efficient to locate evidence about an intervention question in these databases than in the large electronic databases.

Clinical question about diagnosis

- You are an occupational therapist who works in a community health centre. The team that you work in is putting together an initial assessment form for newly referred clients and they wish to include some screening questions that will provide useful information to various members of the team. You are interested in including a brief cognitive screening test, such as the Mini-Mental State Examination (MMSE), as part of this initial assessment but wonder how accurate this test is at predicting cognitive impairment in older people who live in the community. Your question is:

  Does the MMSE accurately detect the presence of cognitive impairment in older community-living people?

- After confirming that there is nothing available at the top three levels of the pyramid, you proceed to the fourth level of the pyramid (syntheses). You conduct a search in the Cochrane Database of Systematic Reviews, but no search results are returned. Since the Cochrane database only recently started adding diagnostic reviews you are not surprised that no relevant reviews are retrieved.

- You then search using PubMed Clinical Queries (with diagnosis selected as the clinical category and a narrow search chosen) with the terms: (MMSE OR Mini-Mental State Examination) AND (cognitive impairment) AND (older OR elder*). This produces 73 hits which you decide is too many to look through. You add the word 'community' to your search string and this produces 22 articles, one of which is exactly what you are after.[11]

Clinical question about prognosis

- You are a recently graduated speech pathologist who has just commenced working in a stroke rehabilitation unit. One of your clients is 2 months post-stroke and has severe dysphagia (difficulty swallowing). His wife asks you how likely it is that his swallowing will get better in the next few months and that he will be able to return to eating a normal diet. As you are new to this area of clinical practice and have little clinical experience to guide your answer, you form the following clinical question:

In adults with dysphagia following stroke, what is the likelihood of recovery within 6 months of the stroke?

- You search using PubMed Clinical Queries (with prognosis selected as the clinical category and a narrow search chosen) with the terms: (dysphag* OR swallow*) AND (stroke OR CVA) and (recover*). This produces 17 hits, one of which is exactly what you are after.[12]

Clinical question about clients' experiences and concerns

- You are a dietician working with children who are obese. The children are having a very difficult time losing weight. You wonder why it is that children who are obese often find it so difficult to lose weight when the lifestyle factors that contribute to the condition are so widely recognised. Your question is:

What are the barriers to losing weight from the child's perspective?

- This question would best be answered by a qualitative research design. Currently, qualitative studies are most likely found on the bottom layer of the pyramid: studies. You start your search using CINAHL (through EBSCOhost) as this can be a useful database to search when looking for qualitative research. You search using the search string: barrier* AND weight AND child*. You also limit the search by using the Clinical Queries feature of CINAHL and select 'qualitative—best balance' as you only want to retrieve qualitative articles.
- Your search produces 15 hits, one of which is directly on target.[13] You notice that one of the other hits is also very relevant, but when you look at the abstract of it you realise that it is actually a synopsis[14] of the original article that has been published in *Evidence-Based Nursing*, which is one of the resources that is at the third layer of the pyramid (synopses). This is great news for you as it means that this original article has been pre-appraised for you and considered to be clinically important and that the synopsis will also contain a clinical bottom line that has been written by a clinical expert in this field!
- Another approach for this search would be to use PubMed, using the Health Services Research Queries feature (accessed by clicking on the Special Queries link on the left-hand menu on the main PubMed page) that was described earlier in this chapter. One of the categories for searching on this page is qualitative research. You choose this category and 'Narrow, specific search' for the scope and enter the same search terms as we used above in CINAHL. The search retrieves 26 citations. The fourteenth article on the list of search results is the same primary article[13] that you found using CINAHL.

Summary points of this chapter

- Using the PICO format to structure your clinical question makes choosing key search terms easy.
- Combining search terms using the Boolean operators (AND, OR) helps to narrow or broaden your search as required, and wildcard and truncation symbols are also useful.
- Organising your literature search using the '5S' pyramid is an effective and efficient approach to finding the best evidence.
- Where to start your search on the '5S' pyramid depends largely on the type of question that is being asked and what resources are available to you.
- Although many online evidence-based resources require a subscription, many great resources are readily available on the internet free of charge.
- Many clinical questions can be answered by searching online for the best evidence.

References

1. Ely JW, Osheroff JA, Ebell MH et al. Obstacles to answering doctor's questions about patient care with evidence: qualitative study. BMJ 2002; 324:710–716.
2. Haynes RB. Of studies, syntheses, synopses, summaries, and systems: the "5S" evolution of information services for evidence-based health care decisions. ACP J Club 2006; 145:A8–A9.
3. Garg AX, Adhikari NK, McDonald H et al. Effects of computerized clinical decision support systems on practitioner performance and patient outcomes. A systematic review. JAMA 2005; 293:1223–1238.
4. Montori VM. Evidence-based endocrinology. Totowa, NJ: Humana Press; 2005.
5. Wong S, Wilczynski N, Haynes RB et al. Developing optimal search strategies for detecting clinically relevant qualitative studies in MEDLINE. Medinfo 2004; 11:311–316.
6. Wilczynski N, Marks S, Haynes RB. Search strategies for identifying qualitative studies in CINAHL. Qual Health Res 2007; 17:705–710.
7. Walters L, Wilczynski N, Haynes RB et al. Developing optimal search strategies for retrieving clinically relevant qualitative studies in EMBASE. Qual Health Res 2006; 16:162–168.
8. McKibbon KA, Wilczynski N, Haynes RB. Developing optimal search strategies for retrieving qualitative studies in PsycINFO. Eval Health Prof 2006; 29:440–454.
9. Pennick VE, Young G. Interventions for treating and preventing pelvic and back pain in pregnancy. Cochrane Database Syst Rev 2007; 2: Art. No.: CD001139. DOI: 10.1002/14651858. CD001139.pub2.
10. Ee CC, Manheimer E, Pirotta MV et al. Acupuncture for pelvic and back pain in pregnancy: a systematic review. Am J Obstet Gynecol 2008; 198:254–259.
11. Gagnon M, Letenneur L, Dartigues J et al. Validity of the Mini-Mental State examination as a screening instrument for cognitive impairment and dementia in French elderly community residents. Neuroepidemiology 1990; 9:143–150.
12. Mann G, Hankey G, Cameron D. Swallowing function after stroke: prognosis and prognostic factors at 6 months. Stroke 1999; 30:744–748.
13. Murtagh J, Dixey R, Rudolf M. A qualitative investigation into the levers and barriers to weight loss in children: opinions of obese children. Arch Dis Child 2006; 91:920–923.
14. Macdonald M. Clinically obese children identified facilitators and barriers to initiating and maintaining the behaviours required for weight loss. Evid Based Nurs 2007; 10:92.

CHAPTER 4

Evidence about effects of interventions

Sally Bennett and Tammy Hoffmann

LEARNING OBJECTIVES

After reading this chapter, you should be able to:

- Understand more about study designs appropriate for answering questions about effects of interventions
- Generate a structured clinical question about intervention for a clinical scenario
- Appraise the validity of randomised controlled trials
- Understand how to interpret the results from randomised controlled trials and calculate additional results (such as confidence intervals) where possible
- Describe how evidence about the effects of intervention can be used to inform practice

This chapter focusses on research that can inform us about the effects of intervention. Let us consider a clinical scenario that will be useful for illustrating the concepts that are the focus of this chapter.

Clinical scenario

You are working in a community health centre and, during a regular team meeting, the general practitioner notes that there are a large number of older people attending the clinic who have had multiple falls. He questions whether there is a need for the delivery of a preventative program for this group. A number of staff have similar concerns and decide to form a small group to look for research regarding the effectiveness of falls prevention programs. In your experience working with people who have a history of falling, you are aware that many of them have low confidence in their ability (this is also known as self-efficacy) to prevent themselves from falling. You are therefore particularly interested in finding evidence about the effectiveness of falls prevention programs that have looked at improving participants' self-efficacy as well as reducing the number of falls that they experience.

This clinical scenario raises several questions about the interventions that might be effective for reducing falls in people who are at risk of falling. Is balance and strength training effective in reducing the risk of falls? Does providing advice about how to modify a person's home to make it safer prevent falls in people who are at risk of falling? Which of these interventions is most effective or are both combined more effective than one intervention alone? How cost-effective are multifactorial falls prevention education programs? These are questions that health professionals might ask when making decisions about which interventions will be most effective and optimise outcomes for their clients.

As we saw in Chapter 1, clinical decisions are made by integrating information from the best available research evidence with information from our clients, the practice context and our clinical experience. Given that one of the most common information needs in clinical practice relates to questions about the effects of interventions, this chapter will begin by reviewing the role of the study design that is used to test intervention effects before moving on to explaining the process of finding and appraising research evidence about the effects of interventions.

Study designs that can be used for answering questions about the effects of interventions

There are many different study designs that can provide information about the effects of interventions. Some are more convincing than others in terms of the degree of bias that might be in play given the methods used in the study. From Chapter 2, you will recall that bias is any systematic error in collecting and interpreting data. In Chapter 2, we also introduced the concept of hierarchies of evidence. The higher up the hierarchy that a study design is positioned, in the ideal world, the more likely it is that the study design can minimise the impact of bias on the results of the study. That is why randomised controlled trials (sitting second from the top of the hierarchy of evidence for questions about the effects of interventions) are so commonly recommended as the study design that best controls for bias when testing the effectiveness of interventions. Systematic reviews of randomised controlled trials are located above them (at the top of the hierarchy) because they can combine the results of multiple randomised controlled trials. This can potentially provide an even clearer picture about the effectiveness of interventions. Systematic reviews are explained in more detail in Chapter 12.

One of the best methods for limiting bias in studies that test the effects of interventions is to have a control group.[1] A control group is a group of participants in the study who should be as similar in as many ways as possible to the intervention group except that they do not receive the intervention being studied. Let us first have a look at studies that do not use control groups and identify some of the problems that can occur.

Studies that do not use control groups

Uncontrolled studies are studies where the researchers describe what happens when participants are provided an intervention, but the intervention is not compared with other interventions. Examples of uncontrolled study designs are case reports, case series and before and after studies. These study designs were explained in Chapter 3. The big problem with uncontrolled studies is that when participants are given an intervention and simply followed for a period of time with no comparison against another group it is impossible to tell how much (if any) of the observed change is due to the effect of the intervention itself. There are some obvious reasons this might occur and these problems need to be kept in mind if you use an uncontrolled study to guide your clinical decision making. Some of the forms of bias that commonly occur in uncontrolled studies are described below.

- **Volunteer bias.** People who volunteer to participate in a study are usually systematically different from those who do not volunteer. They tend to be more motivated and concerned about their health. If this is not controlled for, it is possible that the results can make the intervention appear more favourable (that is, more effective) than it really is. This type of bias can be controlled for by randomly allocating participants as we shall see later in this chapter.
- **Maturation.** A participant may change between the time of pre-test (that is, before the intervention is given) and post-test (after the intervention has finished) as a result of maturation. For example, consider that you wanted to measure the improvement in fine motor skills that children in grade 2 of school experienced as a result of a fine-motor skill intervention program. If you test them again in grade 3, you will not know if the improvements that occurred in fine motor skills happened because of natural development (maturation) or because of the intervention.
- **Natural progression.** Many diseases and health conditions will naturally improve over time. Improvements that occur in participants may or may not be due to the intervention that was being studied. The participants may have improved on their own with time, not because of the intervention.
- **Regression to the mean.** This is a statistical trend that occurs in repeated non-random experiments, where participants' results tend to move progressively towards the mean of the behaviour/outcome that is being measured. This does not occur due to maturation or improvement over time, but due to the statistical likelihood of someone with high scores not doing as well when a test is repeated or of someone with low scores being statistically likely to do *better* when the test is repeated. Suppose, for example, that you assessed 200 children who had attention deficit hyperactivity disorder with

a behavioural test and scored their risk of having poor academic outcomes and that you provided the 30 children who had the poorest scores with an intensive behavioural regimen and medication. Even if the interventions were not effective, you would still expect to observe some improvement in the children's scores on the behavioural test when it is next given due to regression to the mean. When outliers are repeatedly measured, subsequent values are less likely to be outliers (that is, they are expected to be closer to the mean value of the whole group). This always happens and health professionals who do not expect this to occur often attribute any improvement that is observed to the intervention. The best way to deal with the problem of regression to the mean is to randomly allocate participants to either an experimental group or a control group. The regression to the mean effect can only be accounted for by using a control group (which will have the same regression to the mean if the randomisation succeeded and the two groups are similar). How to determine this is explained later in this chapter.

- **Placebo effect.** This is a well-known type of bias where an improvement in the participants' condition occurs because they expect or believe that the intervention they are receiving will cause an improvement (even though, in reality, the intervention may not be effective at all).
- **Hawthorne effect.** This is a type of bias that can occur when participants experience improvements, not because of the intervention that is being studied, but because of the attention that participants are receiving from being a part of the research process.
- **Rosenthal effect**. This occurs when participants perform better because they are expected to and, in a sense, this expectation has a similar sort of effect as a self-fulfilling prophecy.

Controlled studies

By now, it should be clear that having a control group which can be compared to the intervention group in a study is the best way of making sure that bias and extraneous factors that can influence the results of a study are limited. However, it is not so simple as just having a control group as part of the study. The way in which the control group is created can make an enormous difference to how well the study design actually controls for bias.

Non-randomised controlled studies

You will recall from the hierarchy of evidence about the effects of interventions (in Chapter 3) that case-control and cohort studies are located above uncontrolled study designs. This is because they make use of control groups. Cohort studies follow a cohort that have been exposed to a situation or intervention and have a comparison group of people who have not been exposed to the situation of interest (for example, they have not received any intervention). However, because cohort studies are observational studies, the allocation of participants to the intervention and control groups is not under the control of the researcher. It is not possible to tell if the participants in the intervention and control groups are similar in terms of all the important factors and, therefore, it is unclear to what extent the exposure (that is, the intervention) might be the reason for the outcome rather than some other factor.

We saw in Chapter 2 that a case-control study is one in which participants with a given disease (or health condition) in a given population (or a representative sample) are identified and are compared to a control group of participants who do not have that disease (or health condition). When a case-control study has been used to answer a question about the effect of an intervention, the 'cases' are participants who have been exposed to an intervention and the 'controls' are participants who have not.

As with cohort studies, because this is an observational study design, the researcher cannot control the assembly of the groups under study (that is, which participants go into which group). Although the controls that are assembled may be similar in many ways to the 'cases', it is unlikely that they will be similar with respect to both known and unknown confounders. Chapter 2 explained that confounders are factors that can become confused with the factor of interest (in this case, the intervention that is being studied) and obscure the true results.

In a non-randomised experimental study, the researchers can control the assembly of both experimental and control groups, but the groups are not assembled using random allocation. In non-randomised studies, participants may choose which group they want to be in, or they may be assigned to a group by the researchers. For example, in a non-randomised experimental study that is evaluating the effectiveness of a particular public health intervention (such as an intervention that encourages walking to work) in a community setting, a researcher may assign one town to the experimental condition and another town to the control condition. The difficulty with this approach is that the people in these towns may be systematically different to each other and so confounding factors, rather than the intervention that is being trialled, may be the reason for any difference that is found between the groups at the end of the study.

So not only are control groups essential, but in order to make valid comparisons between groups, they must be as similar as possible at the beginning of a study. This is so we can say with some certainty that any differences that are found between groups at the end of the study are likely to be due to the factor under study (that is, the intervention), rather than because of bias or confounding. To maximise the similarity between groups at the start of a study, researchers need to control for both known and unknown variables that might influence the results. The best way to achieve this is through randomisation. Non-randomised studies are inherently biased in favour of the intervention that is being studied, which can lead researchers to reach the wrong conclusion about the effectiveness of the intervention.[2]

Randomised controlled trials

The key feature of randomised controlled trials is that the participants are randomly allocated to either an intervention (experimental) group or a control group. The outcome of interest is measured in participants in both groups before (known as pre-test) and then again after the intervention (known as post-test) is provided. Therefore, any changes that appear in the intervention group pre-test to post-test, but not in the control group, can be reasonably attributed to the intervention. Figure 4.1 shows the basic design of a randomised controlled trial.

You may notice that we keep referring to how randomised controlled trials can be used to evaluate the effectiveness of an intervention. It is worth noting that they can also be used to evaluate the efficacy of an intervention. Efficacy refers to interventions that are tested in ideal circumstances, such as where intervention protocols are very carefully supervised and participant selection is very particular. Effectiveness is an evaluation of an intervention in circumstances that are more like real life, such as where there is a broader range of participants included and a typical clinical level of intervention protocol supervision. In this sense, effectiveness trials are more pragmatic in nature (that is, they are accommodating of typical practices) than efficacy trials.

There are a number of variations on the basic randomised controlled trial design, which partly depend on the type or combination of control groups used. There are many variations on what the participants in a control group in a randomised controlled trial actually receive. For example, participants may receive no intervention of any kind

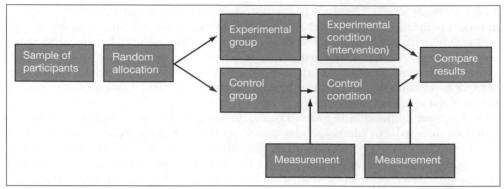

FIGURE 4.1   Basic design of a randomised controlled trial

(a 'no intervention' control), or they may receive a placebo, some form of social control or a comparison intervention. In some randomised controlled trials, there are more than two groups. For example, in one study there might be two intervention groups and one control group or, in another study, there might be an intervention group, a placebo group and a 'no intervention' group. Randomised crossover studies are a type of randomised controlled trial in which all participants take part in both intervention and control groups but in random order. For example, in a randomised crossover trial of transdermal fentanyl (a pain medication) and sustained-release oral morphine (another pain medication) for treating chronic non-cancer pain, participants were assigned to one of two intervention groups.[3] One group was randomised to four weeks of treatment with sustained release oral morphine followed by transdermal fentanyl for four weeks. The second group received the same treatments but in reverse order. A difficulty with crossover trials is that there needs to be a credible wash-out period. That is, the effects of the intervention provided in the first phase must no longer be evident prior to commencing the second phase. In the example we used here, the effect of oral morphine must be cleared prior to the fentanyl being provided.

As we have seen, the advantage of a randomised controlled trial is that any differences that are found between groups at the end of the study are likely to be due to the intervention rather than extraneous factors. But the extent to which these differences can be attributed to the intervention is also dependent on some of the specific design features that were used in the trial, and these deserve close attention. The rest of this chapter will look at randomised controlled trials in more depth within the context of the clinical scenario that was presented at the beginning of this chapter. In this scenario you are a health professional who is working in a small group at a community health centre and you are looking for research regarding the effectiveness of falls prevention programs. To locate relevant research, you start by focusing on what it is that you specifically want to know about.

How to structure a question about the effect of intervention

In Chapter 2, you learnt how to structure clinical questions using the PICO format: Patient/Problem/Population, Intervention/Issue, Comparison (if relevant) and Outcomes.

In our falls clinical scenario, the *population* that we are interested in is elderly people who fall. We know from our clinical experience that people who have had falls in the past are at risk of falling again, so it makes sense to target our search for interventions aimed at people who are either 'at risk' of falling and/or have a history of falling. The *intervention* that we are interested in is a falls prevention program. Are we interested in a *comparison* intervention? While we could compare the effectiveness of one type of intervention with another, for this scenario it is probably more useful to start by firstly thinking about whether the intervention is effective. To do this we would need to compare the intervention to either a placebo (a concept we will discuss later) or to usual care. There are a number of *outcomes* that we could consider important for people who fall. The most obvious outcome of interest is a reduction in the number of falls. However, we could also look for interventions that consider the factors that contribute to falls such as balance problems or, in this scenario, a person's confidence (or self-efficacy) to undertake actions that will prevent them from falling.

Clinical scenario (continued): The question

While there are a number of questions about interventions that can be drawn from the scenario that was presented at the beginning of this chapter, you decide to form the following clinical question: In community-dwelling older people with a history of falling, are falls prevention programs effective in reducing falls and increasing self-efficacy compared to usual care?

How to find evidence to answer questions about the effects of intervention

Our clinical scenario question is a question about the effectiveness of an intervention to prevent falls and to improve self-efficacy. You can use the hierarchy of evidence for this type of question as your guide to know which type of study you are looking for and where to start searching. In this case, you are looking for a systematic review of randomised controlled trials. If there is no relevant systematic review, you should next look for a randomised controlled trial. If no relevant randomised controlled trials are available, you would then need to look for the next best available type of research, as indicated by the hierarchy of evidence for this question type that is shown in Chapter 2.

As we saw in Chapter 3, the best source of systematic reviews of randomised controlled trials is the Cochrane Database of Systematic Reviews, so this would be the logical place to start searching. The Cochrane Library also contains the Cochrane Central Register of Controlled Trials which includes a large collection of citations of randomised controlled trials. If you are looking for randomised controlled trials specifically in the rehabilitation field, two other databases that you could consider searching for this topic are PEDro (www.pedro.org.au/) or OTseeker (www.otseeker.com). These databases were explained in Chapter 3. One of their advantages is that they have already evaluated the risk of bias that might be of issue in the randomised controlled trials that they index.

Now that you have found a research article that you are interested in, it is important to critically appraise it. That is, you need to examine the research closely to determine whether and how it might inform your clinical practice. As we saw in Chapter 1, to critically appraise research, there are three main aspects to consider: 1) its internal validity (in particular, the risk of bias); 2) its impact (the size and importance of any

Clinical scenario (continued): Finding evidence to answer your question

You search the Cochrane Database of Systematic Reviews and there are two reviews concerning falls prevention. One of these reviews evaluated the effect of interventions that were designed to reduce the incidence of falls in the elderly, but not just those who are community-living—it also included those in institutional care and hospital care. The other review focussed on population-level interventions. As neither of these reviews is what you are after, you next search OTseeker and find six articles that are possibly relevant. You are specifically interested in interventions aimed at community-dwelling older people and the title of one of these articles matches this. After reading the abstract, you know that this article describes a randomised controlled trial that has investigated the effectiveness of a program (called the 'Stepping On' program) for reducing the incidence of falls in the community-living elderly.[4] As you found this article indexed in OTseeker, it has been evaluated with respect to risk of bias; however, in order to evaluate whether it also measured self-efficacy as an outcome and to specifically examine the results of the trial and determine whether the findings may be applicable to your clinical scenario, you obtain the full text of the article. You find that it does measure self-efficacy, so you proceed to critically appraise the article. (As most of the trials in OTseeker are pre-appraised, you would normally not need to appraise the risk of bias in the article for yourself. However, as the purpose of this clinical scenario exercise is to demonstrate how to appraise a randomised controlled trial, we will proceed to appraise this article even though it was located in OTseeker.)

Clinical scenario (continued): Structured abstract of our chosen article (the 'stepping on' trial)

Citation: Clemson L, Cumming R, Kendig H et al. The effectiveness of a community-based program for reducing the incidence of falls in the elderly: a randomised trial. Journal of the American Geriatrics Society 2004; 52:1487–1494.
Design: Randomised controlled trial.
Setting: Community venues and follow-up home visits in New South Wales, Australia.
Participants: 310 community-living people aged over 70 years and older (mean age 78.4 years, 74% female) with a history of falling in the past year or who were concerned about falling.
Intervention: A community-based small-group education program that aimed to help older people reduce falls and enhance their self-efficacy in fall-risk situations. Key content that was covered by the program included: lower limb balance and strength exercises, coping with visual impairment, medication management and home and community safety. One session also involved community mobility practice. A cognitive-behavioural approach was used, with practice and application

of behaviours encouraged during and after groups. The program consisted of 2-hour group sessions (held weekly for 7 weeks), an individual home visit (held within 6 weeks of the last group session) and a 3-month group booster session. All intervention was provided by an experienced occupational therapist. Participants in the control group received one or two social home visits from a student.

Outcomes: The primary outcome measure was the occurrence of falls (for which a specific definition was used). There was also a range of secondary outcome measures used. Of particular interest to this clinical scenario, there were two self-efficacy outcome measures that were used. One was the Modified Falls Efficacy Scale, which assesses how confident a person is in their ability to avoid falls when performing basic activities of daily living. The other was the Mobility Efficacy Scale, which assesses how confident a person is in their ability to avoid falls when performing functional tasks that require a greater degree of postural challenge than the tasks assessed by the Modified Falls Efficacy Scale.

Follow-up period: Approximately 14 months (median 420 days).

Main results: The intervention group experienced a 31% reduction in falls relative to the control group.

Conclusion: Cognitive-behavioural learning in a small group environment can reduce falls and the Stepping On program is an option for effective falls prevention.

effect found); and 3) whether or how the evidence might be applicable to your client or clinical practice.

Is this evidence likely to be biased?

In this chapter we will discuss six criteria that are commonly used for appraising the potential risk of bias in a randomised controlled trial. These six criteria are summarised in Box 4.1 and can be found in the Users Guide to the Literature[5] and in many appraisal checklists such as the Critical Appraisal Skills Program (CASP) checklist and the PEDro scale.[6] A number of studies have demonstrated that estimates of treatment effects may be distorted in trials that do not adequately address these issues.[7,8] As you work through

---

BOX 4.1 KEY QUESTIONS TO ASK WHEN APPRAISING THE VALIDITY (RISK OF BIAS) IN A RANDOMISED CONTROLLED TRIAL

1. Was the assignment of participants to groups randomised?
2. Was the allocation sequence concealed?
3. Were the groups similar at the baseline or start of the trial?
4. Were participants, health professionals and study personnel 'blind' to group allocation?
5. Were all participants who entered the trial properly accounted for at its conclusion and how complete was follow-up?
6. Were participants analysed in the groups to which they were randomised using intention-to-treat analysis?

each of these criteria when appraising an article, it is important to consider the direction of the bias (that is, is it in favour of the intervention or control group?) as well as its magnitude. As we pointed out in Chapter 1, all research has flaws, but we do not just want to know what the flaws might be, but whether and how they might influence the results of a study.

Was the assignment of participants to groups randomised?

Randomised controlled trials, by definition, randomise participants to either the experimental or control condition. The basic principle of randomisation is that each participant has an equal chance of being assigned to any group, such that any difference between the groups at the beginning of the trial can be assumed to be due to chance. The main benefit of randomisation is related to the idea that this way, both known and unknown participant characteristics should be evenly distributed between the intervention and control groups. Therefore, any differences between groups that are found at the end of the study are likely because of the intervention.[9]

Random allocation is best done by a random numbers table which can be computer-generated. Sometimes it is done by tossing a coin or 'pulling a number out of a hat'. Additionally, there are different randomisation designs that can be used and you should be aware of them. Researchers may choose to use some form of restriction, such as blocking or stratification, when allocating participants to groups in order to create a greater balance between the groups at baseline in known characteristics.[10] Different randomisation designs are summarised below:

- **Simple randomisation:** involves randomisation of individuals to the experimental or control condition.
- **Cluster randomisation:** involves random allocation of intact *clusters* of individuals rather than individuals (for example, randomisation of schools, towns, clinics or general practices).
- **Stratified randomisation**: in this design, participants are matched and randomly allocated to groups. This method ensures that potentially confounding factors such as age, gender or disease severity are balanced between groups. For example, in a trial that involves people who have had a stroke, participants might be stratified according to their initial stroke severity as belonging to either a 'mild', 'moderate' or 'severe' stratum. This way when randomisation to study groups occurs, researchers can ensure that, within each stratum, there are equal numbers of participants in the intervention and control groups.
- **Block randomisation:** In this design, participants who are similar are grouped into 'blocks' and then assigned to the experimental or control conditions within each block. Block randomisation often uses stratification An example of block randomisation can be seen in a randomised controlled study of a community-based parenting education intervention program designed to increase the use of preventive paediatric

---

Clinical scenario (continued): Was the assignment of participants to groups randomised?

In the Stepping On trial, it is explicitly stated that participants were randomised and that the randomisation was stratified in blocks of four, according to participants' gender and number of falls in the previous 12 months.

healthcare services among low income, minority mothers.[11] Two hundred and eighty-six mother–infant dyads recruited from four different sites in Washington DC were assigned to either the standard social services (control) group or the intervention group. To ensure that there were comparable numbers within each group across the four sites, site-specific block randomisation was used. By using block randomisation, selection bias due to demographic differences across the four sites was avoided.

Was the allocation sequence concealed?

As we have seen, the big benefit of a randomised controlled trial over other study designs is the fact that participants are randomly allocated to the study groups. However, the benefits of randomisation can be undone if the allocation sequence is manipulated or interfered with in any way. As strange as this might seem, a health professional who wants their client to receive the intervention that is being evaluated may swap their client's group assignment so that their client receives the intervention being studied. Similarly, if the person who recruits participants to a study knows which condition the participants are to be assigned to, this could influence their decision about whether or not to enrol them in the study. This is why assigning participants to study groups using alternation methods, such as every second person who comes into the clinic, or assigning participants by methods such as date of birth is problematic because the randomisation sequence is known to the people involved.[9]

Knowledge about which group a participant will be allocated to if they are recruited into a study can lead to the selective assignment of participants, and thus introduce bias into the trial. This knowledge can result in manipulation of either the sequence of groups that participants are to be allocated to or the sequence of participants to be enrolled. Either way, this is a problem. This problem can be dealt with by concealing the allocation sequence from the people who are responsible for enrolling clients into a trial or from those who assign participants to groups, until the moment of assignment.[12] Allocation can be concealed by having the randomisation sequence administered by someone who is 'off-site' or at a location away from where people are being enrolled into the study. Another way to conceal allocation is by having the group allocation placed in sealed opaque envelopes. Opaque envelopes are used so that the group allocation cannot be seen if the envelope is held up to the light! The envelope is not to be opened until the client has been enrolled into the trial (and is therefore now a participant in the study).

Hopefully, the article that you are appraising will clearly state that allocation was concealed, or that it was done by an independent or off-site person or that sealed opaque envelopes were used. Unfortunately though, many studies do not give any indication about whether allocation was concealed,[13,14] so you are often left wondering about this, which is frustrating when you are trying to appraise a study. It is possible that some of these studies did use concealed allocation, but you cannot tell this from reading the article.

Clinical scenario (continued): Concealed allocation

In the Stepping On trial, allocation was concealed. The article states that the randomisation was conducted by a researcher who was not involved in participant screening or assessment.

Were the groups similar at the baseline or start of the trial?

One of the principal aims of randomisation is to ensure that the groups are similar at the start of the trial in all respects, except for whether they received the experimental condition (that is, the intervention of interest) or not. However, the use of randomisation does not guarantee that the groups will have similar known baseline characteristics. This is particularly the case if there is a small sample size. Authors of a research article will usually provide data in the article about the baseline characteristics of both groups. This allows readers to make up their own minds as to whether the balance between important prognostic factors (variables that have the potential for influencing outcomes) is sufficient at the start of the trial. Consider, for example, a study about the effectiveness of acupuncture for reducing pain from migraines compared to sham acupuncture. If the participants who were allocated to the acupuncture group had less severe or less chronic pain at the start of the study than the participants who were allocated to the sham acupuncture group, any differences in pain levels that are seen at the end of the study might be the result of that initial difference and not the acupuncture that was provided.

Differences between the groups that are present at baseline after randomisation have occurred due to chance and, therefore, determining if these differences are statistically significant by using *p* values is not an appropriate way of assessing such differences.[15] That is, rather than using the *p* value that is often reported in studies, it is important to examine these differences by comparing means or proportions visually. The extent to which you might be concerned about a baseline difference between the groups depends on how large a difference it is and whether it is a key prognostic variable, both of which require some clinical judgement. The stronger the relationship between the characteristic and the outcome of interest, the more the differences between groups will weaken the strength of any inference about efficacy.[5] For example, consider a study that is investigating the effectiveness of group therapy in improving communication for people who have chronic aphasia following stroke compared with usual care. Typically, such a study would measure and report a wide range of variables at baseline (that is, prior to the intervention) such as participants' age, gender, education level, place of residence, time since stroke, severity of aphasia, side of stroke and so on. Some of these variables are more likely to influence communication outcomes than others. The key question to consider is: are any differences in key prognostic variables between the groups large enough that they may have influenced the outcome(s)? Hopefully if differences are evident, the researchers will have corrected for this in the data analysis process.

As a reader (and critical appraiser) of research articles, it is important that you are able to see data for key characteristics that may be of prognostic value in both groups. Many articles will present this data in a table, with the data for the intervention group presented in one column and the data for the control group in another. This enables you to easily compare how similar the groups are for these variables. As well as presenting baseline data about **key sociodemographic characteristics** (for example, age and gender), articles should *also* report data about important **measures of the severity of the condition** (if that is relevant to the study—most times it is) so that you can see if the groups were also similar in this respect. For example, in a study that involves participants who have had a stroke, the article may present data about the initial stroke severity of participants, as this variable has the potential to influence how participants respond to an intervention. In most cases, sociodemographic variables alone are not sufficient to determine baseline similarity.

One other area of baseline data that articles should report is the **key outcome(s)** of the study (that is, the pre-test measurement(s)). Let us consider the example presented earlier of people receiving group communication treatment for aphasia to illustrate why this is important. Although such an article would typically provide information about sociodemographic variables and clinical variables (such as severity of aphasia, type of stroke and side of stroke), having information about participants' initial (that is, pre-test) scores on the communication outcome measure that the study used would be helpful for considering baseline similarity. This is because, logically, participants' pre-test scores on a communication measure are likely to be a key prognostic factor for the main outcome of the study, which is communication ability.

When appraising an article, if you do conclude that there are baseline differences between the groups that are likely to be big enough to be of concern, hopefully the researchers will have statistically adjusted for these in the analysis. If they have not, you will need to try and take this into account when interpreting the study.

Clinical scenario (continued): Baseline similarity

In the Stepping On trial, the baseline characteristics shown in Tables 1 and 2 are similar between the study groups and include most of the likely confounders. The authors point out that there is a small difference (6% in the intervention group, 10% in the control group) in the number of participants with a previous hip fracture, but go on to report that there were no differences in the trial results when data were reanalysed after adjusting for history of hip fracture. The baseline scores of the outcome measures are also similar between the two groups.

Were participants, health professionals and study personnel 'blind' to group allocation?

People involved with a trial, whether they be the participants, the treating health professionals or the study personnel, usually have a belief or expectation about what effect the experimental condition will or will not have. This conscious or unconscious expectation can influence their behaviour, which in turn can affect the results of the study. This is particularly problematic if they know which condition (experimental or control) the participant is receiving. Blinding (also known as masking) is a technique that is used to prevent participants, health professionals and study personnel from knowing which group the participant was assigned to so that they will not be influenced by that knowledge.[10] In many studies, it is difficult to achieve blinding. Blinding means more than just keeping the name of the intervention hidden. The experimental and control conditions need to be indistinguishable. This is because even if they are not informed about the nature of the experimental or control conditions (which, for ethical reasons, they usually are) when they sign informed consent forms, participants can often work out which group they are in. Whereas pharmaceutical trials can use placebo medication to prevent participants and health professionals from knowing who has received the active intervention, blinding of participants and the health professionals who are providing the intervention is very difficult (and often impossible) in many non-pharmaceutical trials. We will now look a little more closely at why it is important to blind participants, health professionals and study personnel to group allocation.

A **participant's** knowledge of their treatment status (that is, if they know whether they are receiving the intervention that is being evaluated or not) may consciously or unconsciously influence their performance during the intervention or their reporting of outcomes. For example, if a participant was keen to receive the intervention that was being studied and they were instead randomised to the control group, they may be disappointed and their feelings about this might be reflected in their outcome assessments, particularly if the outcomes being measured are subjective in nature (for example, pain, quality of life or satisfaction). Conversely, if a participant knows or suspects that they are in the intervention group, they may be more positive about their outcomes (such as exaggerating the level of improvement that they have experienced) when they report them as they wish to be a 'polite client' and are grateful for receiving the intervention.[16]

The **health professionals** who provide the intervention often have a view about the effectiveness of interventions and this can influence the way they interact with the study participants and the way they deliver the intervention. This in turn can influence how committed they are to providing the intervention in a reliable and enthusiastic manner, participants' compliance to the intervention and participants' responses on outcome measures. For example, if a health professional believes strongly in the value of the intervention that is being studied they may be very enthusiastic and diligent in their delivery of the intervention, which may in turn influence how participants respond to this intervention. It is easy to see how a health professional's enthusiasm (or lack of) could influence outcomes. Obviously some interventions (such as medications) are not able to be influenced easily by the way in which they are provided, but for many other interventions (such as rehabilitation techniques provided by therapists), this can be an issue.

Study personnel who are responsible for measuring outcomes (the assessors) who are aware of whether the participant is receiving the experimental or control condition may provide different interpretations of marginal findings or differential encouragement during performance tests, either of which can distort results. For example, if an assessor knows that a participant is in the intervention group, they might be a little more generous when scoring a participant's performance on a task than they would be if they thought that the participant was in the control group. Studies should aim to use blinded assessors to prevent measurement bias from occurring. This can be done by ensuring that the assessor who measures the outcomes at baseline and at follow-up is unaware of the participant's group assignment. Sometimes this is referred to as the use of an independent assessor. The more objective the outcome that is being assessed, the less critical this issue becomes. However, there are not many truly objective outcome measures as even measures that appear to be reasonably objective (for example, measuring muscle strength manually or functional ability) have a subjective component and, as such, can be susceptible to measurement bias. Therefore, where it is at all possible, studies should try and ensure that the people who are assessing participants' outcomes are blinded. Ideally studies should also check and report on the success of blinding assessors and, where this information is not provided, you may wish to reasonably speculate about whether or not the outcome assessor was actually blinded as claimed.

However, there is a common situation that occurs, particularly in many trials in which non-pharmaceutical interventions are being tested, that makes assessor blinding not possible to achieve. If the participant is aware of their group assignment, then the assessment cannot be considered to be blinded. For example, consider the outcome measure of pain that is assessed using a visual analogue scale. The participant has to complete the assessment themselves due to the subjective nature of the symptom experience. In this situation, the participant is really the assessor and, if the participant is not blind to which study group they are in, then the assessor is also not blind to group allocation. Research articles often state that the outcome assessors were blind to group allocation. Most articles measure more than one outcome and often a combination of objective and subjective outcome measures are used. So, while this statement may be true for objective outcomes, if the article involved outcomes that were assessed by participant self-report and the participants were not blinded, you cannot consider that these subjective outcomes were measured by a blinded assessor.

Clinical scenario (continued): Blinding

In the Stepping On trial, the primary outcome measure was the occurrence of falls and this was measured by participant self-report. Participants had to fill out a monthly postcard calendar, noting whether they did or did not fall on each day of the month, and post this to the researchers. Participants who reported falling received a telephone call to verify if the fall met the definition of falling that was being used in the trial. As the primary outcome measure was measured by participant self-report and participants were not blinded, technically, the measurement of the primary outcome measure was not done by a blinded assessor. However, participant self-report is an appropriate, and widely used and accepted, measure of collecting data about falling in community-living people and there is not really any other feasible method that enables this data to be collected in a blinded manner. All other outcome measures were assessed, at the 14-month follow-up assessment, by a research assistant who was blind to group allocation. Neither the participants nor the health professionals who provided the intervention were blind to group allocation. For this type of intervention, blinding is not possible for participants or those providing the intervention.

Were all participants who entered the trial properly accounted for at its conclusion and how complete was follow-up?

In randomised controlled trials, it is common to have missing data at follow-up. There are many reasons why data may be missing. For example, some questionnaires may not have been fully completed by participants, some participants may have decided to leave the study or some participants may have moved house and are unable to be located at the time of the follow-up assessment. How much of a problem this is for the study, with respect to the bias that is consequently introduced, depends on *why* participants left the study and *how many* left the study.

It is therefore helpful to know whether all the participants who entered the trial were properly accounted for. In other words, we want to know what happened to them. Could the reason that they dropped out of the study have affected the results? This may be the case, for example, if they left the study because the intervention was making them worse or causing adverse side effects. If this was the case, this might make the intervention look more effective than it really was. Did they leave the study simply because they changed jobs and moved interstate, or was the reason that they dropped out related to the study or to their health? For example, it may not be possible to obtain data from participants at follow-up measurement points because they became unwell or maybe because they improved and no longer wanted to participate. Hopefully, you can now see why it is important to know why there are missing data for some participants.

The more participants who are 'lost to follow-up', the more the trial may be at risk of bias because participants that leave the study are likely to have different prognoses from those who stay in the study. It has been suggested that 'readers can decide for themselves when the loss to follow-up is excessive by assuming, in positive trials (that is, trials that showed that the intervention was effective), that all participants lost from the treatment group did badly, and that all lost from the control group did well, and then recalculating the outcomes under these assumptions. If the conclusions of the trial do not change, then the loss to follow-up was not excessive. If the conclusions would change, the strength of inference is weakened (that is, less confidence can be placed in the study results)'.[5]

When large numbers of participants leave a study, the potential for bias is enhanced. Various authors suggest that *if more than 15–20% of participants leave the study* (with no data available for them), then the results should be considered with much greater caution.[16,17] Therefore, you are looking for a study to have a minimum follow-up rate of at least 80–85%. To calculate the loss to follow-up, you just need to divide the number of participants included in the analysis at the time point of interest (such as the 6-month follow-up) by the number of participants who were originally randomised into the study groups. This gives the percentage of participants who were followed up. In some articles it is straightforward to find the necessary data that you need to calculate this, particularly if the article has provided a flow diagram (see Figure 4.2). It is highly recommended that trials do this and this is explained more fully later in the chapter when the recommended reporting of a randomised controlled trial is discussed. In other articles, this information can be obtained from the text, typically in the results section. In some articles, the only place to locate information about the number of participants who remain in the groups at a particular time point is from the column headers in a results table. And finally, in some articles, despite all of your best hunting efforts, there may be no information about the number of participants who were retained in the study. This may mean that there were no participants lost to follow-up (which is highly unlikely as at least some participants are lost to follow-up in most studies) or the authors of the article did not report the loss of participants that occurred. Either way, as you cannot determine how complete the follow-up was, you should be suspicious of the study and consider the results to be potentially biased.

It is worth noting that where there is loss to follow-up in both the intervention and control groups and the reasons for these losses are both *known* and *similar* between these groups, it is less likely that bias will be problematic.[18] When the reasons for why participants leave the study are unknown, or when they are known to be different between the groups and potentially prognostically relevant, you should be more suspicious about the validity of the study. That is why it is important to consider the reasons for loss to follow-up and if the number of participants lost to follow-up was approximately the same for both of the study groups, as well as the actual percentage of participants who were lost to follow-up.

Clinical scenario (continued): Follow-up of participants

In the Stepping On trial, participants were followed from baseline to 14 months post-randomisation. The flow of participants through the trial is clearly provided in Figure 1 of the article. Loss to follow-up was minimal, with 8% of participants lost to follow-up before the 14-month assessment (therefore 92% follow-up rate). Loss to follow-up for secondary outcome measures was higher (15.5%), but this is still around the 85% follow-up rate that is considered acceptable when evaluating a trial's internal validity.

Were participants analysed in the groups to which they were randomised using intention-to-treat analysis?

The final criterion for assessing risk of bias that we will address in this chapter is whether or not data from all participants were analysed in the groups to which participants were initially randomised, regardless of whether they ended up receiving the treatment. This analysis principle is referred to as intention-to-treat analysis. In other words, participants should be analysed in the group that corresponds to how they were *intended* to be treated, not how they were actually treated.

It is important that an intention-to-treat analysis is performed because study participants may not always receive the intervention or control condition as it was allocated (that is, intended to be received). In general, participants may not receive the intervention (even though they were allocated to the intervention group) because they are either unwell or unmotivated, or for other reasons related to prognosis.[5] For example, in a study that is evaluating the effect of a medication, some participants in the intervention group may forget to take the medication and therefore do not actually receive the intervention as intended. In a study that is evaluating the effects of a home-based exercise program, some of the participants in the intervention group may not practise any of the exercises that are part of the intervention because they are not very motivated. Likewise, in a study that is evaluating a series of small group education sessions for people who have had a heart attack, some participants in the intervention group may decide not to attend some or all education sessions because they feel unwell. From these examples, you can see that even though these participants were in the intervention group of these studies, they did not actually receive the intervention (either at all or only partly). It may be tempting for the researchers who are conducting these studies to analyse the data from these participants as if they were in the control group instead. However, doing this would increase the numbers in the control group who were either unmotivated or unwell. This would make the intervention appear more effective than it actually is because there would be a greater number of participants in the control group who were likely to have unfavourable outcomes. It may also be tempting for researchers to discard the results from participants who did not receive the intervention (or control condition) as was intended. This is also an unsuitable way of dealing with this issue as these participants would then be considered as lost to follow-up, and we saw in the previous criterion why it is important that as few participants as possible are lost to follow-up.

For the sake of completeness, it is important that we point out that it is not only participants who are allocated to the intervention group but do not receive the intervention that we should think about. The opposite can also happen. Participants who are allocated to the control group can inadvertently end up receiving the intervention. Again, intention-to-treat analysis should be used and these participants should still be analysed as part of the control group.

The value of intention-to-treat analysis is that it preserves the value of randomisation. It helps to ensure that prognostic factors that we know about, and those that we do not know about, will still be, on average, equally distributed between the groups. Because of this, any effect that we see, such as improvement in participants' outcomes, is most likely to be because of the intervention rather than unrelated factors.

The difficulty in carrying out a true intention-to-treat analysis is that the data for *all* participants is needed. However, as we saw in the previous criterion about follow-up of participants, this is unrealistic to expect and most studies have missing data. There is currently no real agreement about the best way to deal with this missing data (probably because there is no ideal way) but researchers may sometimes estimate or impute data.[19]

Data imputation is a statistical procedure that substitutes missing data in a data file with estimated data. Other studies may simply report that they have carried out an intention-to-treat analysis or that participants received the experimental or control conditions as allocated without providing details of what was actually done or how missing data were dealt with. In this case, as the reader of the article, you may choose to accept this at face value or to remain sceptical about how this issue was dealt with, depending on what other clues are available in the study report.

> ## Clinical scenario (continued): Intention-to-treat analysis
>
> **In the Stepping On trial, it is stated that data were analysed using intention-to-treat.**

The role of chance

So far in this chapter we have considered the potential for bias in randomised controlled trials. Another aspect that is important to consider is the possibility that the play of chance might be an alternative explanation for the findings. So, a further question that you may wish to consider when appraising a randomised controlled trial is: did the study report a power calculation that might indicate what sample size would be necessary for the study to detect an effect if the effect actually exists? As we saw in Chapter 2, having an adequate sample size is important so that the study can avoid a type II error occurring. You may remember that a type II error is the failure to find and report a relationship when a relationship actually exists.[20]

> ## Clinical scenario (continued): Did the study have enough participants to minimise the play of chance?
>
> **In the Stepping On trial, 310 participants were recruited. A power calculation (with a power of 80% and an alpha of 5%) was performed and it was estimated that 300 participants would be needed to detect a 40% relative reduction in fall rate. Therefore, it appears that an adequate number of participants was recruited into the trial.**

Completeness of reporting of randomised controlled trials

As we have seen in many places throughout this chapter, it can often be difficult for readers of research studies to know whether a study has or has not met some of the requirements to be considered a well-designed and well-conducted randomised controlled trial that is relatively free of bias. To help overcome this problem and aid in the critical appraisal and interpretation of trials, an evidence-based initiative known as the CONSORT (Consolidated Standards of Reporting Trials) statement[12,21] has been developed to guide authors about how to completely report the details of a randomised controlled trial. The CONSORT statement is considered an evolving document and, at the time of writing this chapter, it consisted of a 22-item checklist and a flow diagram (see Figure 4.2). Full details are available at http://www.consort-statement.org/. The CONSORT statement is

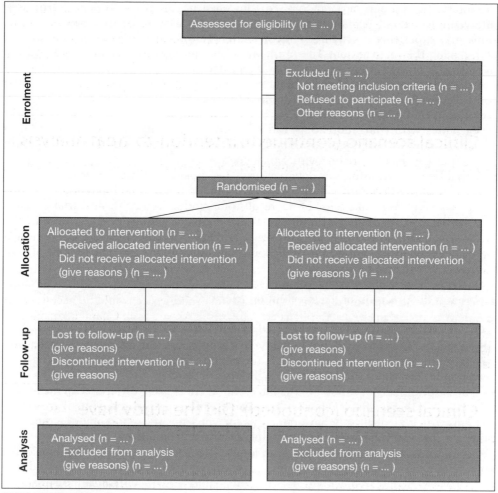

FIGURE 4.2 CONSORT flow diagram

Reproduced with permission from Moher et al, The CONSORT statement: revised recommendations for improving the quality of reports of parallel-group randomised trials. Elsevier; 2001[21]

also used by reviewers of articles when the articles are being considered for publication, and many journals now insist that articles about randomised controlled trials follow the CONSORT statement. This is helping to improve the quality of reporting of trials but, as this is a recent requirement, many older articles do not contain all of the information that you need to know.

After determining that an article about the effects of an intervention that you have been appraising appears to be reasonably free of bias, you then proceed to looking at the importance of the results.

Understanding results

One of the fundamental concepts that you need to keep in mind when you are trying to make sense of the results of a randomised controlled trial is that clinical trials provide us with an ***estimate*** of the ***average*** effects of an intervention. Not every participant in the intervention group of a randomised controlled trial is going to benefit from the intervention that is being studied—some may benefit a lot, some may benefit a little, some may experience no change, some may even be worse (a little or a lot) as a result of receiving the intervention. The results from all participants are combined and the *average* effect of the intervention is what is reported.

Before getting into the details about how to interpret the results of a randomised controlled trial, the first thing that you need to look at is whether you are dealing with continuous or dichotomous data:

- **Variables with continuous data** can take any value along a continuum within a defined range. Examples of continuous variables are age, range of motion in a joint, walking speed and score on a visual analogue scale.
- Variables with **dichotomous data** have only two possible values. For example, male/female, satisfied/not satisfied with treatment and hip fracture/no hip fracture.

The way that you make sense of the results of a randomised controlled trial depends on whether you are dealing with outcomes that were continuous or dichotomous. We will look at continuous data first. However, regardless of whether the results of the study were measured using continuous or dichotomous outcomes, we will be looking at how to answer two main questions:

1. What is the **size** of the intervention effect?
2. What is the **precision** of the intervention effect?

Continuous outcomes—size of the intervention effect

When you are trying to work out how much of a difference the intervention made, you are trying to determine the size of the intervention effect. When you are dealing with continuous data, this is often quite a straightforward process.

- The best estimate for the size of the intervention effect is the **difference in means** (or medians if that is what is reported) **between the intervention and control groups.**

Many articles will already have done this for you and will report the difference. In other articles, you will have to do this simple calculation yourself.

Let us consider an example. In a randomised controlled trial[22] that evaluated the efficacy of a self-management program for people with knee osteoarthritis in addition to usual care, compared with usual care, one of the main outcome measures was pain, which was measured using a 0–10-point visual analogue scale. At the 3-month follow-up, the mean reduction in knee pain was 0.67 (standard deviation [SD] = 2.10) in the intervention group and 0.01 (SD = 2.00) in the control group. This difference was statistically significant ($p = 0.023$). You can calculate the intervention effect size (difference in mean change between the groups) as: 0.67 minus 0.01 = 0.66.

Note that in this study, the authors reported the mean *improvement (reduction in pain) scores* at the 3-month follow-up (that is, the *change* in pain from baseline to the 3-month follow-up). Some studies report **change scores**; other studies report **end scores** (which are the scores at the end of the intervention period). Regardless of whether change scores or end scores are reported, the method of calculating the size of the intervention effect is the same. When dealing with change scores, it becomes the difference of the mean *change* between the intervention and control groups that you need.

Clinical significance

Once you know the size of the intervention effect, you need to decide if this result is clinically significant. As we saw in Chapter 2, just because a study finds a statistically significant result, it does not mean that the result is *clinically* significant. Deciding whether a result is clinically significant requires your judgement (and, ideally, your client's, too) on whether the benefits of the intervention outweigh its costs. Cost should be regarded in the broadest sense to be any inconveniences, discomforts or harms associated with the intervention, in addition to any monetary costs. To make decisions about clinical significance it helps to determine what the smallest intervention effect is that you consider to be clinically worthwhile. Where possible, this decision is one which is reached in conjunction with the client so that their preferences are considered.

To interpret the results of a study, the smallest clinically worthwhile difference (to warrant using a self-management program in addition to standard care) needs to be established. This might be decided directly by the health professional, by using guidelines established by research on the particular measure being used (if available), by consultation with the client or by some combination of these approaches. Frequently health professionals make a clinical judgement based on their experience with a particular measure and by discussion with the client about their preferences in relation to the costs (including both financial costs and inconveniences) involved. Health professionals then need to consider how the smallest clinically worthwhile difference that was determined relates to the effect found in the study. This is handled in a number of different ways in the literature.

One of the earliest methods for deciding important differences using effect sizes was developed by Cohen.[23] Effect sizes (represented by the symbol d) were calculated by taking the difference between group average scores and dividing it by the average of the standard deviation for both groups. This effect size is then compared to ranges classified intuitively by Cohen: 0.2 being a small effect size, 0.5 a moderate effect size and 0.8 a large effect size. This general rule of thumb has consequently been used to determine whether a change or difference was important or not.

Norman and colleagues looked at effect sizes empirically (looking at a systematic review of 62 effect sizes from 38 studies of chronic disease that had calculated minimally important differences) and found that, in most circumstances, the smallest detectable difference was approximately half a standard deviation.[24] They thus recommend that, when no other information exists about the smallest clinically worthwhile difference, an intervention effect should be regarded as worthwhile if it exceeds half a standard deviation. However, the use of statistical standards for interpreting differences has been criticised because the between-patient variability, or number of standard deviation units, depends on the heterogeneity of the population (meaning whether the population is made up of different sorts of participants).[25]

A more direct approach is to simply compare the mean intervention effect with a nominated smallest clinically worthwhile difference. If the mean intervention effect lies below the smallest clinically worthwhile difference, we may consider it to be *not* clinically significant. For our knee osteoarthritis example, let us assume that in conjunction with our client we nominate a 20% reduction of initial pain as the smallest difference that we would consider to be clinically worthwhile in order to add self-management to what the client is already receiving. Our calculations show that a 20% reduction from the initial average pain of 4.05mm experienced by participants in this study would be 0.8mm. If the intervention has a greater effect than 20% reduction in pain from baseline, we may consider that the benefits of it outweigh the costs and may therefore use it with our client(s). In this study, the difference between groups in mean pain reduction (0.66mm) is lower than 0.8mm so we might be tempted to conclude the result may not be clinically significant for this client.

An alternative approach to considering the effect size relative to baseline values that is sometimes used involves comparing the effect size to the scale range of the outcome measure. In this example we would simply compare the intervention effect size of 0.66

in relation to the overall possible score range of 0–10 and see that this between-group difference is not very large and therefore conclude that the result is unlikely to be considered clinically significant.

Note, however, that as this is an *average* effect there may be some clients who do much better than this and, for them, the intervention is clinically significant. Of course, conversely, there may be some clients who do much worse. This depends on the distribution of changes that occur in the two groups. One way of dealing with this is to look for the proportion of clients in both groups who improved, stayed the same, or got worse relative to the nominated smallest clinically worthwhile difference. However, these data are often elusive as they are often not reported in articles.

Another approach to determining clinical significance takes into account the uncertainty in measurement using the *confidence intervals* around the estimate. To understand this approach, we need to first look at confidence intervals in some detail.

Continuous outcomes—precision of the intervention effect

How are confidence intervals useful?

At the beginning of this results section we highlighted that the results of a study are only an *estimate* of the true effect of the intervention. The size of the intervention effect in a study approximates but **does not equal** the true size of the intervention effect in the population represented by the study sample. As each study only involves a small sample of participants (regardless of the actual sample size, it is still just a *sample* of all of the clients who meet the study's eligibility criteria and therefore is small in the grand scheme of things), the results of any study are just an estimate based on the sample of participants in that particular study. If we replicated the study with another sample of participants, we would (most likely) obtain a different estimate. As we saw in Chapter 2, the true value refers to the population value, not just the estimate of a value that has come from the sample of one study.

Confidence intervals are a way of describing how much uncertainty is associated with the estimate of the intervention effect (in other words, the precision or accuracy of the estimate). We saw in Chapter 2 how confidence intervals provide us with a range of values that the true value lies within. When dealing with 95% confidence intervals, what you are saying is that you are **95% certain that the true average intervention effect lies between the upper and the lower limits of the confidence interval.** In the knee osteoarthritis trial that we considered above, the 95% confidence interval for the difference of the mean change is 0.05mm to 1.27mm (see Box 4.2 for how this was calculated). So, we are 95% certain that the true average intervention effect (at 3 months follow-up) of the self-management program on knee pain in people with osteoarthritis lies between 0.05mm and 1.27mm.

How do I calculate a confidence interval?

Hopefully the study that you are appraising will have included confidence intervals with the results in the results section. Fortunately this is becoming more and more common in research articles. If not, you may be able to calculate the confidence interval yourself if the study provides you with the right information to do so (see Box 4.2 for what you need). An easy way of calculating confidence intervals is to use an online calculator. There are plenty available, such as those found at http://glass.ed.asu.edu/stats/analysis/ or http://www.graphpad.com/quickcalcs/index.cfm. If the internet is not handy, you can use a simple formula to calculate the confidence interval for the difference between the means of two groups. This is shown in Box 4.2.

> ## BOX 4.2 **HOW TO CALCULATE THE CONFIDENCE INTERVAL (CI) FOR THE DIFFERENCE BETWEEN THE MEANS OF TWO GROUPS**
>
> A formula[26] that can be used is:
> $$95\% \text{ CI} \approx \text{Difference} \pm 3 \times \text{SD}/\sqrt{n_{av}}$$
> where
> $$\text{Difference} = \text{difference between the two means}$$
> $$\text{SD} = \text{average of the two standard deviations}$$
> $$n_{av} = \text{average of the group sizes}$$
> For the knee osteoarthritis study: Difference = 0.66; SD = (2.10 + 2.00)/2 = 2.05; and n_{av} = (95 + 107)/2 = 101.
> Therefore, the 95% CI ≈ 0.66 ± 0.61
> $$\approx 0.05 \text{ to } 1.27.$$
> When you calculate confidence intervals yourself, they will vary slightly depending on whether you use this formula or an online calculator. This formula is an approximation of the complex equation that researchers use to calculate confidence intervals for their study results, but it is adequate for the purposes of health professionals who are considering using an intervention in clinical practice and wish to obtain information about the precision of the estimate of the intervention's effect. Occasionally you might calculate a confidence interval that is at odds with the p value reported in the paper (that is, the confidence interval might indicate non-significance when in fact the p value in the paper is significant). This might occur because the test used by the researchers does not assume a normal distribution (as the 95% confidence interval does) or because the p value was close to 0.05 and the rough calculation of the confidence interval might end up including zero as it is a less precise calculation.
> *Note:* If the study reports standard errors (SEs) instead of standard deviations, the formula to calculate the confidence interval is:
> $$95\% \text{ CI} = \text{Difference} \pm 3 \times \text{SE}$$

Confidence intervals and statistical significance

Confidence intervals can also be used to determine whether a result is statistically significant. Consider a randomised controlled trial where two interventions were being evaluated and, at the end of the trial, it was found that, on average, participants in both groups improved by the same amount. If we were to calculate the size of the intervention effect for this trial it would be zero, as there would be no difference between the means of the two groups. When referring to the difference between two groups with means, zero is considered a 'no effect' value. Therefore:

- if a confidence interval includes the 'no effect' value, the result is not statistically significant, and the opposite is also true
- if the confidence interval does *not* include the 'no effect' value, the result is statistically significant.

In the knee osteoarthritis trial, we calculated the 95% confidence interval to be 0.05mm to 1.27mm. This interval does *not* include the 'no effect' value of zero, so we can therefore conclude that the result is statistically significant without needing to know the p value although, in this case, the p value (0.023) was provided in the article and it also indicates a statistically significant result.

As an aside, if a result is *not* statistically significant, it is incorrect to refer to this as a 'negative' difference and imply that the study has shown no difference and conclude that the intervention was not effective. It has not done this at all. All that the study has shown is an absence of evidence of a difference.[27] A simple way to remember this is that **non-significance does not mean no effect.**

Confidence intervals and clinical significance

We now return to our previous discussion about clinical significance. Earlier we saw that there are a number of approaches that can be used to compare the effect estimate of a study to the smallest clinically worthwhile difference that is established by the health professional (and sometimes their client as well). We will now explain a useful way of considering clinical significance that involves using confidence intervals to help make this decision.

Before we go on to explain the relationship between confidence intervals and clinical significance, you may find it easier to understand confidence intervals by viewing them on a **tree plot** (see Figure 4.3). A tree plot is a line along which varying intervention effects lie. The 'no effect' value is indicated in Figure 4.3 as the value 0. Effect estimates to the left of the no effect value may indicate harm. Also marked on Figure 4.3 is a dotted line that indicates the supposed smallest clinically worthwhile intervention effect. Anything to the left of this line, but to the right of the no effect value estimate, represents effects of the intervention that are too small to be worthwhile. On the contrary, anything to the right of this line indicates intervention effects that are clinically worthwhile.

In the situation where the **entire confidence interval is *below* the smallest clinically worthwhile effect**, this is a useful result. It is useful because at least we know with some certainty that the intervention is *not* likely to produce a clinically worthwhile effect. Similarly, when an **entire confidence interval is *above* the smallest clinically worthwhile effect**, this is a clear result, as we know with some certainty that the intervention is likely to produce a clinically worthwhile effect.

However, in the knee osteoarthritis trial, we calculated the 95% confidence interval to be 0.05mm to 1.27mm. The lower value is below 0.8mm (20% of the initial pain level that we nominated as the smallest clinically worthwhile effect), but the upper value is above 0.8mm. We can see this clearly if we mark the confidence interval onto a tree plot (see Figure 4.4, tree plot A). This indicates that there is uncertainty about whether there is a clinically worthwhile effect occurring or not.

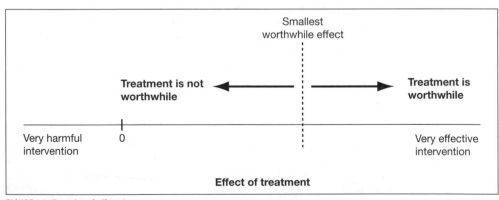

FIGURE 4.3 Tree plot of effect size

When the confidence interval *spans* the smallest clinically worthwhile effect, it is more difficult to interpret clinical significance. In this situation, the true effect of the intervention could lie either above the smallest clinically worthwhile effect or below it. In other words, there is a chance that the intervention may produce a clinically worthwhile effect, but there is also a chance that it may not. Another example of this is illustrated in tree plot B in Figure 4.4, using the data from a randomised controlled trial that investigated the efficacy of a guided self-management program for people with asthma compared with traditional asthma treatment.[28] One of the main outcome measures in this study was quality of life, which was measured using a section of the St George Respiratory Questionnaire. The total score for this outcome measure can range from −50 to +50, with positive scores indicating improvement and negative scores indicating deterioration in quality of life compared with one year ago. At the 12-month follow-up, the difference between the means of the two groups (that is, the

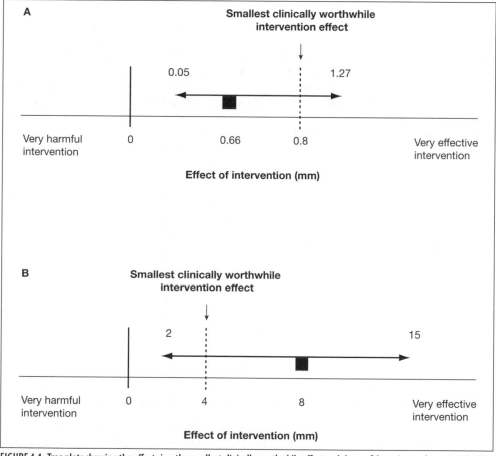

FIGURE 4.4 Tree plots showing the effect size, the smallest clinically worthwhile effect and the confidence interval associated with the effect size

In tree plot A, the estimate of the intervention effect size (0.66) sits below the smallest clinically worthwhile effect of 0.8mm and the confidence interval (0.05mm to 1.27mm) spans the smallest clinically worthwhile effect of 0.8mm. The estimate of the intervention effect size is indicated as a small square, the 95% confidence interval about this estimate is shown as a horizontal line and the dotted line indicates the supposed smallest clinically worthwhile intervention effect.

In tree plot B, the estimate of the intervention effect size (8) is above the smallest clinically worthwhile effect (4) and the confidence interval (2 to 15) spans the smallest clinically worthwhile effect.

intervention effect size) was 8 points (in favour of the self-management group), with a 95% confidence interval of 2 to 15. This difference was statistically significant (*p* = 0.009). Let us assume that we nominate a difference of 4 points to be the smallest clinically worthwhile effect for this example. In this example, the mean difference (8) is above what we have chosen as the smallest clinically worthwhile effect (4), but the confidence interval includes some values that are above the worthwhile effect and some values that are below it. If the true intervention effect was at the upper limit of the confidence interval (at 15), we would consider the intervention to be worthwhile, while if the true intervention effect was at the lower limit of the confidence interval (2), we may not. So, although we would probably conclude that the effect of this self-management intervention on quality of life was clinically significant, this conclusion would be made with a degree of uncertainty.

The situation of a confidence interval spanning the smallest clinically worthwhile effect is a common one and there are two main reasons why it can occur. Firstly, it can occur when a study has a small sample size and therefore low power. The concept of power was explained in Chapter 2. As we also saw in Chapter 2, the smaller the sample size of a study, the wider (that is, less precise) the confidence interval is, which makes it more likely that the confidence interval will span the worthwhile effect. Secondly, it can occur because many interventions only have fairly small intervention effects, meaning that their true effects are close to the smallest clinically worthwhile effect. As a consequence, they need to have very narrow confidence intervals if the confidence interval is going to avoid spanning the smallest worthwhile effect.[16] As we just discussed, this typically means that a very large sample size is needed. In allied health studies in particular, this can be difficult to achieve.

There are two ways that you, as a health professional who is trying to decide whether to use an intervention with a client, can deal with this uncertainty:[16]

- Accept the uncertainty and make your decision according to whether the difference between the group means is higher or lower than the smallest clinically worthwhile effect. However, keep the confidence interval in mind as it indicates the degree of doubt that you should have about this estimate.
- Try to increase the certainty by searching for similar studies and establishing if the findings are replicated in other studies. This is one of the advantages of a systematic review, in particular a meta-analysis, as combining the results from multiple trials increases the sample size. The consequence of this is usually a more narrow (more precise) confidence interval which is less likely to span the smallest clinically worthwhile effect. Systematic reviews and meta-analyses are discussed in detail in Chapter 12.

Clinical scenario (continued): Main results—self-efficacy

In the 'Stepping On' trial, the self-efficacy results are reported as change scores (follow-up score minus baseline score). For the Mobility Efficacy Scale, the mean difference (in the change score) between the two groups was 4.28 points (95% confidence interval = 8.40 to 0.54), which was statistically significant. Note that the confidence interval does not contain zero and therefore this result was statistically significant. We will assume for argument's sake that a 10% change in mobility efficacy would be considered clinically significant. A mean difference of 4.28 points from the initial average mobility efficacy baseline score of 66 points represents a change of only 6% (as 4.28/66 × 100 = 6). This mean difference in improvement of 4.28 (6% change) is smaller than the 10% we were hoping for but for some clients it may still be clinically significant, depending on their values or preferences, as the confidence interval indicates that for some people the mean improvement achieved could be as high as 8.40 (or 12.7% change).

For the Modified Falls Efficacy Scale, the mean difference (in the change score) between the two groups was 1.74 (95% confidence interval = –6.14 to 2.67) which was not statistically significant. Note that the confidence interval does contain zero as the result was not statistically significant. As the result for this outcome was not statistically significant, there is no need to consider the clinical significance of this result as we cannot be convinced that this result did not occur by chance.

Dichotomous outcomes—size of the treatment effect

Often the outcomes that are reported in a study will be presented as dichotomous data. As we saw at the beginning of this results section, these are data for which there are only two possible values. It is worth being aware that data that are measured using a continuous scale can also be categorised, using a certain cut-off point on the scale, so that the data become dichotomised. For example, data on a 10-point visual analogue pain scale can be arbitrarily dichotomised around a cut-off point of 3 (or any point that the researchers choose), so that a pain score of 3 or less is categorised as mild pain and a score of above 3 is categorised as moderate/severe pain. By doing this, the researchers have converted continuous data into data that can be analysed as dichotomous data.

Health professionals and clients are often interested in comparative results, that is, the outcome in one group relative to the outcome in the other group. This overall (comparative) consideration is one of risk. Before getting into the details, let us briefly review the concept of risk. Risk is simply the chance, or probability, of an event occurring. A probability can be described by numbers, ranging from 0 to 1, and is a proportion or ratio. Risks and probabilities are usually expressed as a decimal, such as 0.1667, which is the same as 16.67 percent. Risk can be expressed in various ways.[29] We will consider each of these in turn:

1. relative risk (or the flip side of this, which is referred to as relative benefit)
2. relative risk reduction (or relative benefit increase)
3. absolute risk reduction (or absolute benefit increase)
4. number needed to treat.

Relative risk (and relative benefit)

Consider a hypothetical study that investigated the use of relaxation training to prevent the recurrence of migraines. The control group (n=100) received no intervention and is compared with the intervention group (n=100) who received the relaxation training. Suppose that at the end of the 1-month trial, 30 of the participants in the control group had had a migraine. The risk for recurrence of migraine in the control group can be calculated as 30/100, which can be expressed as 30%, or a risk of recurrence of 0.30. If, in the relaxation group, only 5 participants had had a migraine the risk of recurrence would be 5% (5/100) or 0.05.

The **relative risk** is a ratio of the probability of the event occurring in the intervention group versus the control group.[30] In other words, **relative risk is the risk or probability of the event in the intervention group divided by that in the control group.** So, in the relaxation trial the relative risk would be calculated as:

$$0.05/0.30 = 0.17 \text{ (or } 17\%)$$

This can be expressed as: 'people who were in the intervention group have 17% less risk of having a migraine recurrence at 1 month relative to those in the control group'.

Remember when we were discussing continuous outcomes and explained that the no effect value was zero when referring to the difference between group means? When referring to relative risk, the no effect value (that indicates that there is no difference between groups) is 1. Therefore, a relative risk of less than 1 indicates lower risk—that is, a benefit from the intervention.[30]

If we are evaluating a study that aimed to improve an outcome (that is, make it more likely to occur) rather than reducing a risk, we might instead consider using the equivalent concept of **relative benefit**. For example, in a study that evaluated the effectiveness of phonological training to increase reading accuracy among children with learning disabilities, we could calculate relative benefit as the study was about improving an outcome, not reducing the risk of it happening.

Sometimes a study will report an **odds ratio** instead of relative risk. It is similar, except that an odds ratio refers to a ratio of odds, rather than a ratio of risks and is therefore somewhat harder for health professionals to interpret. The odds ratio is the ratio of the odds of an event for those in the intervention group compared with the odds of an event in the control group. Odds are derived by dividing the event rate by the non-event rate for each group, it is calculated by the following formula where CER is the 'control event rate' and EER refers to the 'experimental event rate':

$$\text{Odds ratio (OR)} = [EER/(1 - EER)] \div [CER/(1 - CER)].$$

Relative risk reduction (or relative benefit increase)

Relative risk reduction is the proportional reduction in an event of interest (for example, headaches) in the intervention group compared with the control group, at a specified time point. Again, there is a flip side of this concept, which is known as relative benefit increase. When appraising an article and using this concept, you need to keep in mind whether you are considering negative or positive outcomes:

- Relative risk reduction (RRR) is used for expressing the reduction in risk of a negative outcome (such as falling).
- Relative benefit increase (RBI) is used for expressing an increase in the probability of a beneficial outcome (such as returning to work).

The formula that can be used for calculating relative risk reduction or relative benefit increase is:

$$(CER - EER) \div CER \times 100.$$

CER is the 'control event rate' and EER refers to the 'experimental event rate'.[29] The control event rate is simply the proportion of participants in the control group who experienced the event of interest. In our study of relaxation training for migraines, this was 30% (or 0.30). Similarly, the experimental event rate is the proportion of participants in the intervention (experimental) group who experienced the event of interest. This was 5% (or 0.05) in the migraine study.

Using our trial of relaxation training for migraines, we will illustrate how the relative risk reduction can be calculated as: $(0.30 - 0.05) \div 0.30 = 0.83$. We could multiply this by 100 to get 83% and report that the relaxation training reduced the migraine rate by 83%.

Alternatively, if you already know the relative risk, then the relative risk reduction can be calculated easily using the formula: $RRR = 1 - RR$. In our example, where the relative risk (RR) is 0.17, the relative risk reduction is 0.83 or 83% (calculated as $1 - 0.17$). This result can be interpreted as an 83% reduction in the relative risk of the outcome in the intervention group compared with the control group.

The main difficulty in the use of relative risk reduction is that it does not reflect the baseline risk of the event. This means that as a reader you are unable to discriminate between small intervention effects and large ones. **Baseline risk** has an important role to play. To understand this you need to think about the risk in different populations. For example, in the general population the risk of migraine might be around 5–10% (depending on factors such as gender, age and so on). Reducing the risk of migraine in a population that has a low risk to start with is very hard to achieve, and any risk reduction that is found would be fairly small (and as you will see in the next section, absolute risk reduction would be smaller still). However, in a population of people who commonly have migraines, the risk of recurrence is much higher and it would, therefore, be easier to achieve a larger relative risk reduction. Interventions that reduce the risk in populations who are at high risk of the event under consideration are likely to be clinically worthwhile.[32]

Another difficulty with the use of the relative risk reduction concept is that it can make results seem more impressive than they really are. Expressing the effects of an intervention in relative terms will result in larger percentages than when the same intervention is expressed in absolute terms. For example, suppose the use of a particular type of mattress reduced the risk of pressure sores from 0.05 to 0.025. In relative terms, the mattress reduces the risk by 50% (calculated by: $0.025 \div 0.05 = 0.5$ or 50%), while in absolute terms it reduces the risk by 2.5% (calculated by: $0.05 - 0.025 = 0.025$ or 2.5%). So we can see that the concept of relative risk reduction can inflate the appearance of intervention effectiveness.

You should also be aware that two studies might have the same relative risk reduction but there may be a large difference in the absolute risk reduction. As we saw in the example above about reducing the risk of pressure sores by using a particular type of mattress, a reduction in risk from 0.05 to 0.025 reduces the relative risk by 50%, while in absolute terms it reduces the risk by 2.5%. However let us say that another study found that the risk of pressure sores in a very high risk group of people was reduced from 0.8 to 0.4 because of the intervention (the mattress). In relative terms, although the mattress reduced the relative risk by 50% (calculated by: $0.8 \div 0.4 = 0.5$ or 50%), the absolute risk reduction is 40%, which is a more clinically valuable result than the absolute risk reduction of 2.5% that the first study found.

Absolute risk reduction (or absolute benefit increase)

Another way of presenting information about dichotomous outcomes is by referring to the absolute risk reduction. The absolute risk reduction is simply the absolute arithmetic difference in event rates between the experimental (intervention) and control groups.[33] Absolute values are simply the value of a number, regardless of its sign (positive or negative sign). The notation used for absolute values is vertical bars either side of the value, for example: $|x|$. The absolute arithmetic difference for risk reduction is calculated as: $|EER - CER|$. As with the previous methods of calculating risk that we have explained, there is a flip side to this concept. This is known as absolute benefit increase and is used when referring to a beneficial outcome (such as being discharged home instead of discharged to residential care).

In our relaxation training study, the absolute risk reduction would be 30% − 5% = 25%. This could be expressed as 'there is an absolute reduction in risk of migraine of 25% in the people who were allocated to the relaxation group compared with those who were in the control group'. A big absolute risk reduction indicates that the intervention is very effective, but how big is big enough to be considered clinically significant? A far more meaningful measure, known as number needed to treat, can be used instead.

Number needed to treat

We saw that the absolute risk reduction of having a migraine in the relaxation training study was calculated as 25%, but is this clinically worthwhile? Number needed to treat (NNT) is a method of making the magnitude of the absolute risk reduction more explicit and is a more clinically useful concept.[30] The number needed to treat is simply the inverse of absolute risk reduction and is calculated as 1 ÷ (EER − CER).[34] It tells you the number of people who would need to be treated to achieve the event of interest once. In the relaxation training study, the number needed to treat is 1 ÷ (0.30 − 0.05) = 4. So, in this example, you would have to treat four people (for one month) with relaxation training to prevent one person from having recurrence of a migraine. Obviously a smaller number needed to treat is better than a large one. An intervention that has a smaller number needed to treat is more effective than an intervention that has a larger number needed to treat.

This concept of number needed to treat makes it easier to consider clinical significance as you can more easily weigh up the benefits of preventing the event in one person against the costs and risks of providing the intervention. The size of the smallest clinically worthwhile effect (that is, the smallest worthwhile number needed to treat) will then depend on the seriousness of the event and the costs and risks of the intervention.

Another handy feature when using number needed to treat is that you can compare two different interventions (that are trying to achieve the same outcome) that have the same number needed to treat but have other features that are different. For example, one of the interventions may have a shorter intervention time and/or result in fewer side effects and/or be more convenient to clients and/or be less expensive. It is important to consider features such as these that a particular intervention has when making a decision about which intervention to use with a client.

Applying results to your clinical situation

Most health professionals find it difficult to translate the results from studies to individual clients or to specific clinical situations as studies usually only tell us about the average effects of the intervention. Further, the participants who took part in the study may be different to the clients that we see, and the intervention may differ to the intervention that we use. However, as a rough guide, if your client is 'healthier' or the situation that you are considering is more optimistic than that in the study, the number needed to treat would be lower, the relative benefit increase would be higher, the mean difference would be larger and so on. If, however, your client is 'worse off' or the situation that you are considering is worse than that in the study, the number needed to treat would be higher, the relative benefit increase would be lower, the mean difference would be smaller and so on. A solution to applying the results of a trial to clients with higher or lower levels of risk has been described by Straus and Sackett[35] and you may wish to read their article to learn more about this.

Dichotomous outcomes—precision of the treatment effect

Confidence intervals are also important to consider when examining dichotomous outcomes as, again, they indicate how much uncertainty is associated with the estimate of the intervention effect (in other words, the precision or accuracy of the estimate). The principles of confidence intervals associated with dichotomous data are similar to those for continuous data but there is one very important difference to consider—what is the appropriate no effect value to use?

- For effect size estimates where **subtraction is involved**, such as mean differences (for continuous outcomes) and absolute risk reductions, the **no effect value is 0**.
- For effect sizes that involve **division** such as risk ratios and odds ratios, the **no effect value is 1**.

Therefore, you can see it is important to consider the *type* of effect measure that you are interpreting in order to reliably interpret the confidence interval. The same general principle applies though—a 95% confidence interval that does *not* include the no effect value indicates that the result is statistically significant. Table 4.1 presents a summary of the dichotomous effect measures, including what the no effect value is, that have been discussed in this section of the chapter.

As we could do with continuous outcomes, if the confidence interval has not been provided by the authors of the article, it can be possible to calculate an approximate confidence interval. This is illustrated in Box 4.3. Again, a simplified version of the more complex equation is used, but the confidence interval that is calculated is sufficient for use by health professionals who wish to use the information to assist in clinical decision making. Once you know the confidence interval for the absolute risk reduction, if you wish you could plot it, the effect estimate and the smallest clinically worthwhile effect on a tree plot in the same way that we did for continuous outcomes in Figure 4.4.

Calculating the confidence intervals for number needed to treat is fairly straightforward as you just use the inverse of the numbers in the confidence interval of the absolute risk reduction.[30] However, understanding how to interpret the confidence intervals for number needed to treat can be complicated, and the article by Altman[36] is recommended to understand this in detail.

Clinical scenario (continued): Main results—falls

In the Stepping On trial, the relative risk was 0.69 (95% confidence interval = 0.50–0.96). As the relative risk is less than 1, it indicates that the intervention decreased the ratio of the risk (event rate) in the intervention group compared to the control group. Also note that the confidence interval does not extend across 1, indicating that this result was statistically significant. The relative risk reduction was 31% (that is, the intervention group experienced a 31% reduction in falls relative to the control group). No raw data are reported in the paper that would allow calculation of the number needed to treat from the results. It has been suggested in the literature that, for a falls intervention to be considered clinically significant, a reduction of at least 30% in the falls rate should be achieved.[37,38] This was achieved in this trial; therefore, the results can be considered clinically significant.

Type of measure	Definition	Formula	No effect value
Relative risk (RR)	The ratio of the probability of the event occurring in the intervention group versus the control group. Expressed as either a decimal proportion or a percentage.	The risk of an event in the intervention group divided by the risk in the control group	1
Relative risk reduction (RRR)	The proportion of the risk that is removed by the intervention. That is, the proportional reduction in an event of interest in the intervention group compared with the control group. Usually expressed as a percentage.	(CER − EER) ÷ CER x 100 *or* 1 − RR	0
Absolute risk reduction (ARR)	The absolute arithmetic difference in event rates between the experimental (intervention) and control groups. Usually expressed as a percentage.	|EER − CER|	0
Number needed to treat (NNT)	The number of people that would need to be treated for the event of interest to occur in 1 person.	1 ÷ ARR *or* 1 ÷ (EER − CER)	Infinity. Refer to article by Altman[36] for an explanation about why this is so.
Odds ratio (OR)	The odds of an event in the intervention group divided by the odds of an event in the control group. Usually expressed as a decimal proportion.	[EER/(1 − EER)] ÷ [CER/(1 − CER)]	1

CER = control event rate; EER = experimental event rate.

TABLE 4.1 Summary of dichotomous effect measures

BOX 4.3 HOW TO CALCULATE THE CONFIDENCE INTERVAL (CI) FOR ABSOLUTE RISK REDUCTION

A formula[32] that can be used is:

$$95\% \text{ CI} \approx \text{Difference in risk} \pm 1\sqrt{n_{av}}$$

where n_{av} = average of the group sizes.

For our study of relaxation training, the 95% confidence interval for the absolute risk reduction would be:

$$\approx (30\% - 5\%) \pm 1\sqrt{100}$$
$$\approx 25\% \pm 0.1$$
$$\approx 25\% \pm 10\%$$

This tells us that the best estimate of the absolute risk reduction achieved from the relaxation training is 35% and that the 95% confidence interval extends from 15% to 35%.

When making sense of the results of a randomised controlled trial, one further issue that you should be aware of is that trials usually report results from many different outcomes. With so much information to process it may be helpful, in some cases, for you to focus your attention on the main outcome(s) of the trial, the outcome(s) of interest to the question that you initially formed and/or the outcome that is of interest to your client. If you have got to this point and determined that the article that you have been appraising not only appears to be reasonably free of bias but also contains some clinically important results, you then proceed to look at whether you can apply the results from the study to your client or clinical situation. This is the third and final step of the critical appraisal process that we described in Chapter 1.

How can we use this evidence to inform practice?

If you have decided that the validity of the study that you are appraising is adequate and that the results are clinically important, the final step of the critical appraisal process is to consider the application of this information to the clinical situation that prompted your original clinical question. To do this, there are a few important questions that should be considered:

- Do the results apply to your client or situation?
- Do the benefits found outweigh any harm, costs and/or inconveniences that are involved with the intervention?
- What other factors might need to be considered when applying this evidence?

Do the results apply to your client or situation?

When considering whether the results apply to your client or situation, you essentially need to assess whether your client is so different from the participants in the study that you cannot apply the results of the study that you have been reading to your client or situation. So, rather than just thinking about the study's eligibility criteria with respect to your client, are the differences problematic enough that the results should not be applied? Further to this, results can sometimes be individualised to a particular client by considering the individual benefit and harm for that client. There is some complexity involved in doing so which is beyond the scope of this book. If you wish to learn about this further, you are advised to read the article by Glasziou and Irwig[39] to understand how this may be done.

Do the benefits found outweigh any harm, costs and/or inconveniences that are involved with the intervention?

Understanding whether benefits outweigh harms or costs requires using information about benefits that is given in terms of size of the intervention effect (for example, mean differences, relative risk reduction, number needed to treat) and comparing this against possible harms or even inconveniences. When information about harm and cost is provided in the article, this is relatively straightforward. However, this type of information is often not provided and some estimate of the costs associated with the intervention might need to be made. Information about harm is obviously more difficult to estimate and other sources might need to be consulted to get a sense of the potential harms involved. This is a grey area of practice in which clinical experience and discussion with clients about their preferences and values become very important.

What other factors might need to be considered when applying this evidence?

A further important question to consider is: what other factors might need to be considered when applying this evidence? When you are thinking about what other factors affect the delivery of an intervention, there are a few key questions that you can ask:

• How much does it cost?
• How many sessions might be involved or how long would the client need to stay in hospital?
• How far would the client (or the health professional) need to travel?
• Are the resources (for example, any equipment that is needed) available to deliver the intervention?
• Do you or other health professionals working with you have the skills to provide the intervention?

A central component of applying research evidence to your client is discussing the information with them. The success of many interventions is dependent upon the health professional successfully providing the client with appropriate information.

Involving the client in the decision-making process is important and this is discussed further in Chapter 14. In Chapter 1 we emphasised the need for integrating information from clients, clinical experience, research and the practice context. To do so is the art of evidence-based practice. Integrating so many pieces of information from many different sources is certainly an art form and one that requires clinical reasoning and judgement. The roles of clinical reasoning and judgement are discussed further in Chapter 15.

Clinical scenario (continued): Using the evidence to inform practice

So what can we conclude from our reading of the article about the Stepping On trial? You know as a health professional that falls are a major cause of accidental injury and death in the elderly, that they are costly in terms of loss of function and quality of life at both the individual and community level and that preventing falls is an important issue. In summary, the trial that evaluated the Stepping On program[4] was a well-constructed trial of a multifaceted educational and behavioural intervention for falls prevention. However the trial design was unable to achieve blinding of participants, health professionals or study personnel, which leads you, as the reader, to be a bit cautious of results reported. For example, the falls data were collected by participant self-report which would not only be subject to error but also to differential bias (that is, there could be systematic differences in the self-reports of people in the intervention compared to those in the control group due to their knowledge about which group they were in). Participants in the intervention group received an individual home visit and a 3-month group booster session whereas participants in the control group did not. This makes you wonder what part the attention (that intervention group participants received) might have played in influencing outcomes. The intervention group experienced a 31% reduction in falls with sustained effects at 14 months that we could consider to be clinically significant. Although the mean difference of 4.28 (95% confidence interval = −8.40 to −0.54) on the Mobility Efficacy Scale was statistically significant, you consider its clinical significance to be uncertain. However, participants' outcomes on the Modified Falls Efficacy Scale, which is an outcome that you were particularly interested in, were not statistically significant. As the reader of this article you need to contemplate how the biases present in this study might have affected these results. You then also need to consider how to apply these results in your situation.

Do the results apply to our client or situation? The group of people that we were concerned about were community-living elderly people who had had multiple falls. The study that we have looked at involved community-living men and women aged 70 years and older who had fallen in the previous year or were concerned about falling, but were not housebound and did not have cognitive impairment. It is likely these results do apply to the group of people that we are concerned about; however, we would need to be aware that the results may not be as relevant for people who have cognitive impairment.

Are the benefits worth the harms and costs? There are no real 'harms' associated with this intervention. No details about costs of the intervention are provided in the article, but we do know that the intervention involved a group program (with approximately 12 participants per group) and a total of 15.5 hours of intervention. A very general idea of costs can be determined from this information. For individual clients, the 'cost' to them can be thought about in terms of the time commitment and travel involved in attending seven community-based sessions. Unfortunately data were not provided which enabled a number needed to treat to be calculated which could have been valuable in helping us to interpret whether the benefits are worth the costs.

Other factors to consider: Other practical factors to consider are the availability of this type of comprehensive program in your clinical vicinity or, if you were to run it at the community health centre, the resources (such as staffing and space) and costs that would be involved. Data about the cost-effectiveness of this study would be valuable to further facilitate your team's decision making about whether to implement this intervention or not.

Summary points of this chapter

- The effects of intervention are best determined through rigorous randomised controlled trials (or better still, systematic reviews of randomised controlled trials), as their methods best reduce the risk of bias.
- Most randomised controlled trials are not free from bias. Key questions that should be asked when appraising the risk of bias in a randomised control trial are: How were participants randomised to groups? Was the allocation sequence concealed? Were the groups similar at baseline? Were participants, health professionals and study personnel blind to group allocation? Was follow-up adequate? Was intention-to-treat analysis used?
- Our understanding of the degree of bias that is present in a study is affected not just by the methods that the researchers used, but also by how well these are reported in the article that describes the study.
- Two factors to consider when making sense of the results of a randomised controlled trial are: 1) the size or magnitude of the intervention effect (this may be provided

as continuous data or dichotomous data); and 2) the precision of the intervention effect (which can best be determined by inspecting the confidence interval for the intervention effect).
- Applying the results of the study requires thinking through whether the results apply to your client or situation, whether benefits outweigh any harm, costs or inconveniences and a range of logistical factors that can affect the delivery of the intervention.

References

1. Portney L, Watkins M. Foundations of clinical research: applications to practice. Upper Saddle River, NJ: Prentice Hall Health; 2000.
2. Deeks J, Dinnes J, D'Amico R et al. Evaluating non-randomised intervention studies. Health Technology Assessment Programme 2003; 7:1–186.
3. Allan L, Hays H, Jensen N et al. Randomised crossover trial of transdermal fentanyl and sustained release oral morphine for treating chronic non-cancer pain. BMJ 2001; 322:1154–1158.
4. Clemson L, Cumming R, Kendig H et al. The effectiveness of a community-based program for reducing the incidence of falls in the elderly: a randomised trial. J Am Geriatr Soc 2004; 52: 1487–1494.
5. Guyatt GH, Sackett DL, Cook DJ. Users' guides to the medical literature. II. How to use an article about therapy or prevention. JAMA 1993; 270:2598–2601.
6. Maher C, Sherrington C, Herbert R et al. Reliability of the PEDro scale for rating quality of randomised controlled trials. Phys Ther 2003; 83:713–721.
7. Shulz K, Chalmers I, Hayes RJ et al. Empirical evidence of bias: dimensions of methodological quality associated with estimates of treatment effects in controlled trials. JAMA 1995; 273: 408–412.
8. Kunz R, Vist G, Oxman A. Randomisation to protect against selection bias in healthcare trials. Cochrane Database Syst Rev 2007: 2: Art. No: MR000012. DOI:10.1002/14651858.MR000012. pub2.
9. Altman DG, Bland JM. Treatment allocation in controlled trials: why randomise? BMJ 1999; 318:1209.
10. Hewitt C, Torgerson D. Is restricted randomisation necessary? BMJ 2006; 332:1506–1508.
11. El-Mohandes A, Katz K, El-Khorazaty M et al. The effect of a parenting education program on the use of preventive paediatric health care services among low-income, minority mothers: a randomised, controlled study. Pediatrics 2003; 111:1324–1332.
12. Altman D, Schulz K, Moher D et al. The revised CONSORT statement for reporting randomised trials: explanation and elaboration. Ann Intern Med 2001; 134:663–694.
13. Pildal J, Chan AW, Hróbjartsson A et al. Comparison of descriptions of allocation concealment in trial protocols and the published reports: cohort study. BMJ 2005; 330:1049.
14. Bennett S, McKenna K, McCluskey A et al. Evidence for occupational therapy interventions: status of effectiveness research indexed in the OTseeker database. Br J Occup Ther 2007; 70: 426–430.
15. Roberts C, Torgerson D. Understanding controlled trials: baseline imbalance in randomised controlled trials. BMJ 1999; 319:185.
16. Herbert R, Jamtvedt G, Mead J et al. Practical evidence-based physiotherapy. Edinburgh: Elsevier; 2005.
17. Dumville J, Torgerson D, Hewitt CE. Reporting attrition in randomised controlled trials. BMJ 2006; 332:969–971.
18. Higgins J, Altman D, eds. Assessing risk of bias in included studies. In: Higgins J, Green S, eds. Cochrane Handbook for Systematic Reviews of Interventions Version 5.0.0 (updated February 2008). The Cochrane Collaboration, 2008. Available: http://www.cochrane-handbook.org (12 Nov 2008).
19. Hollis S, Campbell F. What is meant by intention to treat analysis? Survey of published randomised controlled trials. BMJ 1999; 319:670–674.
20. Ottenbacher K, Maas F. How to detect effects: statistical power and evidence-based practice in occupational therapy research. Am J Occup Ther 1999; 53(2):181–188.
21. Moher D, Schulz KF, Altman DG. The CONSORT statement: revised recommendations for improving the quality of reports of parallel-group randomised trials. Lancet 2001; 357:1191–1194.

22. Heuts P, de Bie R, Drietelaar M et al. Self-management in osteoarthritis of hip or knee: a randomised clinical trial in a primary healthcare setting. J Rheumatol 2005; 32:543–549.
23. Cohen J. Statistical power analysis for the behavioural sciences. 2nd edn Hillsdale, NJ: Lawrence Erlbaum; 1988.
24. Norman G, Sloan J, Wyrwich K. Interpretation of changes in health-related quality of life: the remarkable universality of half a standard deviation. Med Care 2003; 41:582–592.
25. Guyatt G. Making sense of quality-of-life data. Med Care 2000; 39(II): 175–179.
26. Herbert R. How to estimate treatment effects from reports of clinical trials. I: continuous outcomes. Aust J Physiother 2000; 46:229–235.
27. Altman D, Bland J. Absence of evidence is not evidence of absence. BMJ 1995; 311:485.
28. Lahdensuo A, Haahtela T, Herrala J et al. Randomised comparison of guided self-management and traditional treatment of asthma over one year. BMJ 1996; 312:748–752.
29. Guyatt G, Sackett D, Cook D. User's guide to the medical literature: II. How to use an article about therapy or prevention: B. what were the results and will they help me in caring for my patients? JAMA 1994; 271:59–63.
30. Cook R, Sackett D. The number needed to treat: a clinically useful measure of treatment effect. BMJ 1995; 310:452–454.
31. Sackett D, Richardson WS, Rosenberg W et al. Evidence-based medicine. How to practice and teach EBM. New York: Churchill Livingstone; 1997.
32. Herbert R. How to estimate treatment effects from reports of clinical trials. II: Dichotomous outcomes. Aust J Physiother 2000; 46:309–313.
33. Centre for Evidence-Based Medicine. Glossary. Online. 2008. Available: http://www.cebm.net/index.aspx?o=1116 (28 Aug 2008).
34. Laupacis A, Sackett DL, Roberts RS. An assessment of clinically useful measures of the consequences of treatment. N Engl J Med 1988; 318:1728–1733.
35. Straus S, Sackett D. Applying evidence to the individual patient. Ann Oncol 1999; 10:29–32.
36. Altman D. Confidence intervals for the number needed to treat. BMJ 1998; 317:1309–1312.
37. Cumming R. Intervention strategies and risk-factor modification for falls prevention: a review of recent intervention studies. Clin Geriatr Med 2002; 18:175–189.
38. Campbell A, Robertson M, Gardner M et al. Falls prevention over 2 years: a randomised controlled trial in women 80 years and older. Age Ageing 1999; 28:513–518.
39. Glasziou P, Irwig L. An evidence based approach to individualising treatment. BMJ 1995; 311:1356–1359.

CHAPTER 5

Questions about the effects of interventions: examples of appraisals from different health professions

Tammy Hoffmann, John W Bennett, Mark R Elkins, Craig Lockwood, Angela Morgan, Sharon Sanders, Alan Spencer, Luis Vitetta and Caroline Wright

This chapter is an accompaniment to the previous chapter (Chapter 4) in which you learnt how to critically appraise evidence about the effects of interventions. In order to further illustrate the key points from Chapter 4, this chapter contains a number of worked examples of questions about the effects of interventions. As we mentioned in the preface of the book, we believe that it can be easier to learn the process of critical appraisal when you see some worked examples of how it is done, and it is even better when the examples are from your own health profession. Therefore, this chapter (and Chapters 7, 9 and 11) contains examples from a range of health professions. Some of the clinical examples are relevant to more than one health profession. Each example is formatted in a similar manner and contains the following elements:
- a clinical scenario that explains the origins of the clinical question
- the clinical question
- the search terms and databases used to find evidence to answer the clinical question
- a brief description of the article chosen and the reason for its selection
- a structured abstract of the chosen article
- an appraisal of the risk of bias of the evidence
- a summary of the main results of the article that are relevant to the clinical question
- a brief discussion about how the evidence can be used to inform practice.

You will notice that in most of the examples the type of article that has been chosen to be appraised is a randomised controlled trial. You may wonder why this is the case when Chapters 2 and 4 explained that systematic reviews of randomised controlled trials should be the first choice of study design to answer questions about the effects of intervention. There is a good reason behind this. The authors of the examples that are contained in this chapter were asked to not choose (or indeed, specifically search for) systematic reviews if they were available to answer their question. Why? Because it is easier to learn how to appraise a systematic review of randomised controlled trials if you have first learnt how to appraise a randomised controlled trial. This chapter and Chapter 4 are designed to help you learn how to appraise a randomised controlled trial. Once you know how to do this, Chapter 12 will help you to learn how to appraise a systematic review. As you read through these examples, keep in mind that because the suggestions that the authors of these worked examples have provided in the 'how might we use this evidence to inform practice' section have been drawn from only one individual study, in reality, additional studies would need to be located and appraised prior to drawing clear conclusions about what should be done in clinical practice.

When appraising an article, you need to obtain and carefully read the full text of the article. We have not included the full text of the articles that are appraised in the example. However, for each of the examples in this chapter (and Chapters 7, 9 and 11), the authors of the examples have prepared a structured abstract that summarises the article. This has been done so that you have some basic information about each article. As we mentioned in Chapter 1, the more you practise doing the steps of evidence-based practice, the easier it will become. This is particularly true of the critical appraisal step. You may find it useful if you approach these worked examples as a self-assessment activity and try and obtain a copy of the article that is appraised in each of the examples (or just the ones that are relevant to your health profession if you feel more comfortable with that). You can then critically appraise the articles for yourself and check your answers with those that are presented in the worked examples.

One other thing to note about the examples in this chapter (and Chapters 7, 9 and 11) is that the appraisal of articles is not an exact science and sometimes there are no definite right or wrong answers. As with evidence-based practice in general, the health professional's clinical experience has an important role to play, particularly in deciding about issues such as baseline similarity (as we saw in Chapter 4) and clinical significance (as we saw in Chapters 2 and 4). Some of the examples may contain statements that you do not completely agree with and that you, as a health professional, would interpret a little differently. Also, the examples are provided to give you an overall sense of the general process of evidence-based practice. The content that is presented in the examples is not exhaustive (particularly in the 'how do we use this evidence to inform practice' section) and there may be other factors or issues that you, as a health professional, would suggest or consider if you were in that situation. That is OK.

Occupational therapy example

Clinical scenario

You are an occupational therapist who works in a recently opened community adult health centre. In the last few weeks, you have received referrals for a number of clients who have been diagnosed with rheumatoid arthritis in the last one or two years. Most of these clients are female and middle-aged and their arthritis is causing them considerable pain (particularly in the hand) and affecting their ability to perform self-care activities. You are considering running an education group about joint protection techniques and wonder if this will be effective in reducing your clients' pain and improving their function.

Clinical question
In adults with rheumatoid arthritis, is education about joint protection techniques effective in reducing hand pain and improving function?

Search terms and databases used to find the evidence
Database: OTseeker
Search terms: 'rheumatoid arthritis' AND 'joint protection'
   This search retrieved nine results. Only two of these articles specifically evaluated the effectiveness of a joint protection program, with the remainder evaluating the effectiveness of general patient education programs for people with arthritis. The two most relevant articles were both based on the same study, with one describing the 6- and 12-month results, and the other reporting the long-term (4-year) effects of the intervention. You initially choose to appraise the earlier article (the 12-month results) and, if the quality and results of this article are promising, you will then also look at the article that reports the long-term results.

Article chosen
Hammond A, Freeman K. One-year outcomes of a randomised controlled trial of an educational–behavioural joint protection programme for people with rheumatoid arthritis. Rheumatology 2001; 40:1044–1051.

Structured abstract
Study design: Randomised controlled trial.

Setting: Outpatients from the occupational therapy departments of two hospitals in the UK.

Participants: 127 patients with rheumatoid arthritis; aged between 18 and 65 years (mean age 50.5 years, 76% female); diagnosed with rheumatoid arthritis within the last 5 years, a history of wrist or metacarpophalangeal joint pain and inflammation, and experiencing hand pain during activity. Exclusion criteria included no other medical condition that affected hand function.

Intervention: Two small-group education interventions, both of 8 hours duration, were compared. One group attended a standard arthritis education program, which included 2.5 hours of joint protection education. Approximately 15–45 minutes was spent practising joint protection techniques. The other group attended a joint protection education program that used educational–behavioural teaching methods and aimed to enhance self-efficacy and motor learning. Participants in this program spent about two-thirds of their time practising and receiving feedback about hand joint protection methods.

   Outcomes: Primary measures: hand pain experienced during a moderate activity (such as cooking or housework) within the last week (measured using a 100mm visual analogue scale); adherence with joint protection. Secondary measures: functional status (measured using the Arthritis Impact Measurement Scales [AIMS2] with a range of 0–10 where 0 indicated better function), indicators of disease severity, hand status and psychological status.

Follow-up period: 12 months. Assessments were performed at baseline, 6 months and 12 months.

Main results: Compared to participants in the standard group, participants in the joint protection group demonstrated significant improvements in terms of adherence to joint protection, hand pain, general pain, early morning stiffness, self-reported number of disease flare-ups, visits to the doctor for arthritis and the AIMS2 activities of daily living (ADL) scale. Both groups experienced an increase in hand deformity scores.

Conclusion: Among those who attended the joint protection program, significant improvements were found in adherence, pain, disease status and functional ability. It is suggested that joint protection can help to slow the progression of the effects of rheumatoid arthritis, over and above the effects of drug therapy, as the benefits became more apparent with time.

Is the evidence likely to be biased?

- *Was the assignment of participants to groups randomised?*
  Yes. Participants were randomly allocated, using a four-block sequence.
- *Was the allocation sequence concealed?*
  Yes. Allocation occurred using sealed envelopes that had been prepared in advance.
- *Were the groups similar at the baseline or start of the trial?*
  Yes. The baseline characteristics were similar between the two study groups. There is a small difference between the two groups in terms of steroid use (6% of participants in the standard group and 20% of participants in the joint protection group) but this difference is probably not large enough to have affected the results. The baseline scores of the outcome measures were also similar between the two groups.
- *Were participants blind to which study group they were in?*
  No. For this trial, it was not possible for participants to be blinded to group allocation.
- *Were the health professionals who provided the intervention blind to participants' study group?*

No. For this trial, it was not possible for the health professionals who provided the intervention to be blinded to group allocation.

- *Were the assessors blind to participants' study group?*
  Yes, some for measures. Baseline, 6- and 12-month assessments were conducted by an independent assessor who was not informed of group allocation. The assessor was also asked to avoid discussing the education programs with the participants. However, for the outcomes that were measured by participant self-report, the assessment of these outcomes was not blind as participants were not blinded to group allocation.
- *Were all participants who entered the trial properly accounted for at its conclusion and how complete was follow-up?*
  Yes. The follow-up rate was 95.3% at 6 months and 96.8% at 12 months. Reasons are given as to why some participants were not able to be followed up, as well as which group they were in.
- *Was intention-to-treat analysis used?*
  Cannot tell. The authors do not explicitly state that an intention-to-treat analysis was conducted. Therefore, we cannot tell if this was done and so the results could be subject to bias because of this.
- *Did the study have enough participants to minimise the play of chance?*
  Yes. Based on data from a previous study, the authors conducted a power analysis and determined that, with a power of 80% and a significance level of 0.05, 63 participants would be needed in each group.

What are the main results?

For hand pain at 12 months, the effect size is 12.98, which is a statistically significant result. Both the *p*-value (0.02) and confidence interval (CI), which does not include the no effect value of zero, show this. As hand pain was measured using a 100mm visual analogue scale, an effect size (between groups) of 13 is probably large enough to also be considered clinically significant. However, the confidence interval is very wide indicating some imprecision in the result. Thus, for some people the intervention effect may not be large enough to be considered clinically significant, whereas for other people the effect could be quite large and deemed clinically significant.

With respect to function, the ADL subscale of the AIMS2 was used to measure participants' ability to perform self-care and household activities. The effect size for the ADL subscale at 12 months was 0.8, which is statistically significant (confirmed by both the *p*-value and the confidence interval). However, as the AIMS2 is scored on a scale of 0–10, an effect size of 0.8 is small and may not be considered by many to be a clinically significant result. However, if

Outcomes of the clinical question	Mean of joint protection group	Mean of standard group	Difference in mean	95% Confidence interval[a]	P-value
Hand pain at 12 months	33.63	46.61	12.98	1.98 to 23.98	0.02
AIMS2 ADL subscale at 12 months	1.33	2.13	0.8	0.03 to 1.57	0.04

[a]Not provided by authors—calculated using data provided in the article. Confidence intervals may vary slightly depending on the formula used and the extent of the rounding.
AIMS2 = Arthritis Impact Measurement Scales; ADL = activities of daily living.

TABLE 5.1 Hand pain and functional outcome for intervention and control groups at 12 months

we consider that the upper end of the confidence interval is 1.57, it is possible that the effect of this intervention could be clinically significant for some people. As explained in Chapter 4, the decision about clinical significance is a subjective one and depends on a number of factors such as the costs involved and preferences of the individual concerned.

How might we use this evidence to inform practice?

As you are reasonably confident about the validity of the study's results and some of the results were of clinical importance, you proceed to assessing the applicability of this evidence to your clinical scenario. The clients with rheumatoid arthritis that you see are similar to the study participants in a number of ways such as age, gender (predominantly female) and disease duration. The majority of the participants in the study were assessed as having mild or moderate rheumatoid arthritis. You have yet to assess the disease severity in your recently referred clients. Once you do, you will check if their disease severity is comparable to the study participants' before making a decision about whether to implement a joint protection program.

Before making the decision, you will also need to consider whether you and the health centre where you work have the resources available to offer a joint protection program such as the one that was evaluated in the study. You will also need to obtain further, more detailed, information about the content of the program and the teaching strategies that were used. The article mentions that further details may be obtained in another published article, so you will start by obtaining that article and, if you have questions after reading that, you will contact the authors of the article for more information.

Although the study found a statistically and clinically significant effect of the intervention on hand pain, the effect on the other outcome (self-care) that you were particularly interested in may not be conclusively clinically significant. Although it is unlikely that the program would cause any harm and it appears to offer some benefits to participants, there are considerable staffing resources associated with providing the program. You decide to obtain the full text of the article that reports the long-term effects of the joint protection program before making a decision about whether to implement the program at your workplace.

Physiotherapy example

Clinical scenario

As a physiotherapist on the cardiac surgery ward, you attend a conference and hear that some of your peers at another hospital are providing inspiratory muscle training to clients who are undergoing coronary artery bypass graft (CABG) surgery. The training is performed preoperatively in an attempt to reduce the likelihood of pulmonary complications occurring postoperatively. You are unaware of any research that has investigated the use of this intervention in clients undergoing cardiac surgery and decide to search for evidence to decide whether this is something you should institute at the hospital where you work.

Clinical question

Does preoperative inspiratory muscle training in addition to standard care prevent postoperative pulmonary complications in clients who are undergoing CABG surgery?

Search terms and databases used to find the evidence

Database: PEDro (using the 'Advanced Search' option)

Search terms: You decide that *inspiratory muscle training* is likely to be mentioned in the title of the article, although it may be described as *respiratory muscle training*. You therefore enter **spiratory muscle training* in the 'Title' field. You consider that the patient population might be broadly defined in the title using a phrase like *cardiac surgery*, but you expect that it would be defined using *coronary artery bypass graft* or *coronary artery bypass surgery* in the abstract. Therefore you enter *coronary artery bypass* in the 'Abstract & Title' field. You want both of these terms to be present, so you select the option to 'Match all search terms' when searching.

The search returns six records, but this represents only two separate trials as each of these trials had related publications that were retrieved by the search. For the first trial by Hulzebos et al, there is the main publication which is accompanied by a report of pilot data, an English translation of the primary Dutch publication and an analysis of the feasibility of the intervention using data from the trial. For the second trial, there is the main publication and a Hebrew to English translation. Although both trials examine inspiratory muscle training for clients who are undergoing CABG surgery, several features of the main publication of the first trial show that it probably provides less-biased evidence to answer your question. Unlike the second trial, it used concealed allocation, blinded outcome assessment and intention-to-treat analysis, and fewer participants were lost to follow-up. In addition, the sample size of the trial was larger (N = 279 vs 84) and the trial was conducted more recently, so the surgical procedure and standard care in the postoperative period are more consistent with that offered at your hospital. Therefore you decide on the first article.

Article chosen

Hulzebos E, Helders P, Favie N et al. Preoperative intensive inspiratory muscle training to prevent postoperative pulmonary complications in high-risk patients undergoing CABG surgery: a randomised clinical trial. JAMA 2006; 296:1851–1857.

Structured abstract

Study design: Randomised controlled trial.

Setting: University medical centre in Utrecht, the Netherlands.

Participants: 279 clients (mean age 66.9 years; 77.9% male) undergoing CABG surgery at high risk of developing postoperative pulmonary complications, indicated by the presence of two or more of these criteria: age >70 years, productive cough, diabetes mellitus, smoking, chronic obstructive pulmonary disease and body mass index >27. Exclusion criteria included: surgery within 2 weeks of initial contact; a history of stroke; use of immunosuppressive medication for 30 days before surgery; and presence of a neuromuscular disorder, cardiovascular instability or an aneurysm.

Intervention: Participants were randomly assigned to receive either preoperative inspiratory muscle training (n = 140) or usual care (n = 139). The intervention group trained daily (20 minutes), seven times a week (six times without supervision), for at least 2 weeks before the surgery. Both groups received the same postoperative physical therapy and other standard care.

Outcomes: Primary outcome: the incidence of postoperative pulmonary complications, defined according to recognised criteria. Secondary outcome: duration of postoperative hospitalisation, in days.

Main results: Postoperative pulmonary complications occurred in 25 (18%) of the participants in the intervention group and 48 (35%) of the control group, odds ratio 0.52

(95% CI 0.30 to 0.92). Median duration of hospitalisation was 7 days (range 5–41) in the intervention group and 8 days (range 6–70) in the control group ($p = 0.02$).

Conclusion: Preoperative inspiratory muscle training reduced the incidence of pulmonary complications and the duration of postoperative hospitalisation in clients who were at high risk of developing a pulmonary complication after CABG surgery.

Is the evidence likely to be biased?

- *Was the assignment of participants to groups randomised?*
  Yes, participants were appropriately randomised, with a computer-generated number list.
- *Was the allocation sequence concealed?*
  Yes, the number list was sealed in envelopes which were held by an external investigator.
- *Were the groups similar at the baseline or start of the trial?*
  Yes, the baseline characteristics were similar between the two study groups. Although in the table of baseline characteristics the authors of the article have reported a difference between the two groups in terms of median duration of mechanical ventilation (4h in the intervention group vs 5h in the control group), this is technically not a baseline characteristic as it was measured after the intervention had been provided. Additionally, it is unlikely that a difference of this size would be of clinical importance and have affected the results.
- *Were participants blind to which study group they were in?*
  No. For this trial, it was not possible for participants to be blinded to group allocation.
- *Were the health professionals who provided the intervention blind to participants' study group?*
  No. For this trial, it was not possible for the therapists who provided the intervention to be blinded to group allocation.
- *Were the assessors blind to participants' study group?*
  Yes. The investigators who assessed outcomes were blinded to participants' treatment group.
- *Were all participants who entered the trial properly accounted for at its conclusion and how complete was follow-up?*
  Yes. Apart from three participants who died before surgery, all participants were followed up. This is a 98.9% follow-up rate.
- *Was intention-to-treat analysis used?*
  Yes, it is stated that an intention-to-treat analysis was conducted.
- *Did the study have enough participants to minimise the play of chance?*
  Yes. A power calculation was performed but the trial was terminated before this number was reached because safety monitoring determined that statistically and clinically significant results had been achieved at the interim analysis.

What are the main results?

Pulmonary complication: The risk of pulmonary complications is presented appropriately, using an odds ratio with a 95% confidence interval (refer to Table 5.2). The reduction in risk is both statistically and clinically significant. The 95% confidence interval includes only clinically worthwhile reductions in risk. Therefore, the results are sufficiently precise to make clinical recommendations.

This data for the first outcome, pulmonary complications, can be used to estimate two useful statistics. First, let us calculate the absolute risk reduction (ARR), which is simply the risk in the control group minus the risk in the intervention group: 35% − 18% = 17%. Using the formula (95% confidence interval $\approx$ difference in risk $\pm 1\sqrt{n_{av}}$) that was

Outcome	Intervention group	Control group	Odds ratio	95% CI
Pulmonary complications	25 /139 (18%)	48 /137 (35%)	0.52	0.30 to 0.92

TABLE 5.2 Frequency of pulmonary complications in both groups

provided in Box 4.3 in Chapter 4, you also calculate the 95% confidence interval of the ARR to be 9% to 25%. The ARR statistic is useful in clinical practice because, if you decide to implement the intervention, you can use it to explain to clients the value that they can expect from undertaking the inspiratory muscle training regimen. After explaining what a pulmonary complication is and how it can delay recovery, many clients would consider the training program worthwhile to reduce their risk of such a complication from 35% to 18%.

An alternative statistic is the relative risk reduction (RRR). This is calculated by dividing the difference in risk between the two treatment groups, by the risk in the control group:

$$RRR = (\text{Control group risk} - \text{Treatment group risk}) \div \text{Control group risk}$$
$$= (35\% - 18\%) \div 35\% = 49\%$$

When an adverse outcome occurs fairly frequently in a study, the RRR is a useful statistic, but when the outcome is rare, a large RRR may still be found even though the ARR is very small, which can be misleading. Therefore you decide to use ARR instead of RRR.

You then use the absolute risk reduction to calculate the number of people that need to be treated in order to prevent one pulmonary complication.

$$\text{Number neeeded to treat} = 1 \div \text{absolute risk reduction}$$
$$= 1/17\%$$
$$= 5.88$$

The 95% confidence interval of this number needed to treat is 4 to 12. This was calculated by using the inverse of the numbers in the confidence interval of the absolute risk reduction that you calculated earlier (so 1/25 and 1/9). Therefore, for every six high-risk clients that we treat, one pulmonary complication will be prevented that would have otherwise occurred with usual care. However, this number needed to treat could be as low as four or as high as 12.

Duration of hospitalisation: The median duration of postoperative hospitalisation was 7 days (range 5 to 41) in the treatment group and 8 days (range 6 to 70) in the control group, and this difference was statistically significant.

How might we use this evidence to inform practice?

You decide that the trial is valid and that the results are important. Pulmonary complications are dangerous and uncomfortable for the client and they are expensive to treat. Therefore, the effect of this intervention on this outcome alone is clinically worthwhile, and the number needed to treat of six is useful in justifying the introduction of the service. Further justification of the clinical worth of this intervention comes from the other significant outcome, which was a reduction in the duration of hospitalisation. You plan to discuss the results of this study with your head of department as there are resource implications associated with introducing the service, particularly providing an intervention of the same intensity as was provided in the study. However, it is your recommendation that this intervention should be introduced.

Podiatry example

Clinical scenario

You are a podiatrist who works in a private practice. In recent days, you have seen several clients with heel pain which you believe is plantar fasciitis. Your management of this condition usually involves prescribing an orthotic device, which is made in an orthotic laboratory from a cast of the client's foot. Because it takes several weeks for the orthotics to be made, you wonder whether prefabricated orthotics which can be bought over the counter and started immediately are as effective. You decide to search for the evidence.

Clinical question

In clients with plantar fasciitis, are prefabricated orthotic devices as effective as orthotic devices made from a cast of the client's foot and using measurements specific to the client in reducing pain and improving function?

Search terms and databases used to find the evidence

Database: The Cochrane Database of Systematic Reviews, the Database of Abstracts of Reviews of Effects (DARE) and the Cochrane Central Register of Controlled Trials (CENTRAL) in The Cochrane Library. A systematic review of randomised controlled trials or a randomised controlled trial would be the ideal study design to answer this question. Ideally the randomised controlled trial would have 3 arms, allowing comparison of the two types of orthotic devices with each other and a control group.

Search terms: You start by checking for MeSH terms related to the population and intervention of interest and combine these with textword terms using the Boolean operator OR in the 'Search History' and 'Advanced Search' features of The Cochrane Library.

(Fasciitis, plantar (MeSH) OR (heel OR calcan* NEAR spur) OR (plantar OR heel OR calcan* NEAR pain) OR plantar fasciitis) AND (orthotic devices (MeSH) OR orthotic OR orthoses)

This search produced 23 hits, including 4 Cochrane Reviews, 18 trials and 1 economic evaluation. One of the Cochrane Reviews titled 'Interventions for the treatment of plantar heel pain' looks like it may address your question. Reading through the review you find it included only one trial evaluating the impact of orthoses and that this trial compared orthoses with stretching exercises. You also notice that the search for studies was only conducted up to 2002. You go back to your search to see if there are any trials published subsequent to the review that may answer your question. After looking over the titles and abstracts of the trials you are drawn to two articles that compare the effectiveness of different types of orthotic devices. They are both randomised trials conducted in patients with a diagnosis of plantar fasciitis. You select the trial titled 'Effectiveness of foot orthoses to treat plantar fasciitis' to read as it had a longer follow-up (12 months instead of 2 months) and looks at the effect of orthotic devices on both pain and function.

Article chosen

Landorf KB, Keenan A, Herbert RD. Effectiveness of foot orthoses to treat plantar fasciitis. Arch Intern Med 2006; 166:1305–1310.

Structured abstract

Study design: Randomised controlled trial.

Setting: A university podiatry clinic, Melbourne, Australia.

Participants: 136 participants, mean age 48 years, 67% female, with a clinical diagnosis of plantar fasciitis who had experienced symptoms for at least 4 weeks. People with a major orthopaedic or medical condition that may have influenced the condition were excluded.

Intervention: Participants were randomised to receive either: a) 'sham' orthoses which were made of soft foam moulded over an unmodified cast of the foot; b) prefabricated orthoses made from a thicker, firmer density foam moulded over the cast; or c) customised foot orthoses made from semi-rigid polpropylene moulded over neutral position plaster casts with a firm foam heel post.

Outcomes: The primary outcome of the trial was self-reported pain and function at 3 and 12 months, which were measured using the pain and function domains of the Foot Health Status Questionnaire (0–100 measurement scale).

Follow-up period: 12 months.

Main results: This trial found that pain and function improved in all 3 groups over time. Participants receiving prefabricated and customised orthoses showed greater improvement in function than the sham group at 3 months (mean difference of 8.4 points on the function domain between prefabricated and sham orthoses and a mean difference of 7.5 points between customised and sham orthoses). Prefabricated and customised orthoses also reduced pain compared with sham orthoses at 3 months (8.7 points and 7.4 points, respectively), though these differences were not statistically significant. At 12 months, there were no significant differences in pain and function between any of the 3 groups.

Conclusion: Both prefabricated and customised orthoses have similar small short-term benefits for people with plantar fasciitis and negligible long-term effects.

Is the evidence likely to be biased?

- *Was the assignment of participants to groups randomised?*
  Yes. The randomisation sequence was generated using an appropriate method (computer-generated randomisation sequence).
- *Was the allocation sequence concealed?*
  Yes. The allocation was concealed from participants and the investigator enrolling participants in the trial. The allocation sequence appears to be held off-site and, once a participant was enrolled and baseline assessments were completed, the allocation sequence was obtained by telephone or email.
- *Were the groups similar at the baseline or start of the trial?*
  Table 1 in the article shows that study groups were balanced in terms of most of the baseline variables that were measured. One important exception is participant's weight, where the mean weight of participants in the prefabricated orthoses group was approximately 10kg more than the other two study groups. This is a clinically important difference that may influence the outcome. You notice that the results are not adjusted for this difference and keep this in mind. You also notice a considerable difference between the sham and prefabricated groups in the foot function score at baseline, but are satisfied that this has been adjusted for in the analysis.
- *Were participants blind to which study group they were in?*

Cannot tell. Although the article states that it was a 'participant blinded' trial, you cannot tell this for sure. The investigators attempted to 'blind' participants to the orthoses they received by making the devices as similar as possible in terms of colour and shape. Participants were told they would receive soft, medium or hard orthoses. All participants had a cast of the foot taken. However, because the material used for the three devices was different (foam, polyethylene, polypropylene), some participants may have been able to work out which device they had received. Because some participants may not have been blind to which study group they were in and because the study outcomes were measured by participant self-report, you cannot be sure that any treatment effect (or lack of effect) that is reported in this study is not biased. Evaluation of the success of participant blinding was not reported.

- *Were the health professionals who provided the intervention blind to participants' study group?*
  No. Due to the nature of the intervention, the podiatrist who assessed the participants and provided them with their orthoses was not blind to the intervention allocation.
- *Were the assessors blind to participants' study group?*
  Cannot tell. For the same reason that participants may not have been blind to study group allocation, the investigators who were in contact with participants during outcome measurement may also have not been blinded to study group allocation. To prevent study investigators from biasing measures of outcome (and potentially influencing participants' responses), participants completed the Foot Health Status Questionnaire at the beginning of each appointment before they had any interaction with the investigator. However, as the Foot Health Status Questionnaire is a self-report outcome, if participants are not blind to their allocation then the assessment cannot be considered blind either.
- *Were all participants who entered the trial properly accounted for at its conclusion and how complete was follow-up?*
  Yes. The flow of participants through this study is clearly reported in a flow diagram. Five of the 136 participants (4%) were lost to follow-up, three from the sham orthoses group (though one of these withdrew before any baseline measures were conducted or treatment was received) and one each from the prefabricated and customised orthoses groups. The article also reports the number of participants who crossed over to alternative orthoses. This was highest in the sham orthoses group, with two of the 44 participants using alternative orthoses at 3 months and seven (of the 43) at 12 months.
- *Was intention-to-treat analysis used?*
  Yes. The article states that an intention-to-treat analysis was conducted.
- *Did the study have enough participants to minimise the play of chance?*
  Yes. The authors report conducting a power calculation prior to commencing participant recruitment. They determined the number of participants required based on the significance level (risk of type 1 error 5%), statistical power (90%) and an estimated difference in effect between any of the study groups. According to the power calculation, 136 participants were required, which is how many were randomised.

What are the results?

As you are interested in the comparison between prefabricated orthoses and orthoses made from a plaster cast and measurements specific to the client, you look for these results first. The results are presented in the article as the mean difference (and 95% confidence intervals) in pain and function scores between the groups at 3 and 12 months (adjusted for baseline scores). See Table 5.3 for a summary of these results.

Outcome	Mean difference (95% cI) in scores between prefabricated and customised orthoses (adjusted for baseline score)
Pain 3 months 12 months	1.3 (−7.6 to 10.2) 2.3 (−5.6 to 10.1)
Function 3 months 12 months	0.9 (−6.3 to 8.1) 1.2 (−6.1 to 8.5)

TABLE 5.3 Effect of intervention on pain and foot function

Pain: At 3 months, the mean difference in pain between prefabricated and customised orthoses was 1.3 (95% CI −7.6 to 10.2) points on the Foot Health Status Questionnaire pain domain and, at 12 months, it was 2.3 points (95% CI −5.6 to 10.1).

Function: On the function domain, the mean difference between prefabricated and customised orthoses at 3 months was 0.9 points (95% CI −6.3 to 8.1) and, at 12 months, it was 1.2 points (95% CI −6.1 to 8.5).

None of these results are statistically significant (as seen by the confidence intervals which all contain the no effect value of zero). You therefore do not need to consider the clinical significance of these results. The results show that the effects of prefabricated and customised orthoses on pain and function are similar.

The study also presents the effects on foot function as a number needed to treat by dichotomising the data. In the dichotomisation, an improvement in function was considered to have occurred when function increased by more than one-third of the baseline value. The prefabricated foot orthoses produced one additional improved outcome for every six people treated for 3 months and the customised foot orthoses produced one additional beneficial outcome for every four people treated for 3 months.

Other results show that pain and function improved in all study groups over time and that, at 12 months, differences in pain and function between all the groups were small and not statistically significant. However, at 3 months, the prefabricated and customised orthoses group showed greater improvement in pain and function than the sham group. The mean difference in function was statistically significant—a difference of 8.4 (95% CI 1.0 to 15.8) points for prefabricated orthoses vs sham orthoses and a difference of 7.5 (95% CI 0.3 to 14.7) points for customised orthoses vs sham orthoses. Although the authors do not provide any guidance about the amount of difference on the 0–100 scale that would be needed for this to be considered a clinically significant difference, the upper ends of the confidence intervals indicate that these intervention effects may be considered clinically significant to some people depending on their preferences. However, the lower ends of the confidence intervals suggest that it is also possible that some people may not find much benefit from this intervention.

How might we use this evidence to inform practice?

You decide that the trial is valid and that the results are important. Given the similarity in effects of the prefabricated and customised orthoses, it would be reasonable to prescribe a prefabricated device rather than a custom made device for your clients with plantar fasciitis. A major benefit you see in this approach is that the client can start the treatment almost straight away, as opposed to the several weeks it takes for customised devices to be manufactured. However, you think there are other factors to consider. Firstly, several of your clients have had symptoms for only a few weeks. You wonder if they would respond the same way as participants in the trial where the condition was more chronic (symptoms were experienced for a median of 12 months). You also wonder how the results might vary if you use different prefabricated orthoses or customised orthoses manufacturers to those that were used in the study.

The prefabricated orthoses used in the study are easily obtained for a cost of around AUD60. This is considerably cheaper than customised orthoses which can cost anywhere from AUD250 to AUD400. However, prefabricated devices do not last as long as customised devices which are usually made from more durable polypropylene, and may need to be replaced a number of times depending on wear. If, as the results of this study suggest, most people recover from plantar fasciitis by 1 year, then two or three pairs of prefabricated devices over a 12-month period would still be cheaper than customised devices. You know from experience, though, that once people start to wear orthoses they tend to continue long-term and, if this is the case, customised orthoses which last for several years may be more economical. Your experience also tells you that often clients also need to purchase footwear that can accommodate orthotic devices. This, together with the cost of the actual orthoses, can be an issue for some clients. You decide that it is important to discuss the results of this study with your clients, working with them to determine the best management option for their situation.

Speech pathology

Clinical scenario

You are a speech pathologist working in a children's hospital. Ben, a 10-year-old boy, was admitted to hospital with severe traumatic brain injury following a horse-riding accident. He was intubated and ventilated at hospital admission due to difficulty breathing. Two weeks after admission Ben was in a medically stable condition and had been weaned from the ventilator and extubated. He could understand basic commands and speak in two- to three-word phrases at this time, but had severe dysarthria due to persistent breathing difficulties and poor breath support for speech. At two months post-injury Ben was speaking in full sentences, but the dysarthric impairment was persistent. You have previously used an eclectic range of traditional behavioural approaches to treat this form of dysarthria (e.g. using a manometer tube and breathing tasks alongside speech drills). However, you recall hearing about instrumental biofeedback options for dysarthria at a recent conference. You remember that the biofeedback equipment sounded expensive, but wonder whether you should make a case to your manager for buying this equipment to pursue a biofeedback approach for Ben.

Clinical question
Are instrumental biofeedback treatment approaches more effective than traditional behavioural treatment approaches at improving dysarthria associated with underlying respiratory support issues in children?

Search terms and databases used to find the evidence

Database: Medline and CINAHL

Search terms: (dysarthria OR speech) AND (respiration OR breathing) AND ((brain injur* OR (traumatic brain injur*) OR (trauma) OR (acquired brain injur*) AND (child* OR p?ediatric) AND (treatment or intervention)

Only one relevant article was generated by these search terms. You reviewed the title and abstract of the article and determined that the article was appropriate for the clinical question. While the article is a single case study and is classified low on the evidence hierarchy, at the time of searching it was the only article available that was relevant to the clinical question.

Article chosen

Murdoch B, Pitt G, Theodoros D et al. Real-time continuous visual biofeedback in the treatment of speech breathing disorders following childhood traumatic brain injury: report of one case. Paediatr Rehabil 1999; 3:5–20.

Structured abstract

Study design: Quasi-experimental single-case ABAB study design.

Study question: What is the efficacy of traditional (B1) versus instrumental biofeedback (B2) therapy for dysarthria associated with poor respiratory support for speech?

Participant and selection: The study participant was a 12-year-old male who had sustained left parietal lobe damage due to a motor vehicle accident as a cyclist, two and a half years prior to the study commencement. The participant had a chronic mixed spastic-ataxic-flaccid dysarthria with severely impaired respiratory function being the predominant impairment. Inclusion and exclusion criteria were specified.

Assessment: The participant underwent a comprehensive battery of both instrumental and traditional behavioural assessments at baseline (A1), during a 10-week withdrawal phase between treatments (A2) and at the end of the second treatment period (A3). Further monitoring assessments were also conducted at several time points during both B1 and B2. Outcome measures included multiple physiological instrumental measures and perceptual measures across all levels of the speech sub-system (that is, respiration, laryngeal, velopharyngeal and articulatory). All were clinician-rated (that is, no parent or child report) and were impairment-based and focused on the isolated function level of speech production (such as vowel prolongation) or on the single word or sentence level of speech production (for example, the Assessment of Intelligibility of Dysarthric Speech).

Intervention: The main aims of each treatment were to: 1) increase the participant's control of inhalation and exhalation and 2) improve the participant's coordination of phonation and exhalation. Both treatments used a bottom-up intervention approach, with the participant being required to progress along a hierarchy of speech and non-speech tasks. More specifically, traditional therapy involved eight 30- to 45-minute sessions across two weeks, and consisted of a range of tasks largely based on adult treatment approaches that were described in a previous article. These tasks included the use of the U-tube manometer to increase the participant's control of subglottal air pressure via a form of simple traditional visual feedback and description and demonstration of an appropriate breathing pattern for speech. The therapist provided verbal feedback to the participant on issues such as the duration of tasks, depth and speed of inhalation and voice latency.

In relation to the instrumental visual biofeedback, inductance plethysmography (Respitrace system) was used to provide real-time continuous biofeedback of ribcage circumference to the participant during breathing. The participant received eight sessions over two weeks. Tasks involved trying to match a target trace provided at the top of the computer screen through the performance of various non-speech and speech tasks at certain levels. The specific computer feedback enabled the participant to visualise the exact point at which inspiration ended and expiration began, enabling him to try and coordinate phonation with this point. This biofeedback was augmented by the therapist explaining the visual feedback to the participant and instructing him to make adjustments to his breathing and voice onset coordination with expiration.

Main results: The continuous biofeedback treatment was not only effective, but superior to traditional therapy in the modification of speech breathing patterns for a child with persistent dysarthria following severe traumatic brain injury.

Conclusion: A physiological biofeedback treatment approach is potentially useful for the remediation of speech breathing impairment in the paediatric dysarthric population.

Is this evidence likely to be biased?

Given that this was a single case study, it was not appropriate to appraise this article for risk of bias using the criteria that are typically applied to randomised controlled trials.

- Appropriate inclusion and exclusion criteria were applied in participant selection.
- The methodology was appropriate for addressing the research question and methodological strengths included explicit reporting of the baseline assessment characteristics and the reporting of missing data or data that were unable to be analysed.
- The treatment methods were outlined in extensive detail and would enable replication of most components of the study. More prescriptive detail could have been provided about the steps in the progression along the treatment hierarchy, including the number of items administered within each level of the hierarchy.
- A large number of assessment points and assessments were used during baseline assessments and for treatment monitoring. Some level of change in some measures was likely to be found when so many assessments were conducted, which potentially limits the conclusions about treatment efficacy.
- No direct statistical tests were performed to compare treatment outcomes from traditional versus instrumental biofeedback approaches. Rather, multiple quantitative descriptive results were reported for pre- and post-treatment changes that are difficult for the reader to interpret.
- All outcome measures were administered by the treating therapist. This may have introduced rater bias.

What are the main results?

Multiple perceptual and physiological measures were made; however, two key measures included voice onset latencies and phonation time.

Following traditional treatment, the participant's voice onset latencies were reduced (mean = 1.14 seconds, range = 0.5±2 seconds) and phonation time increased (mean = 2.57 seconds, range = 1.5±4 seconds). The authors stated that both of these results were minimal and not convincing evidence of improvement in the participant's control of his breath pattern for speech.

Using visual biofeedback treatment of ribcage excursion, the participant was able to produce a reduced mean voice onset latency of 1 second (range = 0±2 seconds) and to increase mean phonation time to 4.4 seconds (range = 3.5±5 seconds).

How might we use this evidence to inform practice?

In the case of Ben, no firm conclusions are able to be drawn about which treatment method is optimal for dysarthria treatment. This is because the current treatment evidence in this field is limited to a single case study. The participant in the chosen article was also a male and of similar age and aetiology (i.e. traumatic brain injury) to Ben. However, it is difficult to generalise the findings of one case study to other cases, regardless of these similarities. Further research and evidence is required in this field before any one treatment method can be definitively advocated for use in clinical practice. While the authors reported a slight improvement with the use of instrumental biofeedback methods, this approach requires the use of expensive equipment which is not currently available in many settings. The evidence is not strong enough for you, as Ben's speech pathologist, to present a case to your manager of the need to purchase this equipment for client care. Thus, in the absence of the necessary instrumental equipment and the absence of strong evidence for applying a biofeedback approach, you decide that you will continue to use a typical traditional behavioural treatment approach with Ben.

Undertaking the above process of finding and appraising research evidence ensured that you were educated about current research in the field so that you could confidently discuss the treatment literature with Ben and his parents. Importantly, you were able to reassure Ben's parents that the intervention that was being applied was appropriate to continue using. Reading the treatment methodology outlined in the study also encouraged you to reflect upon the structure of Ben's treatment. The study provided a guide as to what may be an appropriate number of treatment sessions for Ben, what the duration of treatment sessions should be and what treatment targets may be useful, and suggested methods for how to progress the client along treatment targets in an hierarchical fashion, moving towards functional speech outcomes.

Medicine example

Clinical scenario

You are a general practitioner who visits a residential aged care facility. Several of the residents have dementia. One 82-year-old male resident with Alzheimer's disease, Mr Jones, has become increasingly aggressive towards staff and his family. His health is otherwise good and he is prescribed no other medications. You consider starting him on a small dose of antipsychotic medication to reduce his aggressiveness as this would make it easier for his family and the staff who care for him, and reduce his overall agitation. Mr Jones's son is his guardian for health matters and feels responsible 'to make the right decision' for his father. He has concerns about the use of this medication. You decide to find out about the level of benefit that could be expected.

Clinical question

In elderly adults with dementia who reside in nursing homes, does treatment with risperidone lessen aggression and paranoid ideation?

Search terms and databases used to find the evidence

Database: PubMed—Clinical Queries (with 'therapy category' and 'narrow search' selected)
Search terms: dementia AND risperidone AND 'nursing home*' AND (aggres* OR agitation)

This search retrieved seven results. Two were randomised trials, but only one of these was directly relevant to the question. The other five articles were secondary analyses of the study that was chosen for appraisal.

Article chosen

Brodaty H, Ames D, Snowdon J et al. A randomised placebo-controlled trial of risperidone for the treatment of aggression, agitation, and psychosis of dementia. J Clin Psychiatry 2003; 64:134–143.

Structured abstract

Study design: Randomised controlled trial.
Setting: 14 nursing homes in Australia and New Zealand whose residents had a DSM-IV diagnosis of Alzheimer's dementia or vascular or mixed dementia.
Participants: 345 nursing home residents were randomised and 337 received at least one dose of the study drug. The mean age of participants was 83 years and 71.8% of them were female. Detailed inclusion criteria including diagnosis of dementia of the Alzheimer's type, vascular dementia or mixed dementia. Extensive list of exclusion criteria such as residents with other types of dementia, other psychiatric disorders or a history of major depression within the last six months or tardive dyskinesia.
Intervention: Participants were allocated to either risperidone (0.25mg to 2mg, with a mean dose of 0.95mg) or a placebo solution for 12 weeks.
Outcomes: Primary outcome measure: total aggression score from the Cohen-Mansfield Agitation Inventory (CMAI). Secondary outcome measures: the Behavioural Pathology in Alzheimer's disease (BEHAVE-AD) rating scale and the Clinical Global Impression of Severity and of Change scales.
Follow-up period: 12 weeks. Assessments were performed at baseline, weeks 4 and 8 and at the endpoint (either week 12 or participant's last visit).
Main results: Participants receiving risperidone showed significant reductions in aggression as measured by the CMAI total aggression score. The intervention group also had significant improvements on the BEHAVE-AD rating scale and the Clinical Global Impression of Severity and of Change scales.
Conclusion: Participants who received low dose risperidone were found to have significantly lower levels of agitation, aggression and psychosis.

Is the evidence likely to be biased?

- *Was the assignment of participants randomised?*
  Yes, participants were randomly allocated, utilising a randomisation code to balance participants across centres.
- *Was allocation concealed?*
  Cannot tell. It is unclear if this was achieved.
- *Were the groups similar at baseline or the start of the trial?*

Yes. The baseline demographics and clinical measures were similar between the two groups. There was an even distribution of comorbid conditions between the two groups. Baseline scores of outcome measures were also well matched across the two groups.

- *Were participants blind to which study group they were in?*
  Yes. Both groups of participants received an oral solution (either a placebo solution or the risperidone solution).
- *Were the health professionals who provided the intervention blind to participants' study group?*
  Yes. A placebo solution was used to match the risperidone solution.
- *Were the assessors blind to participants' study group?*
  Yes. All assessments were conducted by an independent nurse researcher who was unaware of group allocation.
- *Were all participants who entered the trial properly accounted for at its conclusion and how complete was follow-up?*
  The follow-up rate was 68.4% at the end of the trial. Some reasons are given as to why not all participants were able to be followed up, as well as which group they were in.
- *Was intention-to-treat analysis used?*
  Yes. It is explicitly stated that an intention-to-treat analysis was conducted.
- *Did the study have enough participants to minimise the play of chance?*
  Yes. It was estimated that 109 patients per treatment group were needed to detect a clinically significant difference at the 0.05 level with 80% power for the CMAI total aggression score (primary outcome measure). To allow for 30% rate of premature discontinuation, it was estimated that 155 were needed per arm of the study, which was achieved.

What are the main results?

The intention-to-treat analysis showed a statistically significant reduction in aggression on the CMAI at endpoint. Both the *p*-value (<0.001) and confidence interval (which does not include the no effect value of zero) demonstrate this (see Table 5.4). As the minimum score for this outcome measure was 14 and the mean baseline score was 33, this difference between the two groups represents about a 23% reduction in aggression in the intervention group, which could be considered a clinically significant result.

How might we use this evidence to inform practice?

Although you have some concerns about the loss to follow-up and no mention of concealed allocation in this study, the double-blind nature of this trial and attention to other methodological factors mean you are fairly confident about the results. Mr Jones

(Primary) Outcome of interest to clinical question	Risperidone, least squares mean (n=149)	Placebo, least squares mean (n=152)	Difference	95% Confidence interval	P-value
CMAI total aggression (Score range 14–98)	−7.5	−3.1	−4.4	−6.75 to −2.07	<0.001

TABLE 5.4 Effect of risperidone on aggression as measured by the CMAI total aggression score

is a nursing home resident with aggressive behaviour who is similar to the participants who were included in this study. You use this information to involve Mr Jones's son and daughter in discussing the potential benefits of treatment. This is useful in balancing their concerns about some of the risks associated with this medication. As an acknowledgement of their concerns you also explain to them the results of a systematic review about the risk of death from giving antipsychotic medications to people who have dementia.[1] This review concluded that the increased risk of death is small. This facilitates a lengthy discussion with his family and a plan is formed to trial the risperidone at a low dose (0.5mg) for a few weeks to assess its effect on him. You arrange to meet with them again in two weeks to review his response.

Nursing example

Clinical scenario

Working in general practice enables nurses to expand their experiences and engage in primary care outside the acute care model, and that is what attracted you to practise nursing. Within the clinic where you work, there is a focus on mental health, and the clinic was recently funded to establish a new program to assist people with mild to moderate anxiety or depression. With funding available, the format of the services needs to be decided and you are asked to find evidence about the potential of facilitated cognitive behaviour therapy (CBT) in the primary care setting.

Clinical question

In adults with mild to moderate anxiety or depression, is cognitive behaviour therapy facilitated by practice nurses effective in improving anxiety and/or depression?

Search terms and databases used to find the evidence

Database: PubMed—Clinical Queries (specifically selecting the 'therapy' filter)
Search terms: ((cognitive behavior? therapy) OR CBT) AND nurse AND (anxiety OR depression) AND (primary care)

You choose not to truncate 'nurse' as it would result in a huge increase in the number of articles identified but include many that are not focussed on the specifics of a practice nurse. A total of 11 articles are retrieved, and one of these describes both the therapy and the setting of interest to your question in the title. Reading the abstract, you identify that the study also focuses on the specific population that you are interested in.

Article chosen

Richards A, Barkham M, Cahill J et al. PAHSE: a randomised, controlled trial of supervised self-help cognitive behavioural therapy in primary care. Br J Gen Pract 2003; 53:764–770.

Structured abstract

Study design: Randomised controlled trial.
Setting: Primary healthcare teams from general practices in England.

Participants: 140 participants aged 18 years or above (mean age 39.2 years, 84% female) who were consulting their general practitioner for mild to moderate anxiety and/or depression. For each potential participant, general practitioners completed a severity matrix which had four domains—wellbeing, problems, functioning and risk. Clients who were considered to be experiencing slight (or more) distress in the risk domain and/or severe distress in any of the other three domains were excluded from the trial. Clients who were assessed as requiring immediate treatment with antidepressants were also excluded.

Intervention: Practice nurses assisted participants (n=75) to use a self-help book based on cognitive behavioural therapy during three sessions. The first two sessions were one week apart and the third session was three months later. The practice nurse was also available to clients in between sessions as required. Participants in the usual care group (n=64) received usual care from their general practitioner, which may have included the prescription of medications, discussion, counselling or referral to counselling or psychological services.

Outcomes: CORE-OM—a 34-item scale for measuring symptoms, functioning, wellbeing and risk where lower scores equate to reduced problems (total mean score range 0 to 4). EuroQol-5D—a health-related quality of life measurement instrument where higher scores indicate more positive health. The Consultation Satisfaction Questionnaire (total mean score range from 1 to 5).

Follow-up period: 3 months. Assessments were performed at baseline, 1 month, and 3 months.

Main results: Results were analysed by both intention-to-treat analysis and on-treatment analysis. With intention-to-treat analysis, participants in the intervention group achieved similar clinical outcomes to participants in the control group for similar costs and were more satisfied with their care. On-treatment analysis showed that participants in the intervention group were more likely to be below the clinical threshold at 1 month (odds ratio = 3.65; 95% CI = 1.87 to 4.37) than control group participants. This difference was less well marked at 3 months (odds ratio = 1.36; 95% CI = 0.52 to 3.56).

Conclusion: Cognitive behavioural self-help that is facilitated by practice nurses may provide short-term benefit for adults with mild to moderate anxiety or depression.

Is this evidence likely to be biased?

- *Was the assignment of participants to groups randomised?*
  Yes, allocation to groups was undertaken using block randomisation. The process was well described and random number tables were used.
- *Was the allocation sequence concealed?*
  Yes, randomisation occurred independently of the research team, and individual practices were blind to the randomisation strategy
- *Were the groups similar at the baseline or start of the trial?*
  Cannot tell. The authors report that there were no baseline differences between the groups on any demographic or outcome variables, but no details about demographic variables (other than the mean age of the sample and the percentage of participants that were female) are provided.
- *Were participants blind to which study group they were in?*
  No. For this trial, it was not possible for participants to be blinded to group allocation.
- *Were the health professionals who provided the intervention blind to participants' study group?*

No. For this trial, it was not possible for the health professionals who provided the intervention to be blinded to group allocation.

- *Were the assessors blind to participants' study group?*
  No. The outcomes were all based on participant self-report and, as the participants were not blinded to group allocation, therefore the assessment of outcomes was not blind either.
- *Were all participants who entered the trial properly accounted for at its conclusion and how complete was follow-up?*
  No. The follow-up rate was 48.2% at 1 month and 29.5% at 3 months. Data are provided about how participants dropped out of each group, but reasons are not given as to why a large number of participants were not able to be followed up.
- *Was intention-to-treat analysis used?*
  Yes. The authors report conducting an intention-to-treat analysis, but they also report results from an on-treatment analysis.
- *Did the study have enough participants to minimise the play of chance?*
  No. The authors report that 30 participants were required to be retained in each group to provide adequate power. This number of participants was not retained at the 3-month follow-up.

What are the main results?

Table 5.5 shows the CORE-OM scores for both groups at 3 months. This result is not statistically significant as the confidence interval includes zero. You therefore do not need to consider clinical significance. For the CORE-OM scores, the authors report that there were no between-group differences over time. At 3 months, both groups showed statistically significant improvement on the CORE-OM compared to baseline. Mean reduction was 0.34 ($p<0.001$) for the intervention group and 0.41 ($p<0.001$) for the usual care group. This result suggests that, for this main outcome, the facilitated CBT program was similarly effective to usual care.

How might we use this evidence to inform practice?

As the facilitated CBT program was no more effective in reducing levels of anxiety and depression than usual care and you have some major concerns about the validity of the results of this study (particularly because of the very poor follow-up rate which may have introduced substantial bias into this study), you decide that there is not sufficient evidence to recommend that practice nurses should provide a cognitive behavioural self-help strategy for clients who have mild to moderate anxiety or depression. At your next clinic meeting, you plan to present the results of this study and discuss other possible formats for providing assistance to clients who have anxiety and/or depression.

Outcomes	Mean (SD) of intervention group	Mean (SD) of usual care group	Mean difference	95% Confidence interval
CORE-OM score at 3 months	1.24 (0.82)	1.51 (0.87)	−0.27	0.05 to −0.59

TABLE 5.5 CORE-OM scores for both groups at 3 months

Nutrition therapy example

Clinical scenario

As a clinical dietician who works in the orthopaedic ward of a hospital, you are asked to review a 72-year-old lady who was admitted to the accident and emergency department two days ago with a fractured neck of femur. She went to theatre yesterday morning. Today, the orthopaedic team have commenced her on a full ward diet, but due to her thin and malnourished appearance they are concerned that she may develop a pressure ulcer. They have requested a dietician consult for advice about whether supplementary nutritional support may reduce the risk of this occurring.

Clinical question

Does nutritional support prevent pressure ulcer development in people who have undergone surgery for a fractured neck of femur?

Search terms and databases used to find the evidence

Database: Medline (via Ovid)

Search terms: The search was done as an 'advanced Ovid search' and searches were mapped to subject headings. The search terms were: 'hip fracture$/or femoral neck fracture$' AND 'nutritional support/or enteral nutrition' AND 'pressure ulcer$'. The following search limiters were also applied: English language, humans, 65+ and therapy sensitivity.

This search yielded two articles. You obtain the full text of both articles and read them. In one of the articles there were major problems with tolerance of the intervention as it involved a nasogastric tube, so you decide to choose the other article to fully appraise.

Article chosen

Houwing R, Rozendaal M, Wouters-Wesseling W et al. A randomised, double-blind assessment of the effect of nutritional supplementation on the prevention of pressure ulcers in hip-fracture patients. Clin Nutr 2003; 22:401–405.

Structured abstract

Study design: Randomised controlled trial.

Setting: Three medical centres in the Netherlands.

Participants: 103 participants who were post-surgery for a hip fracture and had a pressure ulcer risk score >8 according to the CBO risk-assessment tool. Exclusion criteria included: terminal care, metastatic hip fracture, insulin-dependent diabetes, renal disease (creatinine >176mmol/L), hepatic disease, morbid obesity, need for a therapeutic diet incompatible with supplementation and pregnancy or lactation.

Intervention: Participants in the intervention group (n=51) received 400mL daily of a nutritional supplement enriched with protein, arginine, zinc and antioxidants. Participants in the control group (n=52) received a water-based placebo. The supplement and placebo were commenced post-operatively and continued for 4 weeks or until discharge. Participants in both groups also received a regular diet.

Outcomes: Pressure ulcer development (assessed using a four-stage classification); time of onset, size and location of any pressure ulcer(s) were also recorded.

Follow-up period: 4 weeks or until discharge. Participants were assessed daily by nursing staff.

Main results: There was no difference in the incidence of developing a pressure ulcer between the intervention (55%) and placebo (59%) groups; however, the supplemented group had a lower incidence of stage II ulcers and showed a trend towards later development of a pressure ulcer.

Conclusion: People with hip fracture are prone to developing pressure ulcers at an early postoperative stage. Initiating nutritional support at this stage may delay ulcer development and progression but is unlikely to prevent this process occurring. The authors surmise that nutritional supplementation may be more effective if it is started earlier.

Is the evidence likely to be biased?

- *Was the assignment of participants to groups randomised?*
  Yes, participants were randomised to receive the study or placebo supplement in addition to their regular diet; however, the method of randomisation is not specified.
- *Was the allocation sequence concealed?*
  Cannot tell. The article does not describe how participants were allocated to groups.
- *Were the groups similar at the baseline or start of the trial?*
  The baseline characteristics of participants appear similar between the two study groups. There was also no difference in the median time between the start of supplementation and surgery or admission to hospital between the two study groups.
- *Were participants blind to which study group they were in?*
  Yes. Although participants may have been aware of what they were receiving due to the different taste and viscosity of the two drinks, it is unlikely that this was the case as there was no crossover of drinks between the study groups and participants would have been unlikely to know what each drink tasted like prior to the study.
- *Were the health professionals who provided the intervention blind to participants' study group?*
  Cannot tell. It is stated that nursing staff recorded each participant's daily intake of the supplement, but it is not clear who gave the supplements to the participants in between their regular meals each day.
- *Were the assessors blind to participants' study group?*
  Yes. The authors of the study acknowledge that, although each of the supplements (intervention supplement and placebo supplement) had a different look and taste, both supplements were provided in similar blinded packages to mask this difference. It is therefore unlikely that nursing staff would have been able to tell the difference between the two supplements. The presence of pressure ulcers was assessed daily by nursing staff according to a four-stage classification system based on the European Pressure Ulcer Advisory Panel Guidelines.
- *Were all participants who entered the trial properly accounted for at its conclusion and how complete was follow-up?*
  No. The article does not state if any participants were lost to follow-up or, if so, the reasons for this. However, based on the data provided in Table 4 of the article, it appears that two participants were lost from the intervention group and one from the control group. This would give a 97% follow-up rate.

- *Was intention-to-treat analysis used?*
  Cannot tell. The authors do not explicitly state that an intention-to-treat analysis was conducted; therefore, it is assumed that it was not. There was no mention of percentage error in drinks given, which may mean that there was no error; however, this should also have been stated in the article.
- *Did the study have enough participants to minimise the play of chance?*
  No. This study did not have enough participants to identify a significant difference in outcome between the two groups. A power calculation is described indicating that 350 participants were required in each group to detect a 25% decrease in pressure ulcer incidence. The study only recruited 14% of this required amount.

What are the main results?

As indicated by the confidence intervals and the *p*-values, there were no statistically significant differences in any of the outcomes shown in Table 5.6. Based on the data that are provided in the article, you were able to calculate the absolute risk reduction (ARR), the 95% confidence interval associated with the ARR and the number needed to treat. The development of one pressure ulcer would be prevented for every 27 people who receive the nutritional supplement and the development of one stage II pressure ulcer would be prevented for every 11 people who receive the nutritional supplement.

How might we use this evidence to inform practice?

There are a number of pieces of information which are relevant to this study but are not discussed in the article. For example, were participants using a pressure ulcer relieving mattress prior to and/or after the surgery? What was the immediacy of surgery and had participants been fasted a number of times preoperatively?

It may be difficult to be able to generalise the results of this study to other populations as the sample in the study had specific characteristics, such as a pressure ulcer risk score of around 11, average age of 81years, 81% of the group were female, a well nourished population (average BMI: $23.5–24.5 kg/m^2$) and a haemoglobin of $7.1 g/L$. These specific characteristics may partly explain the low number of participants who were able to be recruited into this study. The consequence of such specific characteristics is that the results can only be translated to clients who have similar characteristics. The client in your clinical scenario differs from the study sample in a number of ways and you do not

Outcomes of interest to clinical question	Supplemented group (n=51)	Placebo group (n=52)	Difference (absolute risk reduction)	95% Confidence interval for ARR	Number needed to treat	P-value
Incidence of pressure ulcer (%)	55.1	58.8	58.8% –55.1% = 3.7%	–10.2% to 17.6%	1/3.7 = 27	0.42
Incidence of stage II ulcer (%)	18.4	27.5	27.5% – 18.4% = 9.1%	–4.8% to 23%	1/9.1 = 10.99	0.34

TABLE 5.6 Development of pressure ulcers after supplementation or placebo

feel confident that you can generalise the results to her. Additionally, the intervention was with a very specific supplement which was enriched with arginine, zinc and antioxidants (Cubitan®, N.V. Nutricia, the Netherlands), and this product is not readily available in your region.

In conclusion, although this study had reasonably good internal validity, it does little to inform the nutritional clinician about changing practices because it was severely underpowered and the sample population had a restricted profile. As such, nutritional practitioners should continue to provide nutritional support based on stronger data in the literature. You are aware of good quality research studies that have demonstrated the positive effects of nutritional supplementation on pressure ulcer development in different clinical populations, particularly for malnourished clients, and wonder if the lack of statistically significant results in this study was due to the fact it was underpowered. Until a larger, sufficiently powered study is conducted with people with hip fractures, your practice will be guided by the research that has been conducted with other clinical populations.

Radiation therapy example

Clinical scenario

You are a radiation therapist who is currently assisting a radiation therapy clinic in preparation for your new advanced practice role in radiation therapy side effect review. One of the clinic clients is Mr Jones who is 58 years old and has a glioblastoma (a brain tumour). He is being treated with palliative high-dose radiation therapy to 60Gy in 30 fractions, over 6 weeks. Prior to starting his treatment, Mr Jones had surgery to de-bulk as much of the tumour as possible. When he attends the weekly radiation oncology review at the clinic with his wife, Mrs Jones says that they have been looking at the internet for other possible treatment options for her husband's terminal brain tumour. She mentions that they have seen some information which suggests that a drug named temozolomide is being used in conjunction with radiation therapy in other hospitals to improve survival and control of the disease. They ask why it is not being used in their case. You decide to look for evidence about the use of this drug, particularly its success with respect to survival post-treatment.

Clinical question

Does the use of concomitant and adjuvant temozolomide with radiation therapy improve survival for people with glioblastoma compared to high-dose palliative radiation therapy alone?

Search terms and databases used to find the evidence

Database: PubMed—Clinical Queries (specifically selecting the 'therapy' filter)
Search terms: (glioblastoma) AND (temozolomide) AND (radiotherapy OR radiation therapy)

The search resulted in 11 articles. Of these, two articles are relevant to your question and compare radiation therapy combined with temozolomide to radiation therapy alone. One of these is a Phase II randomised controlled trial with 130 participants.[2] In this study, overall survival, progression-free survival and toxicity are the primary outcomes. The other publication is a Phase III international multi-centre randomised controlled trial with 573 participants. The primary outcome of this study is overall survival with secondary outcomes being progression-free survival, safety and quality of life. You choose the second article to fully appraise, as it was a Phase III trial and had a larger sample size.

Article chosen
Stupp R, Mason W, van den Bent M et al. Radiotherapy plus concomitant and adjuvant temozolomide for glioblastoma. N Engl J Med 2005; 352:987–996.

Structured abstract
Study design: Phase III, multi-centre, randomised controlled trial.
Setting: Participants were recruited from 85 radiation oncology institutions in 15 countries throughout Europe and Canada.
Participants: 573 participants aged between 18 and 70 years (median age 56 years) with newly diagnosed histologically confirmed glioblastoma. Participants needed a World Health Organisation performance status of 2 or less (indicating that they were relatively fit and self-caring). Additional specific inclusion criteria related to haematologic, renal and hepatic function; serum creatinine and bilirubin levels.
Intervention: Participants in the control group (n=286) received only radiation therapy (60Gy, 30 fractions, 5 days a week for 6 weeks). Participants in the intervention group (n=287) received radiation therapy (same dose and fractionation as the control group) and concomitant temozolomide (75mg/m^2/day, given 7 days a week from the first to the last day of radiation therapy, but for no longer than 49 days). Intervention group participants then had a 4-week break before receiving up to 6 cycles of adjuvant temozolomide (5-day schedule every 28 days) as well as prophylactic antibiotics due to increased chance of infection and prophylactic anti-emetics due to increased chance of nausea/vomiting.
Outcomes: The primary outcome was survival. Secondary outcomes were progression-free survival, safety (toxicity) and quality of life.
Follow-up period: Median follow-up was 28 months. During radiation therapy, participants were seen every week. After the radiation therapy was completed, participants were seen 21–28 days after this, and every 3 months thereafter. Participants in the intervention group received a monthly clinical evaluation while receiving the adjuvant temozolomide therapy and a comprehensive assessment at the end of cycles 3 and 6.
Main results: The median survival was 14.6 months for participants in the intervention group and 12.1 months for those in the control group. The 2-year survival rate was 26.5% in the intervention group and 10.4% in the control group.
Conclusion: Providing temozolomide in addition to radiation therapy for people with newly diagnosed glioblastoma resulted in a statistically significant survival benefit with minimal additional toxicity.

Is the evidence likely to be biased?
- *Was the assignment of participants to groups randomised?*
  Yes. Participants were randomly allocated to either the intervention or control group, although details of the exact method of randomisation are not provided. Participants were stratified according to: performance status, previous surgery and treatment centre.

- *Was the allocation sequence concealed?*
  Cannot tell. The article does not clearly indicate whether allocation to the study groups was concealed. However, it does mention randomisation was undertaken at a large international trials centre, so it is likely that allocation was concealed.
- *Were the groups similar at the baseline or start of the trial?*
  Yes. The article provides details about a large range of participant characteristics and the two groups appear to have been well balanced at baseline.
- *Were participants blind to which study group they were in?*
  No. For this trial, it was not possible for participants to be blinded to group allocation.
- *Were the health professionals who provided the intervention blind to participants' study group?*
  No. For this trial, it was not possible for the health professionals who provided the intervention to be blinded to group allocation.
- *Were the assessors blind to participants' study group?*
  No. Because of the nature and toxic effects of both treatments it was not possible to blind the assessors to the study group. The assessments were performed by qualified radiation oncologists.
- *Were all participants who entered the trial properly accounted for at its conclusion and how complete was follow-up?*
  No. The article does not clearly state if any participants were lost to follow-up. However, given the nature of the treatment and the need for regular medical follow-up and evaluation, it is unlikely that many participants were lost to follow-up. Because of the population (palliative clients) and primary outcome of this study (survival), participants who died would not have been considered as lost to follow-up.
- *Was intention-to-treat analysis used?*
  Yes. The article stated that all analyses were conducted on an intention-to-treat basis, which is important as there were a number of reported deviations from the treatment allocation and treatment protocol.
- *Did the study have enough participants to minimise the play of chance?*
  Yes. This study had 80% power at a significance level of 0.05 to detect a 33% increase in median survival (hazard ratio for death, 0.75), assuming that 382 deaths occurred.

What are the main results?

Survival and disease progression: A total of 480 (84%) participants had died at a median follow-up of 28 months. The authors of the article report that the hazard ratio for death among participants in the intervention group, compared to those in the control group, was 0.63 (95% CI 0.52 to 0.75), which was statistically significant. They also report a 37% relative reduction in the risk of death for participants treated with radiation therapy and temozolomide, compared to participants who received only radiation therapy. Table 5.7 shows the overall survival according to intervention group.

Outcome	Intervention group (n=287) value (95% CI)	Control group (n=286) value (95% CI)
Median overall survival (months)	14.6 (13.2 to 16.8)	12.1 (11.2 to 13.0)
Overall survival at 24 months (%)	26.5 (21.2 to 31.7)	10.4 (6.8 to 14.1)

TABLE 5.7 Overall survival according to intervention group

The median difference between the two groups in length of survival (that is, the median survival benefit) was 14.6 − 12.1 = 2.5 months. During the concomitant temozolomide therapy, 7% of participants had a grade 3 (severe adverse effect) or 4 (life-threatening effect) haematological effect. During the adjuvant temozolomide therapy, 14% of participants had a grade 3 or 4 haematological effect.

How do we use this evidence to inform practice?

You are reasonably satisfied with the validity of the study's results and consider the results to be important and, when you compare the demographic and clinical details of Mr Jones to the study participants, they compare well. Therefore, you decide to consider the side effect profile of temozolomide (which includes fatigue and immunosuppression) before discussing this study with the radiation oncologist for consideration about the potential use of temozolomide in the clinic where you work. The article does not provide data about the effects of the interventions on participants' quality of life. The article describes collecting data about quality of life as a secondary end point but does not report the data in this main article. As this is an important issue to consider, you will search to see if the quality of life data have been published. There are also a number of resource issues related to the use of temozolomide which have to be evaluated in order to ensure that, if the decision is made to use this treatment, there is adequate funding for staff and equipment to support its use. If the clinic decides to implement the use of temozolomide, together with the radiation oncologist, you will make a time to explain the results of the study to Mr and Mrs Jones. This discussion will include both the potential positive effect of temozolomide on the length of survival as well as the risk of adverse events.

Complementary and alternative medicine example

Clinical scenario

You are a clinician in a medical health centre and one of your clients, Mr Andrews, was referred to you by a colleague in your medical centre practice because of your expertise with the use of herbal medicines. Mr Andrews has recently been told that he has type 2 diabetes mellitus. He has had hypertension (high blood pressure) for about 12 months and, since retirement, he has put on a substantial amount of weight. In the past 3 months, he has not lost any weight and has subsequently been put on medication for his diabetes and hypertension. At a follow-up visit with your colleague, he was found to still be hypertensive and the health concern with this clinical picture was explained to him and he subsequently enquired if there were any alternative treatments that could help him to get his blood pressure under control. You are aware of some pilot studies that found that hawthorn extract (a herbal medicine) can be used safely and effectively to treat hypertension and wonder if it is effective in people who also have diabetes.

Clinical question

Is hawthorn effective in reducing hypertension in people who have type 2 diabetes mellitus and are currently taking prescribed hypoglycaemic and hypotensive medications?

Search terms and databases used to find the evidence
Database: PubMed—Clinical Queries (specifically selecting the 'therapy' and 'narrow' filters)
Search terms: hawthorn AND ((hypertens* OR (high blood pressure)) AND diabet*

This search retrieved one article, which seemed to be very relevant, based on its title and abstract. Concerned that you may have missed a relevant article, you repeat the search, this time selecting the 'broad' search. This search results in 21 articles, of which only one is relevant and it is the same article that you had already found.

Article chosen
Walker AF, Marakis G, Simpson E et al. Hypotensive effects of hawthorn for patient with diabetes taking prescription drugs: a randomised controlled trial. Br J Gen Pract 2006; 56:437–443.

Structured abstract
Study design: Randomised controlled trial.
Setting: Outpatients attending general practices in a region of the UK.
Participants: 80 participants (mean age 61.95 years; 69% male) with type 2 diabetes and hypertension (diastolic blood pressure 85–95mmHg and systolic pressure of 145–165mmHg). Exclusion criteria included pregnant women or clients with heart disease or major pathology.
Intervention: Participants in the intervention group (n=40) were given tablets containing 1200mg of hawthorn extract and advised to take one before breakfast and one before their evening meal. Participants in the control group (n=40) received placebo tablets.
Outcomes: The primary outcome was blood pressure. Other data were also collected from fasting blood samples, a wellbeing questionnaire and a food frequency questionnaire that was used to estimate nutrient intake.
Follow-up period: 16 weeks. Participants were assessed at baseline and after 8 and 16 weeks of intervention.
Main results: Participants in the intervention group showed significantly greater reductions in diastolic blood pressure from baseline than participants in the control group. There was no group difference in systolic blood pressure reduction from baseline. No herb–drug interactions were found and minor health complaints were reduced from baseline in both groups.
Conclusion: Hawthorn demonstrated a hypotensive effect in people with diabetes who were taking medication.

Is the evidence likely to be biased?
- *Was the assignment of participants to groups randomised?*
  Yes. Participants were randomly allocated to either the intervention or control group. The researchers used 80 identical pill boxes (numbered 1 to 80), which contained either the hawthorn or placebo tablets, according to the randomisation code.
- *Was the allocation sequence concealed?*
  Yes. The article states that pill boxes were assigned blindly in order of participants' enrolment into the trial. It is also stated that the coding was done by one of the authors who had no direct contact with the participants.
- *Were the groups similar at the baseline or start of the trial?*

Yes. The article provides details about a large range of participant characteristics and the two groups appear to have been well balanced at baseline. There were also no differences in blood pressure between the two groups at baseline.
- *Were participants blind to which study group they were in?*
Yes. Participants were blinded as to whether they were receiving the hawthorn tablets or placebo tablets.
- *Were the health professionals who provided the intervention blind to participants' study group?*
No. It is not clear whether the person who gave the tablets to the participants knew which group each participant was in. However, the possibility of bias being introduced from lack of blinding in the person who is providing the intervention is not of great concern in this study given the type of intervention (tablets) and the use of a relatively objective outcome (blood pressure).
- *Were the assessors blind to participants' study group?*
Cannot tell. It is not explicitly stated if the assessor who measured participants' blood pressure was blind to their group allocation. The article does mention that team members were blind to coding, but does not state who performed the assessments— whether it was a team member or their regular medical practitioner.
- *Were all participants who entered the trial properly accounted for at its conclusion and how complete was follow-up?*
Yes. The overall follow-up rate was 78.8%, with 7 participants lost to follow-up in the intervention group and 8 in the control group. Reasons are given for why participants were lost to follow-up.
- *Was intention-to-treat analysis used?*
Yes. The article stated that an intention-to-treat analysis was conducted but no further details are provided about this.
- *Did the study have enough participants to minimise the play of chance?*
Yes. Prior to the study, the authors used data from a similar participant sample to calculate that they would need to recruit 80 participants to detect a significant difference ($p = 0.05$) between the two groups with a power of 80%.

What are the main results?

Unfortunately, the authors of the article do not provide standard deviations for any of the blood pressure measurements, so it is not possible to calculate the confidence intervals associated with the calculated effect sizes. The authors report that the only statistically significant ($p = 0.035$) between-group difference was for the reduction of diastolic blood

Outcome	Intervention group	Control group	Absolute difference between groups
Mean diastolic BP (mmHg) at 16 weeks	83.0	85.0	2.0
Change in diastolic blood pressure (mmHg) from baseline to 16 weeks	−2.6	0.5	3.1
Mean systolic BP (mmHg) at 16 weeks	148.7	146.6	2.1
Change in systolic blood pressure (mmHg) from baseline to 16 weeks	−3.6	−0.8	2.8

TABLE 5.8 Change in blood pressure in the intervention and control groups

pressure, with participants in the intervention group experiencing a 2.6mmHg reduction in diastolic blood pressure. The mean change in the intervention group was greater than the mean change in the control group; however, you do not consider the size of this effect to be clinically significant.

How might we use this evidence to inform practice?

Although the validity of this study was reasonable, for the outcome that you were interested in the only statistically significant result was not clinically significant. You therefore do not proceed to evaluating the applicability of this evidence to your client. Although the study established the safe use of hawthorn and that there were no herb–drug interactions elicited with medications that are typically prescribed to people who have type 2 diabetes, the effect of hawthorn on blood pressure was not clinically significant. You discuss the results of this study with both your colleague and Mr Andrews and explain that, based on the current evidence, you would not suggest that he commence this intervention as a way of reducing his high blood pressure.

References

1. Schneider L, Dagerman K, Insel P. Risk of death with atypical antipsychotic drug treatment for dementia: meta-analysis of randomised placebo-controlled trials. JAMA 2005; 294:1934–1943.
2. Athanassiou H, Synodinou M, Maragoudakis E et al. Randomised phase II study of temozolomide and radiotherapy compared with radiotherapy alone in newly diagnosed glioblastoma multiforme. J Clin Oncol 2005; 23:2372–2377.

CHAPTER 6

Evidence about diagnosis

Jenny Doust

LEARNING OBJECTIVES

After reading this chapter, you should be able to:

- Generate a structured clinical question about diagnosis for a clinical scenario
- Appraise the validity of diagnostic evidence
- Understand how to interpret the results from diagnostic studies and calculate additional results (such as positive and negative predictive values and likelihood ratios) where possible
- Describe how diagnostic evidence can be used to inform practice

Let us consider a clinical scenario that will be useful for illustrating the concepts of evidence about diagnosis that are the focus of this chapter.

Clinical scenario

You are working in private practice as a physiotherapist. During your Monday clinic, you see a 24-year-old man who twisted his right knee while playing football the day before. He has been suffering with pain and swelling in the knee since the time of the injury and is able to weight bear but with difficulty. You examine his knee and wonder how well does physical examination determine the cause of knee injury?

Diagnosis is essential in all areas of clinical practice and includes the history, physical examination, assessment tools, pathology and imaging tests that may be performed. Health professionals need to understand how each of these elements contributes to the final diagnosis, whether that be the diagnostic label that we use for clients or the various categories and stratifications within the diagnostic label that we use to assist with decisions about management. This chapter will address the process of using diagnostic evidence to assess the clinical examination of the knee. We will start by defining the components of a structured clinical question about diagnosis. Then we will see how to appraise the evidence to determine its likely validity. Subsequent sections of the chapter will review how to understand the results of a diagnostic study and how to use the evidence to inform practice.

Physical signs are a form of diagnostic test. They help health professionals to decide if a client has a disease or not. Like all diagnostic tests, they can be measured against a 'gold standard' test (a test that is known to be highly accurate for the disease being considered) to measure how well they rule in or rule out a diagnosis. Various measures may be used to estimate the accuracy of the test, such as the sensitivity and specificity or the positive and negative likelihood ratios. We will explain these measures later in the chapter.

Study designs that can be used for answering questions about diagnosis

Studies of diagnostic tests generally measure how accurately a test can detect the presence or absence of a disease by comparing the test with a reference test or 'gold standard'. As we saw in Chapter 2, the best type of study to estimate diagnostic accuracy is a 'consecutive cohort study'. This is a study that compares the test of interest with a gold standard test in every client who presents with a similar type of clinical problem in a particular setting over a particular time period. As we saw in Chapter 2, systematic reviews are even better than an individual study or trying to read all the studies that are available. Systematic reviews will be discussed further in Chapter 12.

Other study designs are also possible, such as a convenience sample of clients who have had both the test of interest and the reference test, or studies that compare the test results of the index test and the reference test in clients who are known to have the disease of interest (cases) versus the test results in clients who are known not to have the disease of interest (controls). As these studies do not enroll clients with the whole spectrum of disease that may be seen in clinical practice (for example, they may only include clients who have a 'mild' form of the disease of interest), these study types can lead to biased estimates of diagnostic accuracy. Case-control studies, because they enroll clients who clearly have or do not have the disease, are known to overestimate the diagnostic accuracy of a test.[1]

Diagnostic accuracy studies are often more difficult to find than studies assessing the effectiveness of interventions. As yet, there is no publication type that specifically indexes this type of study in Medline or the other major databases, as there is for randomised controlled trials. A possible approach to searching for diagnostic studies is:

1. In PubMed Clinical Queries, choose the diagnosis and specific options.
2. Type in the name of the test. If the test is used for more than one condition, you may also need to use the name of the target disorder in your search.
   - If you do not find a relevant study, try a sensitive search.
   - If you find too many studies, use the name of the target disorder or the 'gold standard' test in your search.

Clinical scenario (continued): Structuring the clinical question

As with clinical questions about the effectiveness of interventions, we can define the clinical question for diagnostic questions using the PICO format that was outlined in Chapter 2. There are often several possible questions than can be asked, so it is worth spending a few minutes to consider the question you wish to ask more carefully.

In the case of the 24-year-old footballer in the clinical scenario at the beginning of this chapter, you may be considering a meniscal injury, an injury to the anterior cruciate ligament or a soft tissue injury. You may want to define the population in the question broadly, such as in 'all people', or more narrowly, such as in 'adults with a knee injury'. How narrowly you define the question may depend on whether you think that the test may perform differently in different sub-groups of clients. The disorders of meniscal injuries and anterior cruciate ligament injuries are the possible outcomes for the diagnostic test, and in this example we will focus on the physical examination for determining the presence of an anterior cruciate ligament injury. For anterior cruciate injuries, tests include the anterior drawer test, Lachman's test and the pivot shift test[2] (see Figure 6.1). Each of these parts of the physical examination of the knee can be the index tests. The comparator test should be the most accurate method of diagnosing these conditions. In general, the most accurate test for diagnosing intra-articular damage to the knee is arthroscopy. However, magnetic resonance imaging (MRI) is also a highly accurate test for meniscal and ligament injuries of the knee and may be used in some studies because it is less invasive than surgery. Unless clients have a reasonably high probability of the disease or are considering surgery, it is difficult to justify performing surgery in clients to verify the results of physical examination, so many studies will not have used the results of arthroscopy or will only have included clients who are being scheduled for surgery. For this clinical question, both forms of investigation can be considered as the gold standard test.

You decide on the following question: In adults with a knee injury, how well does physical examination, compared with arthroscopy or MRI, determine the presence of anterior cruciate ligament injury?

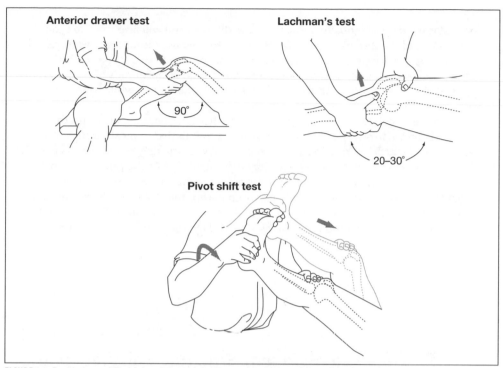

FIGURE 6.1 Description and illustration of the anterior drawer test, Lachman's test, and the pivot shift test

Adapted with permission from Jackson J et al, Evaluation of acute knee pain in primary care, Annals of Internal Medicine, 2003[2]

Anterior drawer test: Place patient supine, flex the hip to 45° and the knee to 90°. Sit on the dorsum of the foot, wrap your hands around the hamstrings (ensuring that these muscles are relaxed), then pull and push the proximal part of the leg, testing the movement of the tibia on the femur. Do these manoeuvres in three positions of tibial rotation: neutral, 30° externally and 30° internally rotated. A normal test result is no more than 6 to 8mm of laxity. *Lachman's test:* Place the patient supine on examining table, leg at the examiner's side, slightly externally rotated and flexed (20 to 30°). Stabilise the femur with one hand and apply pressure to the back of the knee with the other hand with the thumb of the hand exerting pressure placed on the joint line. A positive test result is movement of the knee with a soft or mushy end point. *Pivot shift test:* Fully extend the knee, rotate the foot internally. Apply a valgus stress while progressively flexing the knee, watching and feeling for translation of the tibia on the femur.

Clinical scenario (continued): Finding the evidence to answer your question

As we saw in Chapter 3, one of the best options for finding diagnostic accuracy studies is PubMed Clinical Queries. If you are looking for studies on a particular test, you may select 'diagnosis' and 'specific', and type in the name of the test. This may be enough to find what you want. If you do not find anything with a specific search, you can then look for more studies by selecting 'sensitive' instead of 'specific'. If the test is used for diagnosing more than one disease, you will also need to type in the name of the disease to narrow the search to only the disease that you are considering (for example, ultrasound AND breast cancer). In this scenario, the test is the physical examination of the knee. You could type in the names of the different types of test (such as anterior drawer), but it would take quite a while to search for each separate test.

Using the search terms (knee injury AND physical examination) and with the 'diagnosis' and 'narrow, specific' options selected in PubMed Clinical Queries, your search finds 70 articles. You find a systematic review of the diagnostic accuracy of physical examination to detect anterior cruciate injury.[3] As the purpose of this scenario is to demonstrate how to appraise a diagnostic study, a primary study, rather than a systematic review, will be chosen for appraisal. One of the largest and most recent studies included in the systematic review was an audit of 203 patients who were referred to orthopaedic clinics in Bristol by general practitioners or accident and emergency departments.[4]

Clinical scenario (continued): Structured abstract of the chosen article

Citation: Boeree N, Ackroyd C. Assessment of the menisci and cruciate ligaments: an audit of clinical practice. Injury 1991; 22:291–294.[4]

Question: Can clinical assessment of the knee accurately target which clients need arthroscopy, without the need for alternative methods of investigation?

Design: The reliability of clinical assessment of the menisci and cruciate ligaments of the knee was evaluated by evaluating participants using magnetic resonance imaging (MRI).

Setting: Clients of orthopaedic clinics in Bristol, United Kingdom.

Participants: 203 clients (mean age 32.7 years, 76% male) who were seen during a 2-year period in orthopaedic clinics. Of these, 169 clients were referred by their general practitioner and 34 were from accident and emergency departments.

Test: Clinical assessment of the knee (included clinical symptoms and physical signs such as Lachman's test, the anterior draw sign and the pivot shift test).

Diagnostic standard: MRI of the knee.

Main results: Physical signs proved insufficiently sensitive in detecting abnormalities. Overall, the accuracy of clinical diagnosis was 80.8% for the anterior cruciate ligament, 62.9% for the medial meniscus and 74.9% for the lateral meniscus.

Conclusions: Investigations that are accurate enable arthroscopy to be used for those who are likely to obtain therapeutic benefit. Use of clinical judgement alone would have resulted in an 89% increase in arthroscopic procedures. MRI or arthrography investigations appear to be cost-effective methods of avoiding unnecessary hospitalisation and morbidity.

Is this evidence likely to be biased?

As we saw in Chapter 4, for studies about the effectiveness of interventions it is important to critically appraise the diagnostic test studies that you find to determine whether the study is adequate to inform your clinical practice. As with the other types of study designs, the main elements to consider are: 1) internal validity (in particular, the risk of bias); 2) the results (the estimates of diagnostic accuracy); and 3) whether or how the evidence might be applicable to your client or clinical practice.

We will use the Critical Appraisal Skills Program (CASP) checklist for appraising a diagnostic test study to explain how to assess the likelihood of bias in this type of study. The key questions to ask when appraising the validity of a diagnostic study are summarised in Box 6.1. The checklist begins with two simple screening criteria that, if not met, indicate that the article is unlikely to be helpful and that further assessment of potential bias is probably unwarranted.

BOX 6.1 KEY QUESTIONS TO ASK WHEN APPRAISING THE VALIDITY (RISK OF BIAS) OF A DIAGNOSTIC STUDY

1 Was there a clear question for the study to address?
2 Is the comparison with an appropriate reference standard?
3 Did all participants get the diagnostic test and the reference standard?
4 Could the results of the test of interest have been influenced by the results of the reference standard or vice versa?
5 Was there a clear description of the disease status of the tested population?
6 Was there sufficient description of the methods for performing the test?

Was there a clear question for the study to address?

The first criterion on the checklist is whether there was a clear question for the study to address. For diagnostic evidence, the study should clearly define the population, the index and comparator tests, the setting and the outcomes considered.

Clinical scenario (continued): Did the study address a clearly focussed issue?

The study examined the accuracy of the clinical examination of the knee in people who were referred to an orthopaedic outpatient clinic compared with the results of an MRI examination of the knee in determining injuries of the anterior cruciate ligament and the medial and lateral meniscus. This is slightly different to our clinical question, which concerned adults with a knee injury. Not all of the participants in the study had a knee injury. It is unclear from the article what proportion of participants had such an injury, although it appears that these data were recorded as part of the study. It is important to think through the question clearly before searching for the answer so you can think how this might affect your interpretation of the results of the studies that you find.

Comparison with an appropriate reference standard

The second criterion is whether there was a comparison with an appropriate reference standard. The reference standard should, in general, be the most accurate method available to diagnose the target disorder(s). If the reference test used in the study is not 100% accurate, the diagnostic accuracy of the index test may be either over- or underestimated. Sometimes, the reference standard will be a combination of a number of tests. For example, a test for diagnosing heart failure may be tested against the combined results of clinical examination and echocardiography. If the index test is included in the reference standard (this is called **incorporation bias**), the diagnostic accuracy of the test is likely to be overestimated.

Clinical scenario (continued): Comparison with an appropriate reference standard

The most accurate method for diagnosing knee injuries is from arthroscopy. However, clearly this is too invasive a test to be used in all clients and it would be unethical to perform this test in clients where the clinical examination indicated no need for arthroscopy. The authors of the chosen study had previously demonstrated that MRI is a relatively accurate investigation for assessing the anterior cruciate ligament and therefore used MRI to assess the diagnostic accuracy of the clinical examination of the knee.[5] Although MRI is slightly less accurate than arthroscopy, and is therefore not a perfect gold standard test, it can be used for all the participants in the study, so for pragmatic and ethical reasons is used as the reference standard in this study.

Did all participants get the diagnostic test and the reference standard?

As we explained earlier in this chapter, the best type of study to estimate diagnostic accuracy is a 'consecutive cohort' of clients. That is, every client who presents with a similar type of clinical problem in a particular setting over a particular time period receives both tests and the results are compared. In some studies, not all the clients who receive the test that is being evaluated receive the reference test, or only those clients who have received both tests are included in the study. This is particularly common when the reference test is harmful or invasive. It results in a biased spectrum of clients. Receiving the gold standard test generally overestimates the sensitivity and underestimates the specificity of the test. This type of bias is known as **verification bias**. Sensitivity and specificity will be explained in the results section of this chapter.

Sometimes verification bias is unavoidable. For example, in the clinical question we are considering (the diagnosis of anterior cruciate ligament tears), the gold standard is arthroscopy. However, as we explained earlier, it would be unethical to perform arthroscopy in clients where no abnormality is suspected after clinical examination (the index test). Therefore, it is not possible to perform the gold standard in all clients. In these cases, it may be necessary to use two gold standards, such as arthroscopy for clients with an abnormality on clinical testing and clinical follow-up for clients who initially show no abnormality on clinical testing.

A common form of verification bias occurs when the authors of a study use client records to select clients to include in the study who have had both the index test and the reference test. For example, in this study it appears that clients were included in the study if they attended an orthopaedic clinic and had both a physical examination and an MRI scan. Clients who had both a suspected anterior cruciate ligament injury and an MRI scan are likely to be a different spectrum of clients to all clients who present to an orthopaedic clinic with a suspected anterior cruciate ligament injury. When client records are used to select clients for a study they are likely to be different to the type of clients who present to a clinic with a particular clinical problem and are therefore likely to give a biased estimate of the accuracy of the diagnostic test.

Clinical scenario (continued): Did all participants get the diagnostic test and the reference standard?

The study included 203 clients who had suspected meniscal or cruciate ligament injuries who had been further investigated with an MRI study. The study does not state how many clients were examined in clinics for the above conditions and not investigated with an MRI study. Therefore, there is the possibility of verification bias in this study.

Could the results of the test of interest have been influenced by the results of the reference standard or vice versa?

The results of the index test and the reference test should each be decided without knowledge of the results of the other test. That is, the person who interprets the test should be blinded to the results of the other test. Knowledge of one test result may bias the reading of the other, particularly where the reading is subjective, such as physical examination or the interpretation of imaging results.

Clinical scenario (continued): Could the results of the test of interest have been influenced by the results of the reference standard or vice versa?

Imaging tests are generally performed after the physical examination, so it is likely that the index tests were not influenced by the reference standard. However, it is not clear from the study report whether the clinical examination was performed independently of any previous investigation, such as X-ray reports. It is not reported in the study whether the MRI was performed independently of the physical examination. If the results of the physical examination were included on the radiological request forms, this could have resulted in a bias in the interpretation of the MRI results.

Clear description of the disease status of the tested population

The test should be investigated in a clinical setting that is as close as possible to the clinical setting in which it will be used. The spectrum of clients included in the study can affect the sensitivity or specificity or both, and therefore may affect the observed accuracy of the test. For example, if the study is conducted in a tertiary referral centre (as compared to a general practitioner's office, for example), clients may have more severe symptoms and this may affect the sensitivity and/or the specificity of the physical examination.

Clinical scenario (continued): Clear description of the disease status of the tested population

The study describes the participants as clients who were referred to the orthopaedic clinic for suspected meniscal and anterior cruciate ligament injuries who had been investigated with MRI imaging. The internal validity of the study may be compromised if not all clients who were seen for these suspected disorders were investigated with an MRI. This is not reported in the study, so it is difficult to assess this from the information that is provided in the article.

Sufficient description of the methods for performing the test

Both the index test and the reference standard test should be described in sufficient detail so that it is possible to: 1) reproduce the test and 2) determine if the test is performed adequately and is similar to the test being conducted in your own clinical setting.

If you have got to this point and determined that the article about diagnosis that you have been appraising is valid, you then proceed to looking at the importance and applicability of the results.

Clinical scenario (continued): Sufficient description of the methods for performing the test

The study reports that 'in the examination of the anterior cruciate ligament, the physical signs that were studied included Lachman's test, the anterior drawer sign and the pivot shift (jerk) test'. [4] No further details of either the physical examination techniques or the methods for performing the MRI were given. The reader would need to consider if these tests are standard enough that no further details are required.

What are the results?

Sensitivity and specificity

There are a number of ways that the results of diagnostic accuracy studies may be reported. Diagnostic studies often report sensitivity and specificity results. The most useful results for you as a health professional are the positive and negative predictive values which we will explain in the next section. However, as many articles report sensitivity and specificity results it can be useful to have an understanding of them.

- The **sensitivity** of a test measures how well a test performs in detecting a disease in people who have the disease. It is the probability that a test is positive in people who have a disease (true positives/[true positives + false negatives]). Using data from our clinical scenario article,[4] this is represented graphically in Figure 6.2.
- The **specificity** of a test measures how well a test performs in determining that disease is *not* present in people who do not have the disease. It is the probability that a test is negative in people who do not have the disease (true negatives/[true negatives + false positives]). Using data from our clinical scenario article,[4] this is represented graphically in Figure 6.2.

Box 6.2 shows how to calculate sensitivity and specificity. It is difficult to convert sensitivity and specificity to the probability that the client does or does not have the disease. It is therefore difficult to apply these values clinically, which is why it is important to understand the concepts of positive and negative predictive values. These are explained in the following section.

BOX 6.2 **MEASURING DIAGNOSTIC ACCURACY: SENSITIVITY AND SPECIFICITY**

Using data (see Table 6.1) about the diagnostic accuracy of Lachman's test for detecting anterior cruciate ligament injuries of the knee from our clinical scenario article[4] as an example:

The sensitivity of Lachman's test

= true positives/(true positives + false negatives)

= 37/(37 + 22)

= 37/59

= 63%

The specificity of Lachman's test

= true negatives/(true negatives + false positives)

= 130/(130 + 14)

= 130/144

= 90%

	Anterior cruciate ligament injury present	Anterior cruciate ligament injury not present	Total
Lachman's test positive	True positives 37	False positives 14	51
Lachman's test negative	False negatives 22	True negatives 130	152
Total	59	144	203

TABLE 6.1 The sensitivity and specificity of Lachman's test for detecting anterior cruciate ligament injury as reported by Boeree and Ackroyd[4]

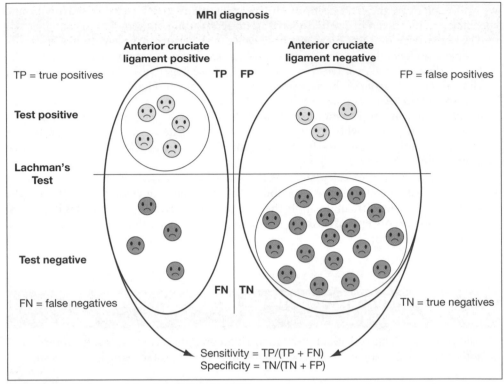

FIGURE 6.2   Graphical representation of sensitivity and specificity

Positive and negative predictive values

As we said earlier, the most useful results for you as a health professional are the positive and negative predictive values:

- The **positive predictive value** tells you the probability that a client has the disease if he or she has a positive test result. The closer that this number is to 100%, the better the test is at ruling in disease. Its calculation (true positives/[true positives + false positives]) is represented graphically in Figure 6.3, using data from our clinical scenario article.[4]
- Conversely, the **negative predictive value** tells you the probability that a client does not have the disease if he or she has a negative test result. The closer that this number is to 100%, the better the test is at ruling out disease. Its calculation (true negatives/ [true negatives + false negatives]) is represented graphically in Figure 6.3, using data from our clinical scenario article.[4]

The difficulty with positive and negative predictive values is that you need to know the pre-test probability of disease (or the likelihood of having the disease before having the test) in order to be able to calculate the positive and negative predictive values. This is different to sensitivity and specificity results, which do not change with the pre-test probability (prevalence) of disease. When the percentage of people in the sample who have the disease increases, the positive predictive value will increase and the negative predictive value will decrease.[6] When using positive and negative predictive values to guide your

BOX 6.3 **MEASURING DIAGNOSTIC ACCURACY: POSITIVE AND NEGATIVE PREDICTIVE VALUES**

As a health professional, what you want to know is if you receive a positive or a negative test result for a client, what is the probability that he or she has the disease? These values are the positive and negative predictive values of the test. However, most diagnostic accuracy studies report the sensitivity and the specificity of a diagnostic test. To calculate the probability of a disease after a positive or negative test result requires the calculation of the positive and negative predictive values and also needs to consider the prevalence (or pre-test probability) of disease.

Using some of the data from our clinical scenario article[4] as an example: Lachman's test had a sensitivity of 63% and a specificity of 90%. The study reports that 59 of the 203 participants included in the study had an anterior cruciate ligament injury. The **prevalence or pre-test probability** in this study is therefore 59 ÷ 203 = 29%. The **positive predictive value** = the probability of having an anterior cruciate ligament injury with a positive Lachman's test

= true positives/(true positives + false positives)

= 37/(37 + 14)

= 37/51

= 73%

The **negative predictive value** = the probability of not having an anterior cruciate ligament injury given a negative test result

= true negatives/(true negatives + false negatives)

= 130/(130 + 22)

= 130/152

= 86%

To help people remember whether tests rule in or rule out disease, the following mnemonics were created:

- **SpPIN** (Specificity-Positive-In) = if a test has a high specificity and the result is positive, it rules the disease in.
- **SnNOUT** (Sensitivity-Negative-Out) = if a test has a high sensitivity and the result is negative, it rules the disease out.

Note that this is a generalisation and that the positive and negative predictive values depend on both sensitivity and specificity and the prevalence of the disease.[7] Even though Lachman's test has a relatively high specificity, it is not a good example of a SpPIN. A positive test result is only a moderate predictor of the disease being present. *Note:* When the pre-test probability is low, for example in screening programs, even tests with high sensitivity and specificity will have a low positive predictive value; that is, most positive test results will be false positives.

decision about whether to use a diagnostic test or not, it is particularly important that you look at the spectrum of clients that were included in the diagnostic accuracy study and ensure that this matches with the sort of clients that you see in your practice. Box 6.3 explains how to calculate positive and negative predictive values and the pre-test probability of disease.

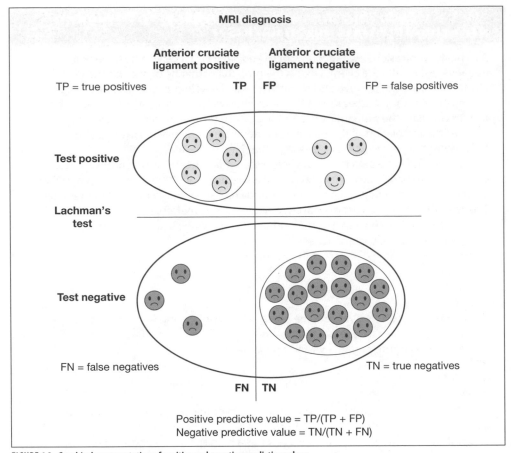

FIGURE 6.3 Graphical representation of positive and negative predictive values

Positive and negative likelihood ratios

Another pair of values than can be used to report results is the **positive/negative likelihood ratios**. Box 6.4 shows how likelihood ratios can be calculated. These results have the advantage of being relatively stable across different clinical settings, but also give an indication of how well the test rules in or rules out disease (refer to Box 6.4).

Clinical scenario (continued): What are the results?

A summary of the pooled results for each of the physical examination tests in our chosen article is presented in Table 6.2. Using the positive likelihood ratios, we can see that all three of the physical examination tests for anterior cruciate ligament injury are moderately good at detecting an injury if present. Looking at the negative likelihood ratios, we can see that if Lachman's test or the anterior drawer sign is negative, it is moderately helpful for ruling an anterior cruciate ligament injury out, but a negative pivot shift test does not rule out this injury.

BOX 6.4 MEASURING DIAGNOSTIC ACCURACY: POSITIVE AND NEGATIVE LIKELIHOOD RATIOS

The positive likelihood ratio is the probability that a test is positive in people with the disease divided by the probability that the test is positive in people without the disease.

Using some of the data from our chosen article as an example:

The **positive likelihood ratio** for Lachman's test = (true positives/people who have the disease) ÷ (false positives/people who do not have the disease)

= 37/59 ÷ 14/144

= 6.4

The negative likelihood ratio is the probability that a test is negative in people with the disease divided by the probability that the test is negative in people without the disease.

The **negative likelihood ratio** for the Lachman's test = (false negatives/people who have the disease ÷ (true negatives/people who do not have the disease)

= 22/59 ÷ 130/144

= 0.41

If the article only reports the sensitivity and specificity of the tests, another way to calculate likelihood ratios is:

Positive likelihood ratio (LR+) = sensitivity/(100 – specificity)

Negative likelihood ratio (LR–) = (100 – sensitivity)/specificity

When interpreting likelihood ratios, as a rough guide:

- A positive likelihood ratio > 2 indicates a test that helps rule in disease.
- A positive likelihood ratio > 10 is an extremely good test for ruling in disease.
- A negative likelihood ratio of < 0.5 indicates a test that helps rule out disease.
- A negative likelihood ratio of < 0.1 is an extremely good test for ruling out disease.

How changes in the cut-off affect test performance

For many diseases, there is no clear threshold between the presence and absence of a disease. For example, blood pressure and blood glucose levels exist on a spectrum and the cut-offs that have been chosen to define hypertension or diabetes are, to some extent, arbitrary. In cases where the cut-off for normal/abnormal levels can be raised or lowered, this will affect the test characteristics, and the choice of cut-off will involve a trade-off between the sensitivity and specificity of the test. If higher values indicate more abnormal test results, as the cut-off is raised, the sensitivity will increase and the

	Sensitivity	Specificity	Positive likelihood ratio	Negative likelihood ratio
Anterior drawer test	56%	92%	6.7	0.48
Lachman's test	63%	90%	6.4	0.41
Pivot shift test	30%	96%	8.8	0.72

TABLE 6.2 Estimates of the diagnostic accuracy of the anterior drawer test, Lachman's test and pivot shift test for the diagnosis of anterior cruciate ligament injuries[4]

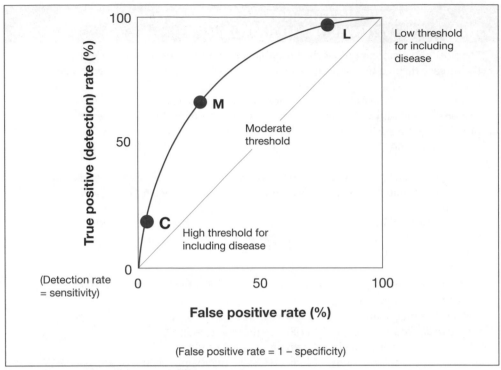

FIGURE 6.4   Receiver operating characteristic (ROC) curve

specificity will decrease. A receiver operating characteristic (ROC) curve (see Figure 6.4) plots this trade-off between sensitivity and specificity with changes in the cut-off. The curve demonstrates the trade-off between sensitivity and specificity of a test as the cut-off point changes.

How can we use this evidence to inform practice?

As part of our judgement about whether to use the results of this study in our own practice, we need to think about how likely it is that the test performs in a similar way in our own clinical setting to the diagnostic accuracy in this study.[8] We need to consider:

1. Is the spectrum of clients in the diagnostic study similar to the spectrum of clients in the clinical setting in which you are working?
2. Is the prevalence of disease in the diagnostic study similar to the prevalence in the clinical setting in which you are working?
3. Is the method for using the index test similar in the diagnostic study and the clinical setting in which you are working? This includes both the method for performing the index test and the person performing the test. In the clinical scenario chosen, the physical examination was performed by orthopaedic consultants and registrars. Will this alter the diagnostic accuracy of the physical examination?
4. Is the method for using the reference test similar in the diagnostic study and the clinical setting in which you are working?
5. Is the study defining the target disorder in the same way as in your own clinical setting?

Clinical scenario (continued): Using the evidence to inform practice

Our chosen study shows that the anterior drawer sign, Lachman's test and the pivot shift test are all moderately good at ruling in an anterior cruciate ligament injury, and Lachman's test and the anterior drawer sign are moderately good at ruling such an injury out.

Could the quality of the study have biased the results?

There are some reasons why we may doubt the results of this study. It seems likely that not all clients with a normal physical examination received the MRI reference test (which will overestimate sensitivity and underestimate specificity). It is also possible that the MRI test was interpreted without blinding to the results of the physical examination test results. Because of these possible biases, it is likely that these signs are even less accurate than estimated by this study.

Could other factors impact on the results, for example the setting of the study?

The study was conducted in an outpatient orthopaedic clinic and many of the clients had been referred to the clinic by a primary care physician. This may also impact on the sensitivity and specificity of the results seen in this study. There is also a limitation with the external validity of the study. External validity was explained in Chapter 2 and refers to the generalisability of the results of a study. The study assessed the diagnostic accuracy of the physical examination in clients who were referred to an orthopaedic clinic and examined by orthopaedic consultants and registrars. This may not be an accurate estimate of the same tests performed in another clinical setting.

Should I use these tests?

Even though these tests have only a moderate discriminatory value, the alternative diagnostic tests (arthroscopy or MRI) are more expensive and have potential harmful effects. Establishing the diagnosis will be primarily of importance in cases where surgery is being considered. If the client is someone for whom the consequences of the injury may be high (such as an elite athlete) or the client has particularly severe symptoms and may benefit from surgery, he or she may benefit from further investigation, such as an MRI. Clients with low demands, however, may be treated conservatively, whatever the findings of the clinical examination. If there is no resolution of symptoms within a reasonable time frame, the client may then require further investigation.

Other types of diagnostic test studies

So far, we have considered diagnostic test accuracy. These results measure how valid a test is. Not all diagnostic test studies measure diagnostic accuracy. Some studies measure the reliability of a test; that is, whether you get the same test result when the test is done by different health professionals or by the same health professional at different times. The first are usually called studies of inter-observer reliability and the latter studies of intra-observer reliability.[9] The agreement between different operators of the test (or different groups of operators) can be assessed using measures of agreement such as Cohen's kappa scores. These scores measure the agreement that is seen beyond that expected by chance.

Summary points of this chapter

- The diagnostic accuracy of a test (whether that be part of the clinical history, physical examination or a pathological or radiological investigation) is best assessed by a study of the test against a 'gold standard' reference test in a consecutive series of clients presenting with a clinical problem.
- Some of the main risks of bias in a diagnostic accuracy study are: 1) only a selected portion of the clients getting both the index test and the reference test and 2) the results of the two tests not being interpreted independently to the other test or blinded to the results of the other test.
- The most common methods for reporting the results of a diagnostic accuracy study are the sensitivity and the specificity of a test. However, the most useful results for a health professional are the positive and negative predictive values of a test or the positive and negative likelihood ratios.
- Along with the assessment of the risk of bias in a diagnostic accuracy test, it is also necessary to think how the results may be affected by the setting of the study and the types of clients included in the study.
- Using the results of a diagnostic accuracy study can help you decide if the test is useful at ruling in or ruling out the diagnosis, or both.

References

1. Rutjes A, Reitsma J, Di Nisio M et al. Evidence of bias and variation in diagnostic accuracy studies. CMAJ 2006; 1744:469–476.
2. Jackson J, O'Malley P, Kroenke K. Evaluation of acute knee pain in primary care. Ann Intern Med 2003; 139: 575–588.
3. Scholten R, Opstelten W, van der Plas C et al. Accuracy of physical diagnostic tests for assessing ruptures of the anterior cruciate ligament: a meta-analysis. J Fam Pract 2003; 52:689–694.
4. Boeree N, Ackroyd C. Assessment of the menisci and cruciate ligaments: an audit of clinical practice. Injury 1991; 22:291–294.
5. Boeree N, Watkinson A, Ackroyd C et al. Magnetic resonance imaging of meniscal and cruciate injuries of the knee. J Bone Joint Surg Br 1991; 73:452–457.
6. Peat J, Barton B, Elliott E. Statistics workbook for evidence-based healthcare. Chichester: Wiley-Blackwell; 2008.
7. Pewsner D, Battaglia M, Minder C et al. Ruling a diagnosis in or out with "SpPIn" and "SnNOut": a note of caution. BMJ 2004; 329:209–213.
8. Deeks J. Using evaluations of diagnostic tests: understanding their limitations and making the most of available evidence. Ann Oncol 1999; 10:761–768.
9. Byrt T, Bishop J, Carlin J. Bias, prevalence and kappa. J Clin Epidemiol 1993; 46:423–429.

CHAPTER 7

Questions about diagnosis: examples of appraisals from different health professions

Chris Del Mar, Sally Bennett, Mark R Elkins, Craig Lockwood, Angela Morgan, Sharon Sanders, Michal Schneider-Kolsky and Jemma Skeat

This chapter is an accompaniment to the previous chapter (Chapter 6) where the steps involved in answering a clinical question about diagnosis were explained. In order to further help you learn how to appraise the evidence for this type of question, this chapter contains a number of worked examples of questions about diagnosis from a range of health professions. The worked examples in this chapter follow the same format as the examples that are in Chapter 5. In addition, as with the worked examples that were written for Chapter 5, the authors of the worked examples in this chapter were asked not to choose a systematic review, but to instead find the next best available level of evidence to answer the clinical question that is in the worked example. This was done for the same reason that was given in Chapter 5—it is easier to learn how to appraise a systematic review of test accuracy studies if you have first learnt how to appraise a study about test accuracy. Chapter 12 will help you to learn how to appraise a systematic review.

Occupational therapy example

Clinical scenario

You are a paediatric occupational therapist who works in private practice. You often work in local schools with children who have a range of developmental disorders. You frequently use the Bruininks–Oseretsky Test of Motor Proficiency to identify children who may have developmental coordination disorder. Due to the busy nature of your practice and the time it takes to administer the Bruininks-Oseretsky (often 45–60 minutes), you would like to know more about a test that you have recently heard about called The Motor Performance Checklist as it is only a 12-item measure and was designed for identifying children with motor performance difficulties such as developmental coordination disorder.

Clinical question
Among children with motor performance problems, is The Motor Performance Checklist as accurate as the Bruininks-Oseretsky Test of Motor Proficiency for identifying developmental coordination disorder?

Search terms and databases used to find the evidence
Database: PubMed—Clinical Queries (with 'diagnosis category' and 'narrow search' selected)
Search terms: (The Motor Performance Checklist)
The PubMed clinical queries diagnosis 'specific' filter automatically combines this phrase with the term 'specificity' in the title or abstract. An alternative search approach would have been to enter this phrase in the CINAHL database and combine it with the term 'specificity'. This search retrieves four titles. The second title is obviously relevant so you obtain the full text of the article.

Article chosen
Gwynne K, Blick B. Motor performance checklist for 5-year-olds: a tool for identifying children at risk of developmental co-ordination disorder. J Paediatr Child Health 2004; 40:369–373.

Structured abstract

Study design: This study used a cross-sectional design to compare a new measure of motor performance with a 'gold standard' test for identifying children with developmental coordination disorder.

Setting: The study was conducted in schools in Sydney, Australia.

Participants: All 5-year-old children in a random sample of seven schools from 59 primary schools in the northern beaches sector of Sydney were invited to participate. Of the total population of children in the participating schools, 141 (60%) participated in the study (mean age 5 years and 5 months; 54% male). The prevalence of developmental coordination disorder in the study population was 4.2%.

Description of test: The Motor Performance Checklist is a 12-item instrument for identifying children at risk of developmental coordination disorder.

Diagnostic standard: The Bruininks-Oseretsky Test of Motor Proficiency Long Form. A composite standard score of 40 (one standard deviation below the mean) was used as the Bruininks-Oseretsky Test of Motor Proficiency Long Form cut-off/failure point to direct children to occupational therapy.

Main results: The checklist was found to have a sensitivity of 83% and a specificity of 98%. Positive predictive validity was found to be 72% and negative predictive validity 99%.

Conclusion: The Motor Performance Checklist has the potential to aid in identifying children who are in need of referral to community occupational therapy services.

Is the evidence likely to be biased?

- *Did all participants get the diagnostic test and the reference standard?*
  Yes. The study report states that all children were tested using both measures. The reference standard used for this study was the Bruininks-Oseretsky Test of Motor Proficiency Long Form. It is a well-validated and frequently used measure for assessing motor performance difficulties in children.
- *Could the results of the test of interest have been influenced by the results of the reference standard or vice versa?*
  No. A nurse was trained to administer the Motor Performance Checklist and an occupational therapist blinded to the Motor Performance Checklist results administered the Bruininks-Oseretsky Test of Motor Proficiency.
- *Is the disease status of the tested population clearly described?*
  Yes. The study included children from a random sample of seven out of 59 primary schools in a district of Sydney, Australia. The article states that the population from which the sample was drawn was fairly homogenous with 11% from non-English-speaking backgrounds. Twenty percent of the population had a tertiary education. There was an approximately even distribution between male (54%) and female (46%) children who participated in the study.
- *Were the methods for performing the test described in sufficient detail?*
  No. Nurses who administered the Motor Performance Checklist were trained in its use for the purpose of this study and a reference to an article that describes the test procedure in detail is provided. However, the actual testing conditions were not clearly described. As the Bruininks-Oseretsky Test of Motor Proficiency is a standardised test it would had to have been carried out as per the standardised instructions.

What are the main results?

In this study, 6 (4.2%) children were identified by the Bruininks-Oseretsky Test of Motor Proficiency as having developmental coordination disorder. This study presents the sensitivity, specificity, predictive values and likelihood ratios for identifying developmental coordination disorder using the Motor Performance Checklist (see Table 7.1) compared with the Bruininks-Oseretsky Test of Motor Proficiency Long Form using a cut-off score of 40 points.

The Motor Performance Checklist has high specificity, which means that there would be very few false positives. The sensitivity of 83% is also reasonably high, meaning not many children who had developmental coordination disorder would be missed (few false negatives). The positive predictive value looks at the data in a different way: how to interpret the results for a given client whose true diagnosis we do not know when we have the test result. A positive predictive value of 72% means that we know the chance of a child having developmental coordination disorder after their score on the Motor Performance Checklist is positive is 72%. Similarly, based on the negative predictive value, the chance of their *not* having it after a negative test is better, at 99%. In other words, a negative test seems better at telling us the true diagnosis than a positive one. As you saw in Chapter 6, two things contribute to the predictive values: the quality of the test (how well it performs as described by the sensitivity and specificity) and the prevalence of the disorder. In this example only approximately 4% of children had the condition. This means that we can only generalise the predictive values to other populations that have similar condition prevalences.

Assessment	Sensitivity	Specificity	Positive predictive value	Negative predictive value	Positive likelihood ratio	Negative likelihood ratio
The Motor Performance Checklist	83%	98%	72%	99%	41.5	0.17

TABLE 7.1 Ascertaining developmental coordination disorder

Another way to deal with this is to use likelihood ratios, which use a clever algebraic approach enabling us not to have to rely on prevalence to describe the usefulness of a test, yet also employ both sensitivity and specificity. Thus the positive likelihood ratio is the likelihood of a positive test result in a child with the condition compared with the same likelihood in one without the condition. In this study the positive likelihood ratio is 41.5 [calculated as sensitivity ÷ (100 − specificity)]. Using the approximate guide values that were presented in Chapter 6, a positive likelihood ratio over 10 indicates that the test is extremely good for ruling in the presence of developmental coordination disorder if it is present. The negative likelihood ratio was 0.17 [calculated as (100 − sensitivity) ÷ specificity] which, again using the values presented in Chapter 6, indicates that it is a test that can also help rule out the presence of developmental coordination disorder.

How might we use this evidence to inform practice?

Although this study may be prone to some types of bias that are common in cross-sectional studies it was otherwise well-designed and you are reasonably confident about the results. There are three factors about this study to think about, though. First, the ability of The Motor Performance Checklist to identify children with developmental coordination disorder was restricted in this study to children who were 5 years old. Testing this measure with children from 4 to 10 years is needed as this is the age range that this assessment was designed to be used with. Second, the study reports a low prevalence of developmental coordination disorder and the authors state this is lower than reported in the literature. This means that, in populations with a higher prevalence of developmental coordination disorder, the positive predictive value (or the chance of the test being correct) will be greater than reported in this study. Finally, the brevity of this measure is appealing and the article also reports on the concurrent validity and reliability of this measure, which are other psychometric test properties that must be considered when considering using an assessment with clients. You think back to your original dilemma. Can you use The Motor Performance Checklist for identifying children with developmental coordination disorder? The results of this study are limited to children 5 years of age so, until further research is done that involves children of other ages, it may have limited, yet useful, value to your clinical practice.

Physiotherapy example

Clinical scenario

As a physiotherapist in an outpatient clinic, a 25-year-old male cricketer presents with right shoulder pain. The pain began without any acute injury and is aggravated by repetitive throwing and catching. The location of the pain and your standard physical examination make you suspect, among other possible diagnoses, that he may have a lesion of the posteroinferior portion of the labrum of his shoulder. You are only aware of manual tests to diagnose superior labral lesions and wonder if there is a formal test for posteroinferior lesions. Also, you have recently read a systematic review that examined a range of widely used manual tests for shoulder pathology.[1] The review indicated that several of the tests have limited diagnostic accuracy compared to the 'gold standard' of observation of the pathology during surgery. You decide to search for a study of the diagnostic accuracy of any test for posteroinferior labral lesions.

Clinical question
In athletes with shoulder pain, is there a manual test for diagnosing posteroinferior lesions of the labrum and what is its diagnostic utility?

Search terms and databases used to find the evidence
Database: PubMed—Clinical Queries (with 'diagnosis category' and 'narrow search' selected)
Search terms: posteroinferior (labral OR labrum)

The search returns four records. One of these articles seems very promising: a comparison of the ability of two manual tests to diagnose posteroinferior labral tears, with surgical observation as the gold standard. It looks highly relevant but you are concerned that your search is too narrow. You repeat the search, selecting the 'broad, sensitive search' option. This returns 17 records, but none of these is as relevant as the original article that you found.

Article chosen
Kim S, Park J, Jeong W et al. The Kim test: a novel test for posteroinferior labral lesion of the shoulder—a comparison to the jerk test. Am J Sports Med 2005; 33:1188–1192.

Structured abstract

Study design: Cohort study.

Setting: Department of Orthopaedic Surgery at a hospital in Korea.

Participants: 172 adults awaiting arthroscopic examination for undiagnosed shoulder pain. Exclusion criteria were septic arthritis, fracture of the greater tuberosity, arthroscopic capsular release due to frozen shoulder, frozen shoulder and previous surgery.

Description of tests: For the Kim test, the client sits with the trunk against a backrest and the arm abducted to 90°. The examiner applies axial force along the humerus at the elbow to compress the glenohumeral joint and elevates the arm by 45°. With the other hand, the examiner applies downward and backward force to the upper arm. Sudden onset of pain indicates a positive test. For the jerk test, the client sits with the arm abducted to 90° and internally rotated 90°. The examiner stands behind and supports the scapula with one hand. With the other hand, axial force is applied at the elbow and maintained while the arm is horizontally adducted. Sharp pain indicates a positive test. Each test was performed by two independent examiners.

Diagnostic standard: Arthroscopic examination of the glenohumeral joint and subacromial space.

Main results: Thirty (17%) of the 172 participants had a posteroinferior labral lesion. The Kim test had sensitivity of 80% and specificity of 94%. The positive predictive value of the Kim test was 0.73 and the negative predictive value was 0.96. The jerk test had sensitivity of 73% and specificity of 98%. The positive predictive value of the jerk test was 0.88 and the negative predictive value was 0.95. The sensitivity in detecting a posteroinferior lesion increased to 97% when the two tests were combined.

Conclusion: The two tests, particularly in combination, have worthwhile clinical utility in the diagnosis of posteroinferior labral lesions.

Is the evidence likely to be biased?

*   *Did all participants get the diagnostic test and the reference standard?*
    Yes. All participants received the diagnostic tests of interest and the reference standard.
*   *Could the results of the test of interest have been influenced by the results of the reference standard or vice versa?*
    No. The results of the two manual tests (the tests of interest) could not have been influenced by the result of the reference standard (arthroscopic examination) because the manual tests were performed before the arthroscopy. The results of the arthroscopy could not have been influenced by the results of the manual tests because the surgeon was blinded.
*   *Is the disease status of the tested population clearly described?*
    Yes. The description of the study population is reassuring: eligible clients were recruited consecutively from an orthopaedic surgical clinic. All participants entered the study with preliminary clinical diagnoses that were potentially consistent but not definitive of the diagnosis of interest.
*   *Were the methods for performing the test described in sufficient detail?*
    Yes. The diagnostic tests of interest are described in sufficient detail for you to replicate them in your clinical practice.

What are the main results?

Thirty (17%) of the 172 participants had a posteroinferior labral lesion. The article presents the sensitivity, specificity, positive predictive value and negative predictive value of the two tests, which are shown in Table 7.2. You also use these results to calculate the positive and negative likelihood ratios (see Table 7.2).

Test	Sensitivity	Specificity	Positive predictive value	Negative predictive value	Positive likelihood ratio	Negative likelihood ratio
Kim test	80%	94%	0.73	0.96	13.3	0.21
Jerk test	73%	98%	0.88	0.95	36.5	0.28

TABLE 7.2 Results of the Kim test and jerk test

The positive predictive value of the Kim test indicates that, on average, 73% of people with a positive test result actually have a posteroinferior labral lesion. The positive predictive value of the jerk test indicates that, on average, 88% of people with a positive result actually have a posteroinferior labral lesion. Using the approximate guide values that were presented in Chapter 6, as both of the positive likelihood ratios are over 10, this indicates that these tests are very helpful for ruling in a posteroinferior labral lesion if it is present. Also, as the negative likelihood ratios are <0.5, this suggests that these tests are moderately helpful in ruling out a posteroinferior labral lesion.

How might we use this evidence to inform practice?

You are satisfied that the study is valid and the results are clinically useful. The study population was reasonably similar to the client to whom you are considering applying the tests, although in your practice not all clients are severe enough to be scheduled for arthroscopy, so the prevalence of posteroinferior labral lesions is likely to be lower. The tests can be performed quickly and without requiring specialised equipment. However, before applying these tests, you should consider other diagnoses. The client's description of the location of the pain suggests that the posteroinferior labrum is involved. Furthermore, the following tests are negative: the apprehension test (for detecting anterior shoulder instability), the impingement test (for detecting rotator cuff inflammation or impingement), the horizontal adduction test (for assessing acromioclavicular joint impingement) and tests for superior labral lesions as mentioned in the clinical scenario. In doing this, you confirm that a posteroinferior labral lesion is the diagnosis that you primarily suspect. You decide to apply the Kim test and the jerk test to your client and use the results of these tests to guide the diagnosis and subsequent management of your client.

Podiatry example

Clinical scenario

You are a podiatrist working in a community health centre and you have just seen a 28-year-old male plumber with a diffuse scaling rash which covers most of his instep area, extending towards the digits of his right foot. It has been present for about 8 weeks, is itchy and there are some vesicles in the instep area. Several weeks ago he tried a topical steroid cream bought from the pharmacy. According to the client, the rash did not really improve and he stopped applying the cream. You suspect a fungal infection, suggest an antifungal cream that is available over the counter, and discuss foot hygiene with him. You wonder how accurate the diagnosis of tinea pedis (a fungal foot infection) is, based on clinical presentation.

Clinical question

In a person with suspected tinea pedis is clinical presentation as accurate as microbiological confirmation for establishing the diagnosis?

Search terms and databases used to find the evidence

Database: PubMed—Clinical Queries (with 'diagnosis category' and 'narrow search' selected)

Search terms: Tinea OR 'athletes foot'

   You click on 'Details' to check how PubMed has processed your search and notice that it has automatically searched the Tinea MeSH term. This search retrieves 33 titles, so you start looking through them. Several studies look promising but, when you read through their abstracts, you find that they are either comparing different laboratory methods for diagnosing mycoses or are case-control studies. You know that case-control studies can overestimate the accuracy of diagnostic tests, so you reject these. There is one study that, on the basis of the abstract, appears to compare the clinical diagnosis of tinea pedis with laboratory methods but the operating characteristics of the tests are not reported. You are really only then left with one possible study. This study investigated the diagnostic value of signs and symptoms compared to culture for diagnosing dermatomycosis in general practice. You consider whether this study, which appears to have looked at the diagnosis of fungal infection on any hairless part of the body, could be relevant to your clinical situation. As there do not appear to be any studies that have looked specifically at the clinical diagnosis of tinea pedis, you obtain the full text of this study.

Article chosen

Lousbergh D, Buntinx F, Piérard G. Diagnosing dermatomycosis in general practice. Fam Pract 1999; 16:611–615.

Structured abstract

Design: This study compared clinical examination, microscopy of a potassium hydroxide preparation and cyanoacrylate surface skin scraping (CSSS) for detecting fungal infection of the skin with culture as the reference standard.

Setting: General practices in Belgium.

Participants: 148 consecutive general practice patients with erythematosquamous lesions of the glabrous skin (hairless skin). Participants whose lesions had already been treated with antifungal therapy were excluded.

Description of tests: Scales were collected from the border of the lesion for microscopic testing using a potassium hydroxide preparation (KOH test) and culture. A strip biopsy (CSSS) was also made from the same site. Each participant's general practitioner also noted their diagnosis, based on each participant's characteristics, and local signs and symptoms.

Diagnostic standard: Culture of scales collected from the border of the lesion.

Main results: 18% of participants had a positive fungal culture. The sensitivity of the clinical diagnosis was 81% (95% confidence interval [CI] 60% to 93%) and the specificity was 45% (95% CI 36% to 54%). The likelihood ratio of clinical examination was 1.47 (95% CI 1.15 to 1.88) for a positive test result and 0.43 (95% CI 0.19 to 0.96) for a negative test result. The most accurate diagnostic method was CSSS, which had a likelihood ratio of 5.17 for a positive test result and 0.43 for a negative test result.

Conclusion: In people with erythrosquamous skin lesions, clinical diagnosis has low diagnostic accuracy for detecting dermatomycosis.

Is this evidence likely to be biased?

- *Did all participants get the diagnostic test and the reference standard?*
  Yes. It appears that all participants received the index tests and the reference standard test (culture is the accepted reference standard).
- *Could the results of the test of interest have been influenced by the results of the reference standard or vice versa?*
  Cannot tell. The article does not clearly state that the index test results were interpreted blind to the results of the reference standard test. You think it is likely, however, that direct microscopy of the scales collected using the traditional method and the strip biopsy would have been performed before the results of the reference standard became available (cultures were examined after 4 weeks incubation) and that interpretation of the results of the KOH and CSSS tests would be without knowledge of the results of the culture. It also appears that signs and symptoms and general practitioner diagnosis were obtained before the results of the culture would have been available from the laboratory. You are also not sure whether the results of the culture were interpreted without knowledge of the results of the index tests.
- *Is the disease status of the tested population clearly described?*
  No. There is no information that you can use to judge whether the spectrum of participants included in this study is similar to those you see in your practice. There is no information about the severity or the duration of the lesions or their location. Demographic and clinical features of the participants in this study are also not reported.
- *Were the methods for performing the test described in sufficient detail?*
  Yes. The microscopy and culture of the samples was done by a laboratory which would need to adhere to certain standards for the tests that they conduct. There is a reasonable description of how the CSSS was performed but you think that more information about how the skin samples for the KOH test and culture were collected would be helpful. For example, what was used to collect the sample, how was it stored and was the lesion cleaned with alcohol before collection?

What are the main results?

In this study, 26 cultures (18%) were considered positive. The study presents the sensitivity, specificity, predictive values and likelihood ratios for the clinical diagnosis of dermatomycosis (see Table 7.3).

Table 7.3 shows clinical examination has moderate sensitivity and low specificity for diagnosing dermatomycosis in general practice. The positive likelihood ratio of 1.47 is of no diagnostic value, suggesting only a minimal increase in the likelihood of dermatomycosis with a positive clinical diagnosis. The likelihood ratio for a negative test (0.42) suggests that it is of some value in ruling out fungal infection, representing a small decrease in the likelihood of disease when a negative clinical diagnosis is made.

How might we use this evidence to inform practice?

The results of this study suggest that a positive clinical diagnosis of fungal infection on hairless skin of the body is of little help in determining that a person has dermatomycosis. You have some doubts about the validity of the study as the methods of the study were not reported in sufficient detail for you to accurately judge the level of bias that may be present. You also have some concerns about how generalisable the study is to your situation, but you have been unable to find any other studies which answer your question. As this

Test	Sensitivity (95% CI)	Specificity (95% CI)	Positive predictive value (95% CI)	Negative predictive value (95% CI)	Positive likelihood ratio (95% CI)	Negative likelihood ratio (95% CI)
Clinical examination	81% (60 to 93%)	45% (36 to 54%)	24% (16 to 34%)	92% (81 to 97%)	1.47 (1.15 to 1.88)	0.42 (0.19 to 0.96)

TABLE 7.3 Using clinical examination to diagnose dermatomycosis

study was carried out in general practices, you think that the population is more likely to be similar to yours than if the study had recruited people from dermatology specialist clinics; however, with the limited information that is provided in the article, it is difficult to be sure about this. You reflect on your management of your client and wonder if you should have referred him for further testing. Further testing would mean that the client would need to see his general practitioner as pathology tests are not covered by Medicare when they are referred by a podiatrist. The study that you just reviewed found that the KOH test and the CSSS test provide additional diagnostic value if a positive clinical diagnosis (from clinical examination) is made. Given the potential for bias in this study, you think it would be wise to conduct a search for other studies that have compared the test characteristics of direct microscopy with these diagnostic methods. You also need to check if the CSSS method is readily available in the geographical area of your practice. In any case, you think that the probability that your client has tinea is quite high and that suggesting antifungal treatment without further testing was a reasonable approach. The antifungal treatments that are available are reasonably cheap, easy to obtain and use and generally well tolerated. You advise your client to see his general practitioner for further testing if the rash does not clear.

Speech pathology example

Clinical scenario

You are a junior speech pathologist working in a rotational position at a tertiary adult hospital. Mr Pitt, a 33-year-old man with Friedrich's ataxia (a neurodegenerative genetic disorder) has been referred to you with recurrent aspiration. He was first diagnosed with the disorder at the age of 16 and had relatively good health until his motor function deteriorated, leaving him wheelchair dependent with moderate dysarthric speech. Despite this, he is a bright and witty young man with intact language skills. He has just completed a University degree in art history. Recently he developed severe swallowing difficulties and has had two successive admissions to hospital with aspiration pneumonia in the last nine months. On his first admission, he was referred to speech pathology for a swallowing assessment by videofluoroscopy (VFS). This demonstrated aspiration on thin fluids. The previous therapist recommended a modified diet of nectar-thick fluids only, using a chin-tuck posture.

However, the problem has not resolved when you see him during his second hospital admission. You wonder what investigations you should use this time and into the future, as many more will probably be needed as he deteriorates. VFS involves large X-ray doses. You consider using fibre-optic endoscopic evaluation of swallowing (FEES), which does not have this problem, but you are not sure if it is sensitive enough.

Clinical question
How do VFS and FEES compare for detecting aspiration in adults with dysphagia?

Search terms and databases used to find the evidence
Database: PubMed—Clinical Queries (with 'diagnosis category' and 'narrow search' selected)

Search terms: Dysphagia AND aspiration AND videofluoroscopy AND (fiberoptic endoscopy)

This search results in one article which was not relevant to your question. You repeat your search, this time selecting the 'broad, sensitive' search. This results in five articles, two of which appear to be relevant to your clinical question. One of these studies compared the two procedures and provided primary data. However, the procedures were conducted on separate days rather than simultaneously (which is a weaker method that is more open to bias). The remaining article is more recent and appears to be the most appropriate to answer your clinical question as it directly compared VFS and FEES which were conducted simultaneously for each participant.

Article chosen
Kelly A, Drinnan M, Leslie P. Assessing penetration and aspiration: how do videofluoroscopy and fiberoptic endoscopic evaluation of swallowing compare? Laryngoscope 2007; 117:1723–1727.

Structured abstract
Study design: Prospective single-blind study design.

Study question: Does the type of instrumental evaluation (VFS vs FEES) influence the speech-language pathologist's rating of penetration and aspiration?

Participants: *Participants with dysphagia*—15 consecutive participants referred to speech-language pathology for dysphagia assessment at one UK hospital. They presented with a wide range of primary diagnoses (such as bilateral vocal fold palsy, previous stroke and skull base tumour, cervical spine degeneration, base of tongue carcinoma). Participants were excluded if they were nil by mouth or judged to be at high risk of aspiration of all oral intake. *Speech-language pathologist raters*—20 therapists were invited to participate, 17 consented and the ratings of 15 were included in the final analyses. All were experienced in performing and interpreting FEES and VFS (with a mean of 6 years of experience for VFS, based on performing and interpreting approximately once per week each year, and a mean of 4.9 years for FEES).

Data collection: *Dysphagia assessments*—All participants underwent both FEES and VFS simultaneously on one occasion. Two therapists, one radiologist and one radiographer performed the examinations. Each participant swallowed two test boluses: 5mL liquid from a cup and 15mL yoghurt from a standard dessert spoon. Both boluses were dyed with 1mL of blue food dye to enable clear visualisation of the bolus. All participants swallowed the boluses in the same order. Thirty recording clips (15 VFS and 15 FEES) were recorded in random order onto two compact discs with the order randomly changed for the second. *Rating*—Each rater used the Penetration–Aspiration Scale to rate all swallows for both procedures (scale ranges from 1 = material does not enter the airway to 8 = material enters the airway, passes below the vocal folds and no effort is made to eject). Each 'clip' was to be viewed no more than twice. The 30 clips on one disc were rated first and then the clips on the second disc were rated one week later.

Main results: The Penetration Aspiration Scale scores were significantly higher (mean difference in scores was 1.15 points) for the FEES recordings than for the VFS recordings.

Conclusion: Penetration aspiration is perceived to be greater (more severe) from FEES than VFS images.

Is this evidence likely to be biased?

This study does not compare a new test with a gold standard test and, therefore, is not designed to determine test accuracy as is the case in many of the other examples in this chapter. Therefore, the same criteria for considering validity are not used here. Instead, more general questions for determining the potential for bias are used in this example. The focus is on the examination of bias in the participants and raters, methods and analysis.

- **Participants.** People with dysphagia: minimal inclusion and exclusion criteria were applied in participant selection and the 15 participants recruited to the study were extremely heterogeneous in age, diagnosis, treatment history and severity of swallowing difficulty. This makes it difficult to generalise the findings of this study to any particular population with dysphagia. Speech-language pathology raters: raters' experience in performing and rating FEES/VSF was only quantified for 14 of the 17 original participants. While the mean years of experience appears high (6 for VSF and 4.9 for FEES), the standard deviation (4.5 for VSF and 4.3 for FEES) shows that there was wide variation in the actual experience level of these 14 raters.
- **Methods.** Strengths include all participants undergoing VFS and FEES simultaneously, the use of a well-validated and commonly used aspiration–penetration rating tool, the randomisation of VFS versus FEES procedures, the use of a large number of raters from a number of different institutions (15 raters from 12 different institutions), the use of a week-long period between ratings of both discs to minimise recall bias, blinding raters to participants' age and aetiology and to the other raters' responses, and the inclusion of both inter- and intra-rater reliability ratings.
- **Replicability.** The assessment methods were well detailed and would enable replication of the study. For example, details were provided about the FEES and VFS procedure, including specific information about the ratio of food/fluid to barium in the bolus administered and the exact type of barium used.
- **Statistical analyses.** Both five-way analysis of variance (ANOVAs) and logistic regression were used to examine the variables that had the greatest impact on ratings of aspiration–penetration. The variables investigated were: the examination (FEES vs VFS), bolus type (liquid or yoghurt), rating order (first or second), rater and participant. The analyses were limited by the small number of participants and the heterogeneity of the participant sample. The total number of swallows rated across the group was high (n=1800) and the number of raters used was considerable (n=15). However,

given that the same 15 individuals were producing each of the swallows, the swallows were all highly-related and were therefore not independent data points, potentially reducing the statistical power of the study. The small and diverse participant sample also limits the ability to directly generalise these findings to any particular population with dysphagia.

What are the main results?

Both penetration and aspiration in patients with dysphagia were rated more severely by experienced health professionals using FEES than using VFS. The authors concluded that FEES and VSF should not be used interchangeably in clinical practice, as they do not lead to equivalent interpretations of swallowing function/dysfunction.

How might we use this evidence to inform practice?

After appraising the article, you come to a number of conclusions. Firstly, you realise that, although the Penetration Aspiration Scale scores were higher for the FEES than for the VFS recordings, the article does not provide information about the sensitivity or specificity of the results in relation to a gold standard for detecting aspiration, and you decide to look for further research in this area. Secondly, FEES and VSF are not interchangeable and swapping between them for a single client may provide a misleading view of the client's changes over time. However, since FEES is more appropriate for repeated use for a client like Mr Pitt, and this is only his second instrumental swallowing assessment, you will consider using FEES from this point onwards, in order to ensure a homogenous interpretation of Mr Pitt's swallowing over time. Thirdly, it is not clear which test is best at predicting aspiration pneumonia. Finally, you do not know whether Mr Pitt's type of dysphagia (neurological degenerative) is best predicted by the FEES test as any sub-group analysis was limited by the small sample of widely differing types of dysphagia.

Medicine example

Clinical scenario

You are a general practitioner working with a primary care team. One of the issues for the team is dealing with the standard way of screening for renal disease (albuminuria) in diabetes of pregnancy, which is becoming a more frequent problem. The standard method is a 24-hour collection of urine from which the lab estimates the albumin excreted. However this method is a problem because it is very inconvenient for women who dislike having to collect it (especially a problem if they have to urinate while out of the home) and bring a large bulky container to the clinic. Yet the information is vital as the presence of microalbuminuria predicts the rate of pre-eclampsia well in women with diabetes of pregnancy. The nurses in the practice are certain that adherence to the 24-hour urine collections is not good, with missing urines leading to underestimates of albuminuria. 'Isn't the usual screening, which is just measuring the urine albumin-to-creatinine ratio, as we do for pregnant women without diabetes, just as good?' one of the nurses asked at a staff meeting.

Clinical question

In women with diabetes of pregnancy, how accurate is the urine albumin-to-creatinine ratio compared to the 'gold standard' of 24-hour excretion of albumin when screening for albuminuria?

Search terms and databases used to find the evidence

Database: PubMed—Clinical Queries (with 'diagnosis category' and 'broad, sensitive' search selected)

Search terms: albuminuria diabetes pregnancy

This search retrieved 30 titles. The sixth article listed was the most relevant to the question and the full text of the article was available online (a 'free' journal article, http://care.diabetesjournals.org/cgi/reprint/29/4/924).

Article chosen

Justesen T, Petersen J, Ekbom P et al. Albumin-to-creatinine ratio in random urine samples might replace 24-h urine collections in screening for micro- and macroalbuminuria in pregnant woman with type 1 diabetes. Diabetes Care 2006; 29:924–925.

Structured abstract

Study design and participants: All women with diabetes in pregnancy who were admitted to the hospital's obstetrics department before 14 weeks of gestation were invited to participate and 119 were enrolled in the study. The urine samples were collected between gestational weeks 7 and 22.

Setting: A university hospital in Denmark.

Description of test: Two random samples of urine collected at different times were used to estimate the albumin-to-creatinine ratio. The cut-off point was >2.5mg albumin/ mmole of creatinine.

Diagnostic 'gold standard': 24-hour urine collections were tested for albumin. The cut-off point was >30mg albumin/24 hours.

Main results: The albumin-to-creatinine ratio had a sensitivity of 94% and a specificity of 100%. Its positive predictive value was 100% and the negative predictive value was 99%.

Conclusion: The simpler and more convenient test (two samples of urine rather than the 24-hour collection) performs well.

Is the evidence likely to be biased?

- *Did all participants get the diagnostic test and the reference standard?*
  Yes. The article describes that all eligible women used both tests.
- *Could the results of the test of interest have been influenced by the results of the reference standard or vice versa?*
  No. The tests were analysed by the laboratory, and were probably automated, which could not have allowed one result to have influenced the other.
- *Is the disease status of the tested population clearly described?*
  Yes. The women were clearly defined. Their mean age was 30 (±4) years, they had had diabetes for a mean of 16 (±7) years and their HbA_{1c} (glycated haemoglobin level) was 7.6 (±1%).
- *Were the methods for performing the test described in sufficient detail?*
  Yes. The cut-off points are described. Details of the biochemical tests are described in detail and this will enable people to replicate them.

What are the main results?

Table 7.4 shows how the 119 women tested for both tests and Table 7.5 shows a summary of the test accuracy for the test that used two random urine samples. These results show that testing for albuminuria had a high specificity, which means that there would be very few false positives. (There were none in this sample, but the numbers were small enough to lend some uncertainty which is expressed by the 95% confidence interval.) The sensitivity was also high at 94%, suggesting that few women with albuminuria would be missed—that is, few false negatives. (In this sample there was only one.) A positive predictive value of 100% means that we know the chance of a woman having albuminuria after having two random samples of urine test positive is 100%. Similarly, based on the negative predictive value, the chance of a woman *not* having it after a negative test is 99%.

The positive likelihood ratio is the ratio of the probability of the test being positive among women with albuminuria divided by that of those who do not have albuminuria. The negative likelihood ratio is the ratio of the probability of the test being negative among women who do not have albuminuria divided by that of those who do. In this study the positive likelihood ratio is ∞, because dividing the sensitivity of 94% by [100 – specificity (100%)] would give an infinitely large number. In other words, the test is extremely good for ruling in the presence of albuminuria if it is present. Using the values presented in Chapter 6, the negative likelihood ratio of 0.06 indicates that it is a test that is extremely good for ruling out the presence of albuminuria.

How might we use this evidence to inform practice?

The simpler test seems to perform so well that your team decides to use it at the practice instead of the slightly more accurate one, judging that the extra convenience of the two random urine samples is much more likely to be adhered to than the cumbersome, embarrassing and inconvenient 24-hour urine collection gold standard.

	Gold standard (24-hour urinary excretion)	
Mean of two random urine samples albumin:creatinine ratio	≤30mg/24 hours	>30mg/24 hours
≤2.5mg/mmole	103	1
>2.5mg/mmole	0	15
	103	16

TABLE 7.4 Results for 24-hour urine collection and two random urine samples for all participants

Diagnosis	Sensitivity (95% CI)	Specificity (95% CI)	Positive predictive value	Negative predictive value	Positive likelihood ratio	Negative likelihood ratio	Post-test probability
Albuminuria	94% (70 to 100%)	100% (94 to 100%)	100%	99%	∞	0.06	6%

∞ = an infinitely large number

TABLE 7.5 Summary of the test accuracy for the test that used two random urine samples

Nursing example

Clinical scenario

You are a nurse working in a hospital emergency department which has an established chest pain evaluation unit to assist in rapid diagnosis and intervention for cardiac clients. Specific protocols were implemented on establishment of the unit to guide practice and assist in the diagnosis and prioritisation of clients with acute, undifferentiated chest pain. A recent conference presentation suggested that serial monitoring in chest pain units was not clinically beneficial. Adding to your interest in this information is the admission of a 64-year-old male for assessment of chest pain. He also has hyperlipidaemia and is a cigarette smoker. He had a normal initial electrocardiograph (ECG) but had low tolerance of serial monitoring as it increased his anxiety levels. As you are a qualified cardiac nurse, you have a specific interest in participating in the unit review of chest pain diagnostic protocols and begin considering whether the research literature can provide evidence on the diagnostic validity of specific elements of the protocols that your chest pain unit uses, particularly for the diagnosis of clinical myocardial infarction.

Clinical question

In adults admitted to a chest pain unit, which elements of serial diagnostic testing are the most sensitive and specific predictors of clinical myocardial infarction?

Search terms and databases used to find the evidence

Database: PubMed—Clinical Queries (with 'diagnosis category' and 'narrow search' selected)

Search terms: (chest pain unit) AND (diagnostic test*)

This search yields five results. From their titles, two of these appear to be potentially relevant studies. You read their abstracts and find that one study clearly addresses the issue of diagnostic elements in chest pain unit protocols and is a good fit with your clinical question.

Article chosen

Goodacre S, Locker T, Arnold J et al. Which diagnostic tests are most useful in a chest pain unit protocol? BMC Emerg Med 2005; 5:6.

Structured abstract

Study design: Cohort study.

Study question: What is the diagnostic accuracy (sensitivity, specificity and likelihood ratios) of four tests for acute coronary syndrome at presentation? The study also aimed to determine the prognostic value of these tests but this component of the study is not relevant to the clinical question and will not be described.

Setting: Chest pain unit that is part of the emergency department of an urban teaching hospital in the UK.

Participants: Diagnostic test results were prospectively recorded for all clients who were assessed in the unit during a specified time period. There were a total of 706 participants (mean age 53.6 years; 61% male). Patients are assessed in the unit if they present with acute chest pain and have a normal or non-diagnostic ECG, no comorbidities that require admission, no serious alternative cause for chest pain and pain that is potentially compatible with cardiac ischaemia.

Description of tests: Serial electrocardiograph (ECG) recording and ST segment monitoring every hour for 2 to 6 hours; biochemical cardiac markers (blood tests for evidence of damage to heart muscle)—CK-MB (mass) at 2 or 6 hours after symptom onset and troponin T assay at least 6 hours after symptom onset; exercise treadmill test.

Main results: Sensitivities for acute coronary syndrome with myocardial infarction and acute coronary syndrome with myocyte necrosis, respectively, were: serial ECG/ST segment monitoring, 33% and 23%; CK-MB (mass), 96% and 63%; and troponin T (0.03ng/mL threshold), 96% and 90%.

Conclusion: Serial ECG/ST segment monitoring has little diagnostic value in people with normal or non-diagnostic initial ECG, with the small number of diagnostic values recorded confounded by a high level of false positive results. CK-MB (mass) can rule out acute coronary syndrome with clinical myocardial infarction but not myocyte necrosis.

Is this evidence likely to be biased?

* *Did all participants get the diagnostic test and the reference standard?*
  Yes. The article reports that diagnostic performance of all tests (except for the treadmill) was compared with the reference standard for diagnosis of acute coronary syndrome on presentation. The routine diagnostic methods used in the chest pain unit were based on the recommendations of the British Cardiac Society and findings of a systematic review.
* *Could the results of the test of interest have been influenced by the results of the reference standard, or vice versa?*
  Yes. The authors state that the reference standard for diagnosis was not independent of the tests that were being evaluated.
* *Is the disease status of the tested population clearly described?*
  Yes. The disease severity of the population is clearly described. To be assessed by the chest pain unit clients were required to have chest pain, a normal or non-diagnostic ECG and absence of comorbidities. Presenting symptoms were clearly described and contraindications to chest pain unit admission and comorbidities associated with increased risk of acute coronary syndrome were also detailed.
* *Were the methods for performing the test described in sufficient detail?*
  Yes. The methods of diagnostic testing are clearly described, with parameters for frequency, positive findings and test protocol methods described in detail.

What are the main results?

From the sample of 706 participants, 30 (4.2%) were diagnosed with acute coronary syndrome with myocardial infarction and 30 (4.2%) with acute coronary syndrome with myocyte necrosis. Table 7.6 presents the sensitivity, specificity, positive and negative predictive values and positive and negative likelihood ratios for the diagnosis of acute coronary syndrome with clinical myocardial infarction at presentation. The ability of these tests to diagnose acute coronary syndrome with myocyte necrosis or clinical myocardial infarction at presentation is further analysed in the article, but these results are not presented here.

As can be seen in Table 7.6, serial ECG recording and ST monitoring had a low sensitivity (ability of the test to detect the disease in people who have the disease). The sensitivity of this test was much lower than any of the other tests presented. Similarly, the positive predictive value (the probability that a client has the disease if the test is positive) was also much lower than the other tests. Using the approximate guide values that were presented in Chapter 6, a test with a positive likelihood ratio greater than 10 is an extremely good test for ruling in the disease. This was not the case for the serial ECG and ST monitoring but was evident in the results of the other three tests that are presented in Table 7.6. Similarly, a test with a negative likelihood ratio less than 0.5 demonstrates a test that helps rules out the disease, with a ratio of less than 0.1 indicating that the test is even more capable of doing this. On this basis, serial ECG and ST monitoring does not achieve this. These results indicate that serial ECG and ST monitoring may not be as useful as the other tests for the diagnosis of acute coronary syndrome with clinical myocardial infarction at presentation. Another result of interest is that the lower threshold of Troponin T (>0.03 ng/mL) improved the sensitivity of this test.

How might we use this evidence to inform practice?

The characteristics of participants in this study appear similar to the client in your clinical scenario. Although he is slightly older than the mean age reported in the study, he fits within the age range described in the study. Additionally, his comorbidities of hyperlipidaemia and the fact that he is a smoker are similar to characteristics of the sample of participants. The diagnostic testing methods described in the article are congruent with the current practice in your unit hence there is ready applicability to your unit and client, with no significant cost or resource implications to consider. With these similarities in mind, the low sensitivity, positive predictive value and positive likelihood ratio of serial ECG recording and ST segment monitoring suggest that you can review the diagnostic protocol currently used and consider a move away from serial ECG recording and ST segment monitoring, particularly for clients who have a normal or non-diagnostic initial ECG such as the client described in the clinical scenario. This decision would be strengthened by considering other research that addresses the same issue.

	Sensitivity (95% CI)	Specificity (95% CI)	Positive predictive value (95% CI)	Negative predictive value (95% CI)	Positive likelihood ratio (95% CI)	Negative likelihood ratio (95% CI)
Serial ECG & ST monitoring (N=690)	33.3% (19.2 to 51.2%)	95.3% (93.4 to 96.7%)	24.4% (13.8 to 39.3%)	96.9% (95.3 to 98.0%)	7.1 (3.8 to 13.1)	0.700 (0.5 to 0.9)
Delta CK-MB (mass) (N=601)	95.7% (79.0 to 99.2%)	98.4% (97.0 to 99.1%)	70.0% (53.4 to 83.9%)	99.8% (99.0 to 100%)	61.4 (39.1 to 118.1)	0.04 (0.006 to 0.3)
Troponin T >0.1ng/mL (N=686)	83.3% (66.4 to 92.7%)	98.8% (97.7 to 99.4%)	75.8% (59.0 to 87.2%)	99.3% (98.3 to 99.7%)	70.4 (34.1 to 140.8)	0.169 (0.07 to 0.4)
Troponin T >0.03ng/mL (N=686)	96.4% (82.3 to 99.4%)	95.9% (94.1 to 97.2%)	50.0% (37.1 to 62.9%)	99.8% (99.1 to 100%)	23.5 (16.1 to 34.2)	0.037 (0.005 to 0.26)

TABLE 7.6 Sensitivity, specificity, positive and negative predictive values and positive and negative likelihood ratios for the diagnosis of acute coronary syndrome with clinical myocardial infarction at presentation

Medical imaging example

Clinical scenario

As the newly appointed chief radiographer of a metropolitan public hospital which has a large gastroenterology unit you are relieved to learn that the department has recently upgraded much of its medical imaging equipment and now offers a full digital imaging service including a 64-slice computed tomography (CT) scanner. As you review the range of CT examinations that have been performed since its installation, you are surprised at the small number of referrals for CT colonography. This is in contrast to what occurred in the hospital where you previously worked, in which there was a move towards giving symptomatic and selected screening clients access to CT colonography in preference to them having to undergo a colonoscopy. You discuss this matter with the Director of Medical Imaging. The Director is sympathetic with your desire to ensure that referrers are aware of the full diagnostic capabilities of the imaging modalities that are available to them. However, before having any broader discussion with the referring health professionals, it is agreed that you will investigate if there is research evidence that supports the broader use of CT colonography in preference to colonoscopy.

Clinical question

What are the sensitivity and specificity of CT colonography, compared to colonoscopy, in the detection of small polyps and lesions in symptomatic people?

Search terms and databases used to find the evidence

Database: PubMed—Clinical Queries (with 'diagnosis category' and 'narrow search' selected)

Search terms: (computed tomography colonography) AND (polyps OR lesions) AND symptomatic

The search yields 11 articles. Based on the abstracts, three articles appear to be potentially relevant and one of these used a similar patient population to the one in your clinic, so you retrieve the full text of this article.

Article chosen

Roberts-Thomson IC, Tucker GR, Hewett PJ et al. Single-center study comparing computed tomography colonography with conventional colonoscopy. World J Gastroenterol 2008; 14:469–473.

The article is available online at: http://www.wjgnet.com/1007-9327/14/469.asp.

Structured abstract

Design: A cohort study comparing sensitivity and specificity of CT colonography with colonoscopy.

Setting: A metropolitan teaching hospital in Australia.

Participants: 227 patients (mean age 60 years; 51% male) presenting with appropriate indications for colonoscopy. Exclusion criteria included inflammatory bowel disease and major coexisting medical disorders.

Description of tests: CT colonography was performed with a multi-slice helical CT scanner with 2-mm collimation that was reconstructed into intervals of 1.0–1.5mm. Colonic distension was achieved by insufflation of carbon dioxide and the use of intravenous Buscopan. Participants were scanned in both supine and prone positions during a single breath hold. Images were read in two-dimensional format with the use of a targeted three-dimensional format when necessary.

Diagnostic standard: Colonoscopy.

Main results: The sensitivity of CT colonography was 71% (95% CI 52% to 85%) for polyps ≥6mm in size. Specificity was 67% (95% CI 56% to 76%) for polyps ≥6mm in size.

Conclusion: CT colonography is well accepted by patients and carries a low risk of adverse effects. However, it is not sensitive enough for widespread application in symptomatic patients.

Is this evidence likely to be biased?

- *Did all participants get the diagnostic test and the reference standard?*
  Yes. All participants received the CT colonography and the colonoscopy. Both tests were performed on the same day. Of the 227 patients recruited, 202 were successfully evaluated with both procedures. Twenty-five (11%) of participants were excluded from analysis participation due to incomplete colonoscopy or poor bowel preparation, both of which are factors that cannot be predicted.
- *Could the results of the test of interest have been influenced by the results of the reference standard or vice versa?*
  No. Colonoscopists were blinded to the CT colonography results prior to the colonoscopy but were segmentally unblinded during the procedure (that is, CT colonography results of the right colon were made available after the colonoscopy of the right colon had been done, and then the same occurred for the left colon). This ensured that all findings reported by CT colonography could be verified during the colonoscopy in real time and any discrepancies clarified by the colonoscopy while the participant was sedated.
- *Is the disease status of the tested population clearly described?*
  Yes. The article states that participants were symptomatic patients with appropriate indications for colonoscopy such as rectal bleeding, abdominal pain and/or change in bowel habits. Some participants also had a family history of colorectal cancer, previous colonic polyps or recent positive faecal occult blood test.
- *Were the methods for performing the test described in sufficient detail?*
  Partially. The procedure for each of the tests was described in reasonable detail. The type of bowel preparation for the CT colonography was not standardised and determined by the colonoscopist, with little detail provided about this.

What are the main results?

Table 7.7 shows the sensitivity, specificity and positive and negative likelihood ratios of CT colonography when analysed according to polyp size. These results show that CT colonography had low to moderate sensitivity and specificity, although this improved when the polyps were larger (≥6mm). According to the positive likelihood ratio, only when polyps are ≥6mm is CT colonography likely to be of some diagnostic value, suggesting a minimal increase in the likelihood of ruling in the presence of polyps if positive. Similarly, the negative likelihood ratios indicate that only when polyps are ≥6mm is CT colonography likely to be able to help rule out polyps when negative.

Polyp size	Sensitivity (95% CI)	Specificity (95% CI)	Positive likelihood ratio	Negative likelihood ratio
<6mm	42% (30 to 55%)	63% (52 to 73%)	1.13	0.92
≥6mm	71% (52 to 85%)	67% (56 to 76%)	2.15	0.43

TABLE 7.7 Sensitivity, specificity and positive and negative likelihood ratios of CT colonography when analysed according to polyp size

How might we use this evidence to inform practice?

The study participants were selected from clients who were referred for a colonoscopy on the basis of symptoms suggestive of colonic pathology and are well matched with the types of clients that you encounter in your clinic in terms of age and indications for colonoscopy. Clients in which CT colonography might be indicated include elderly people who are contraindicated for colonoscopy and those with known bowel obstruction. In such clients, CT colonography can overcome some of the problems associated with colonoscopy. However, the results are dependent on polyp size which limits the usefulness of CT colonography as a screening tool for clients with small (<6mm) lesions. Given that the sensitivity and specificity of CT colonography are not yet sufficient to implement it on a routine basis, you propose to recommend its use only among suitable clients who could benefit from this procedure. Relative costs and complications of the procedures must also be considered.

References

1. Hegedus E, Goode A, Campbell S et al. Physical examination tests of the shoulder: a systematic review with meta-analysis of individual tests. Br J Sports Med 2008; 42:80–92.

CHAPTER 8

Evidence about prognosis

Mark R Elkins

LEARNING OBJECTIVES

After reading this chapter, you should be able to:

- Generate a structured clinical question about prognosis for a clinical scenario
- Appraise the validity of prognostic evidence
- Understand how to interpret the results from prognostic studies and calculate additional results (such as confidence intervals) where possible
- Describe how prognostic evidence can be used to inform practice
- Clearly explain prognostic information to a client

Let us consider a clinical scenario that will be useful for illustrating the concepts of evidence about prognosis that are the focus of this chapter.

Clinical scenario

Mrs Wilson is a 68-year-old woman with osteoarthritis affecting her knees and left hip. Her local doctor has referred her to an orthopaedic surgeon regarding her right knee. The pain in her right knee has been worsening for the past 6 months, making it difficult to manage stairs. The surgeon has recommended a total knee arthroplasty (knee replacement). Mrs Wilson also has mild chronic obstructive pulmonary disease. She takes no medication for this and has not smoked for almost 30 years. Mrs Wilson cares for her husband who has Parkinson's disease. He recently fractured his arm in a fall at home, but has recovered well. Mrs Wilson has not decided whether to proceed with the total knee arthroplasty.

The clinical scenario above raises several questions about the future of the client's condition. What change in pain and mobility can Mrs Wilson expect if she chooses not to undergo the surgery? If she decides not to have the operation now, for how long will she remain a suitable candidate for surgery? Assuming the surgery is performed, many more questions are raised. How long will it take for the immediate symptoms associated with the surgery to resolve? Will complications occur? How much improvement in mobility can she expect after the surgery? How long will it take to achieve this level of mobility? Will surgical revision of the joint replacement become necessary and, if so, when? These types of questions will be the focus of this chapter on prognosis.

Prognosis is about predicting the future—the future of a client's condition. While it is impossible for anyone to predict the future with absolute certainty, we can use evidence from the past to make informed and sensible predictions about the future. These evidence-based predictions about the future can be useful in many ways. They can help reassure clients by removing some doubt about the future, especially if their expectations are unjustifiably pessimistic. Predictions about natural recovery can help you and your client to jointly decide whether interventions need to be considered at all. Sometimes an intervention is chosen that is typically applied only once, as with joint replacement or organ transplant. In such cases, the optimal time to apply the intervention can be determined by predictions about the rate of deterioration before it and the rate of recovery after it. Predictions about the average course of a particular condition can also be adjusted for individual clients. This adjustment is possible when other features about a client or the client's health or management besides the primary diagnosis have been shown to affect outcomes.

This chapter will address the process of using prognostic evidence to make these predictions and incorporating them into clinical practice. We will start by defining the components of a structured clinical question about prognosis. Then we will see how to appraise the evidence to determine its likely validity. Subsequent sections of the chapter will review how to understand the results of a prognostic study, how to use the evidence to inform practice and how to explain prognostic information clearly to clients.

How to structure a prognostic question

You will recall from Chapter 2 that clinical questions can be structured using the PICO format: patient/problem, intervention/issue, comparison (if relevant) and outcomes. When our question was about the effect of intervention, the comparison was an important component. The effect of an intervention was always estimated by comparison against this component, even if it was a 'no-intervention' or usual care control. Questions about prognosis, instead, are questions about expected outcomes, not questions about what has caused those outcomes. Therefore, the comparison component is not used in questions about prognosis. Let us look at each of the remaining components in more detail.

Patient/problem

The patient/problem component can simply be specified as previously described, for example, '*In clients with coronary heart disease …*', '*Among children with epilepsy …*' or, from our scenario, '*In adults with osteoarthritis of the knee …*'. Sometimes, the prognosis for typical clients with the condition is quite different to the prognosis for clients with some extra characteristic. For example, the prognosis for clients with cystic fibrosis who become infected with the bacteria *Burkholderia cepacia* is worse than for those who do not.[1] Characteristics that influence outcomes are known as **prognostic factors**. If you suspect that some characteristic of your client might be a prognostic factor, this can be incorporated into the patient/problem component. Let us assume for a moment that Mrs Wilson, the client in our scenario at the beginning of this chapter, is mildly obese. This may be a prognostic factor, so we could incorporate this into our clinical question: *In adults with osteoarthritis of the knee who are obese* …. In addition to comorbidities like obesity, prognostic factors can also relate to the severity of the condition, for example, '*In clients with coronary heart disease (New York Heart Association Functional Class IV) …*'. The New York Heart Association functional classification is a simple way of describing the extent of heart disease. It places clients in one of four categories based on the severity of their symptoms and how much they are limited during exercise. The history of the condition can also be a prognostic factor, for example, '*Among children who have had their first epileptic seizure …*'.

Intervention/issue

The next component of the question is the intervention/issue. If you are interested in the natural course of a condition, then you can simply add the term 'untreated' to your clinical question, for example, '*In children with untreated nocturnal enuresis …*'. This will remind you when you search for evidence that you are interested in prognostic evidence about untreated clients. It is logical to assume that a client's prognosis may be affected by receiving an intervention, especially if the intervention has been shown to be effective. Therefore, a clinical question about prognosis should specify what intervention a client has received or is receiving for their condition. In fact, some questions are only relevant to a population that has received an intervention, such as in these two examples, '*In clients undergoing surgical skin grafts for major burns, what is the risk of postoperative complications?*' and '*Among clients who no longer stutter at the end of a course of intensive therapy, what is the probability that their stuttering will relapse in the next year?*'

Outcomes

The last component of a clinical question about prognosis is outcomes. It is important to consider outcomes that will have the greatest impact on the client's goals and priorities. The prognosis can also change over time. For example, among alcoholic women who are able to stop drinking alcohol and remain abstained from it, the average improvements in memory and psychomotor speed at 1 year are minimal, while by 4 years they have usually returned to within the normal range.[2] Therefore, it is sometimes worthwhile adding a time frame to the outcome component of your clinical question.

Clinical scenario (continued): Structuring the clinical question

There are many prognostic questions that can be drawn from our scenario. Let us assume that Mrs Wilson has had further discussions with her orthopaedic surgeon and has now decided to go ahead with the surgery. Her primary concern is arranging care for her husband while she is incapacitated by the surgery. Mrs Wilson is keen to know how long it will take for her to regain the function in her knee, particularly her ability to walk independently. Mrs Wilson is eligible for 2 weeks of respite care and the Wilsons' son is able to take 4 weeks off work to assist with the care of his father. From this scenario, a suitable prognostic question would be: In clients undergoing total knee arthroplasty for osteoarthritis, what improvement in walking ability would be expected after 6 weeks?

Clinical scenario (continued): Finding the evidence to answer your question

You start by looking for a prospective cohort study in PubMed Clinical Queries, filtering your search with the 'prognosis' and 'narrow' options selected and using the search terms: osteoarthritis AND ('total knee' OR TKA OR TKR) AND walking ability. You have included TKA and TKR in your search terms as total knee arthroplasty is sometimes abbreviated as TKA and is sometimes referred to as total knee replacement or its abbreviation, TKR. This search results in nine articles. A quick scan of the titles confirms that several of the articles are probably relevant. One of these is very close to what we require, but the earliest point at which outcomes are measured is 6 months after the surgery. Another appears to be exactly what we require as it provides data about mean walking ability from 1 week to 1 year after the surgery.[3] Throughout the rest of this chapter, we will refer to this study as the 'knee arthroplasty study'.

The results of your search—only nine articles with a substantial proportion seeming relevant—suggests that the search may be too narrow. Using the 'broad' search option or adjusting the search terms may help. A third strategy is to click on the 'Related Articles' link next to the most relevant article we have retrieved. This triggers a search in which PubMed seeks the most similar articles it can find to the one you have indicated. In this instance, 102 articles are retrieved. A scan of the titles, and of the abstracts for the most promising titles, identifies very similar types of articles but nothing more suitable than the best article that you chose from the original search.

Clinical scenario (continued): Structured abstract of our chosen article (the 'knee arthroplasty study')

Citation: Kennedy D, Stratford P, Riddle D et al. Assessing recovery and establishing prognosis following total knee arthroplasty. Phys Ther 2008; 88:22–32.

Question: In clients undergoing a primary knee replacement for osteoarthritis, what is the pattern of improvement in lower limb function and walking ability from 1 week to 1 year after surgery?

Design: Inception cohort followed prospectively for 1 year.

Setting: Tertiary care orthopaedic facility in Toronto, Canada.

Participants: Eighty-four clients with osteoarthritis (mean age 66 years, 52% female) undergoing primary total knee arthroplasty. Participants needed to be able to communicate in written and spoken English. Exclusion criteria were any neurological, cardiac or psychiatric disorders or other medical conditions that would substantially compromise physical function.

Prognostic factors: Gender, pre-operative lower limb function and pre-operative 6-Minute Walk Test distance.

Outcomes: Lower Extremity Functional Scale—a self-reported, 20-item scale of lower extremity function that includes activity limitation and participation restriction concepts and is scored from 0 (lowest function) to 80 (highest function). Six-Minute Walk Test—a submaximal exercise test in which participants walk the greatest distance they can in 6 minutes on flat ground with standard encouragement.

Main results: In general, there was a deterioration in both scores at the immediate postoperative measurement. From this point, there was rapid improvement in both scores initially, with progressively slower gains in improvement with increasing time postsurgery. Gender and pre-operative function were prognostic factors for each outcome. For the Lower Extremity Functional Scale, assuming the average preoperative function of the cohort, females had scores of 18 at 1 week, 38 at 6 weeks, and 53 at 6 months. Males had scores of 25 at 1 week, 43 at 6 weeks, and 60 at 6 months. For the 6-Minute Walk Test, assuming the average preoperative function of the cohort, females achieved 200m at 1 week, 330m at 6 weeks, and 470m at 6 months. Males achieved 250m at 1 week, 440m at 6 weeks, and 580m at 6 months. All the 6-month values were maintained to 1 year.

Conclusions: For both outcomes, the rate of improvement was greatest immediately following surgery. Roughly half of the postoperative improvement was observed in the first 6 weeks. This brought clients to an adequate level of function for typical daily activities. Almost all of the remaining improvement had occurred by 6 months, with both outcomes then being maintained until the end of the year.

Is this evidence likely to be biased?

We will use questions drawn from the Critical Appraisal Skills Program (CASP) and associated checklists for appraising a cohort study to explain how to assess the likelihood of bias in a prognostic study. Note, however, that the checklist for cohort studies is not only intended for use with longitudinal single-group studies, but also with other study

---

BOX 8.1 KEY QUESTIONS TO ASK WHEN APPRAISING THE VALIDITY (RISK OF BIAS) OF A PROGNOSTIC STUDY

1. Was there a representative and well-defined sample?
2. Was there an inception cohort?
3. Was exposure determined accurately?
4. Were the outcomes measured accurately?
5. Were important prognostic factors considered and adjusted for?
6. Was the follow-up of participants sufficiently long and complete?

---

designs such as case-control studies. Therefore, not all the questions that are raised in the checklist will be explained in this chapter. The key questions to ask when appraising the validity of a prognostic study are summarised in Box 8.1. The checklist begins with two simple screening criteria that, if not met, indicate that the article is unlikely to be helpful and that further assessment of potential bias is probably unwarranted.

Did the study address a clearly focussed issue?

The first criterion on the checklist is whether the study addressed a clearly focussed issue. For prognostic evidence, the article should clearly define the population, potential prognostic factors and the outcomes considered.

Clinical scenario (continued): Did the study address a clearly focussed issue?

The knee arthroplasty study meets this criterion, as shown in the question it seeks to answer: In clients undergoing a primary knee replacement for osteoarthritis, what is the pattern of improvement in lower limb function and walking ability from 1 week to 1 year after surgery?

Appropriate study type

The second criterion is that the method used was appropriate to answer the question posed by the authors. In Chapter 2, we saw that longitudinal studies, particularly prospective cohort studies, provide the best evidence about prognosis. Even better than that is a systematic review of prospective cohort studies. However, currently there are so few systematic reviews of prognostic studies in this area that it is probably not realistic for you to expect to find one.

Although prospective cohort studies are typically the study type that you should use to answer prognostic questions, you should be aware that prognostic information can also be generated by other study designs. For example, if you are interested in the natural history of a condition, then the outcomes of an untreated control group in a randomised controlled trial can provide this information. Conversely, case-control studies or case series, where all cases receive a particular treatment, give prognostic information about a treated cohort.

Clinical scenario (continued): Appropriate study type

The researchers in the knee arthroplasty study wanted to find prognostic data and they used the ideal study design for this: a prospective, longitudinal study of an inception cohort of clients undergoing primary total knee arthroplasty. Therefore, we can move on to the more detailed criteria on the CASP checklist.

Representative and well-defined sample of participants

The next criterion on the checklist is whether the cohort was recruited in a way that ensured it was representative of the larger population of interest. This criterion is important as a study's estimate of prognosis will be biased if the study's sample is systematically different from (and therefore not representative of) the larger population of interest. It is important that a study clearly defines its inclusion and exclusion criteria as this can help in recruiting a representative sample. Clearly defined criteria help make it clear to everyone (researchers, participants, you) just what the target population of the study was. A representative sample is also more likely to be obtained if the study recruits all of the eligible clients who presented at the recruitment site into the study. When appraising a study, look for a statement in the article that describes either recruiting 'all clients' or recruiting 'consecutive cases'. Recruiting all eligible clients prevents bias in the data that could arise if some eligible clients avoided recruitment and these clients differ in some systematic way from those who were recruited. The greater the proportion of eligible clients that are recruited into the study, the more representative of the target population the sample is likely to be.

Clinical scenario (continued): Representative and well-defined sample

In the knee arthroplasty study, the researchers were unable to achieve consecutive recruitment because of the outbreak of severe acute respiratory syndrome (SARS) in Toronto during their data collection period. However, we are not too concerned about this as it is unlikely to have caused recruitment of an unrepresentative sample. Additionally, the inclusion and exclusion criteria of the study are clearly defined. We conclude that the cohort is likely to be representative of the target population.

The problem with retrospective studies

As we saw in Chapter 2, cohort studies can either be prospective or retrospective, with retrospective studies being lower down the hierarchy of evidence for prognostic questions. The reason for this is that studies that identify clients retrospectively are more likely to have recruitment bias. This is because it is relatively common for clients with a particular characteristic to be systematically missed. As an extreme example, one retrospective study examined 81 clients with infections after total knee arthroplasty.[4] Clearly, we cannot use this cohort to determine the likelihood of joint infection, because this cohort was selected to ensure that 100% of clients had an infection. It is also inappropriate to use the cohort to determine, for example, the likelihood of independent mobility 1 year after total knee arthroplasty, as the mobility of individuals with infections may differ from that of all individuals who undergo knee arthroplasty. In other retrospective studies, the cohort is selected because they presented for treatment. For example, another study examined 1012 clients who presented for treatment of knee complaints after any previous knee injury.[5] The severity of the changes in bone and cartilage were compared to details in their health records to identify prognostic factors for the progression of osteoarthritis. Note that this study does not capture people who sustain a knee injury but do not present for treatment of knee complaints later, such as those who develop very mild or no osteoarthritis. The data from this study could therefore lead to excessively pessimistic predictions about the likely severity of osteoarthritis after knee injury. Instead, what is needed is a study in which clients are identified at the time of knee injury and followed for decades to assess the development of osteoarthritis.[6]

Inception cohort

Although it is not explicitly mentioned on the CASP checklist (but rather is covered by the question 'Was the cohort recruited in an acceptable way?' on the checklist), one of the things that will help you to determine whether the cohort was recruited in an acceptable way and a key issue that affects the validity of a cohort study (by minimising selection bias) is whether there was an inception cohort. In other words, were participants recruited at a similar well-described point in the course of the disease? It is important that this was done because a group of people with the same condition may vary in their prognoses because of how long they have had the condition. Consider the scenario of a disease that is sometimes fatal, with the deaths that do occur usually being within 2 years of its onset. If we consider the prognosis for short-term mortality, it is likely to be worse in newly diagnosed clients than in those who have had the disease for 5 years. This is because the 5-year survivors have survived the 'danger period' and now have a short-term mortality that is similar to people without the disease. This means that, in a cohort study that recruited people with this disease, the average prognosis could be greatly affected by the proportions of participants who are newly diagnosed and participants who are chronic (that is, diagnosed some time ago) that are recruited. Some studies recruit from sources, such as client support groups, that can bias recruitment towards these survivors, which makes any prognostic estimate favourable when this is really not an accurate estimate for this disease.

Avoiding this bias is solved by recruiting participants at a consistent and defined point in their disease. When this point is very early in the disease process, the cohort is called an 'inception' cohort. Some studies recruit participants at diagnosis. However, the point of diagnosis is not always at an early or a uniform point in the disease process. This is particularly the case for chronic conditions, for example rheumatoid arthritis or low back pain. You must therefore consider carefully whether a true inception cohort has been identified when recruitment occurs at diagnosis.

Clinical scenario (continued): Inception cohort

In the knee arthroplasty study, the participants were not recruited at the inception of their osteoarthritis, but we still have an inception cohort. They were recruited at their inception into our target population of clients undergoing total knee arthroplasty for osteoarthritis.

Determination of exposure

The next criterion on the checklist is whether exposure was determined accurately. The term 'exposure' can be confusing when referring to a simple prognostic cohort study as it is more commonly considered in case-control studies. For a simple prognostic cohort study, we can think of it as whether we have accurately determined eligibility criteria (that is, the main condition or disease or event that we are interested in determining the prognosis of). In the knee arthroplasty study, the criterion amounts to whether we have accurately determined whether our clients have undergone a total knee arthroplasty for osteoarthritis. While there is probably little chance of confusion about whether someone has undergone this procedure, the diagnosis of osteoarthritis may be more prone to error. This is relevant given that other prognostic studies have shown that some outcomes after total knee arthroplasty is performed because of *rheumatoid* arthritis differ markedly from those outcomes that occur when the total knee arthroplasty is performed because of osteoarthritis. [7]

Clinical scenario (continued): Determination of exposure

The knee arthroplasty article states that the study was conducted at a Centre of Excellence for knee replacement that is one of the largest centres in Canada that performs this procedure. While we cannot be completely certain, we can probably expect that the diagnoses were made correctly.

Accurate measurement of outcomes

Accuracy is not only important in the application of eligibility criteria, but also in the measurement of outcomes. Researchers should specify and clearly define their outcomes at the start of the study. We must consider whether the outcome measures have been **validated**—that is, do they measure what they claim to measure? The article that you are appraising should provide details about the validity of the outcome measures that were used. The CASP checklist also suggests that we consider whether the outcomes are objective (for example, a fall) or subjective (for example, pain). Although it is not always possible, outcomes should be measured using **objective criteria** where possible. As the subjectivity of the outcome measures increases, the risk of bias increases. In this situation, where the outcomes are subjective and require a degree of judgement on the part of the person who is doing the assessing of the outcome, it becomes important that the **assessor is blinded to the prognostic factors** that each client has. However, it can be difficult to blind assessors to certain prognostic factors of each client, such as age and gender. Prognostic factors are explained in more detail in the following section.

When prognostic studies report dichotomous outcomes, the criterion of accuracy is that the events have been clearly defined and a reliable system for identifying them has been implemented. Otherwise, some events might have occurred but not been recorded. For example, consider a cohort study of clients who commenced non-invasive ventilation for acute respiratory failure and reported the number of clients that died during that hospital admission. As this study involved hospitalised clients, the death of a client would have been recorded in the client's medical record, so we could be confident about the accuracy of this outcome. Now consider a cohort study that followed up elderly clients who had received an intervention (such as home assessment and modification) to prevent falls and evaluated whether the clients sustained a musculoskeletal injury in the year following the intervention. This dichotomous outcome (did or did not sustain musculoskeletal injury) is more difficult to measure accurately than the outcome of death in the above cohort study. Even if musculoskeletal injures were well defined and explained to clients, such injuries may not have been reported if a client misjudged whether the injury was musculoskeletal or forgot that it occurred.

Clinical scenario (continued): Measurement of outcomes

The knee arthroplasty article cites supportive data regarding the reliability, validity and ability to detect change for the Lower Extremity Functional Scale and the 6-Minute Walk Test. In terms of subjective versus objective outcomes, it is reassuring that there is one subjective continuous outcome measure and one objective continuous outcome measure that each measures the same concept— walking ability. It is even more reassuring that the results of the two measures are in agreement. The article does not mention whether assessors were blind to participants' prognostic factors so we will assume that they were not.

Confounding factors and prognostic factors

We saw in Chapter 2 how confounding factors are anything that can become confused with the outcome of interest and bias the results. Although the CASP checklist only refers to confounding factors, it can also be useful to consider a reasonable range of possible prognostic factors that may influence the outcome of interest in the study and check if the study has considered (and also measured) these factors. A **prognostic factor** is any characteristic that can influence the outcome of interest and is associated strongly enough with the outcome that it can accurately predict the eventual development of the outcome. Note that this does not necessarily mean that the prognostic factor causes the outcome. Prognostic factors can include demographic characteristics (such as age), disease-specific characteristics (for example, severity of a head injury) or whether the client has any comorbid conditions (that is, other conditions, for example hypertension or diabetes).

Many prognostic studies will report results for various subgroups of participants who differ because of the presence of a certain prognostic factor (or factors), and the prognosis that is reported for each subgroup will probably be different. When a study reports subgroup results like this, you need to check if the researchers did an adjusted analysis. By this we mean, did they check that these subgroup differences and predictions are not the result of another important prognostic factor? Information about any adjusted analysis that was done is usually presented in the data analysis section of an article. It is beyond the scope of this book to explain the statistical methods that are involved with adjusted analysis. If you are interested in understanding this, we suggest that you consult an additional statistical resource.

Sufficiently long and complete follow-up of participants

There are two elements to this criterion and you should assess whether the study meets both elements. You must use your knowledge about the condition of interest to judge whether the follow-up period was long enough for clinically important changes or events to occur. Consider a cohort study to determine the proportion of tracheostomised clients who can manage a speaking valve as soon as ventilatory support is weaned. The outcome from each participant can be determined within minutes. Therefore, a very short follow-up period is sufficient in this situation. Conversely, a cohort study of very low birth weight infants may need to follow participants for a decade or more to accurately assess the extent of neuro-developmental delay.

As we saw with randomised controlled trials in Chapter 4, the greater the loss to follow-up, the greater the opportunity for bias in the results, especially if there is something systematic about those who drop out. Some experts suggest using the '5 and 20' rule: a loss to follow-up of less than 5% is unlikely to influence the results much, while a loss greater than 20% starts to seriously threaten a study's validity.[8] Using the same rule-of-thumb guide (where a study that has at least 80–85% follow-up is unlikely to be seriously biased) that we discussed in Chapter 4 when explaining how to evaluate the adequacy of follow-up in a randomised controlled trial is another simple way to determine whether follow-up in a prognostic study was sufficiently complete. As with randomised controlled trials, a study should also state the reasons why participants were lost to follow-up. It can also be helpful if a study provides a comparison of prognostic factors for participants who were lost to follow-up and those who were not. This information can help you to determine whether there were certain types of participants who were selectively lost to follow-up.

Clinical scenario (continued): Follow-up of participants

In the knee arthroplasty study, there was so little change in the outcomes in the second 6 months of the follow-up period that it appears that a 1-year follow-up in total was long enough for all clinically important postoperative improvement to be captured. For data on a long-term dichotomous outcome (such as the time to revision of the total knee arthroplasty) to be collected, a follow-up period of 15 or 20 years would be required.[9] A potential complication following total knee arthroplasty is deep vein thrombosis, but the greatest risk of this occurring is during the period of reduced mobility postoperatively.[10] Therefore, the follow-up period of 1 year was adequate to detect this outcome if it were to occur (which it did in one participant). The period of follow-up is inadequate to pick up long-term surgical revisions due to prosthetic wear, but it will identify early revisions due to postoperative complications such as infection. There is no data provided in the article about the number of participants who were lost to follow-up, so you are unable to assess the adequacy of follow-up.

If you have got to this point and determined that the article about prognosis that you have been appraising is reasonably valid, you then proceed to look at the importance and applicability of the results.

What are the results?

Prognostic data can be presented in several ways and the results of the study may have been measured using continuous or dichotomous outcomes. In a similar manner to how we approached understanding the results of a randomised controlled trial in Chapter 4, when understanding prognostic results we will be looking at how to answer two main questions:

1. How **likely** are the outcomes over time?
2. How **precise** are the estimates of likelihood?

Likelihood of the outcomes over time

Regardless of the way the outcome was measured, the prognosis often changes over time. Thus, prognostic data are usually only relevant to a particular time period. For continuous outcomes, the expected value (usually the mean value) of the outcome at a certain point in time is what is usually reported. For example, *men with aphasia after their first stroke showed an average improvement of 12.3 on the Aphasia Quotient 1 year after the stroke.*[11] The Aphasia Quotient is a measure of the severity of aphasia, rated from 0 (worst) to 100 (best). Scores above 93.8 are considered normal (non-aphasic). Where the pattern of change in the outcome is of interest, the outcome may be graphed over time (see Figures 8.2 and 8.3 for graphs related to the knee arthroplasty clinical scenario).

Dichotomous outcomes can be reported as the proportion of clients who experienced the event at a particular time (that is, the risk of the event). For example, *among women who develop postnatal depression, 62% are likely to still have depression 3 months later.*[12] Alternatively, the same information can be reported as the risk for an individual client: *for a woman who develops postnatal depression, the risk of having depression 3 months later is 62%.* Where the change in risk over time is of interest, this may be graphed as a survival curve.

Survival curves are often used to present prognostic data and they show how the likelihood of an event changes over time. Figure 8.1 shows a survival curve from a study that examined the long-term risk of dislocation following total hip arthroplasty (replacement).[13] In this particular survival curve, the cumulative risk of hip dislocation

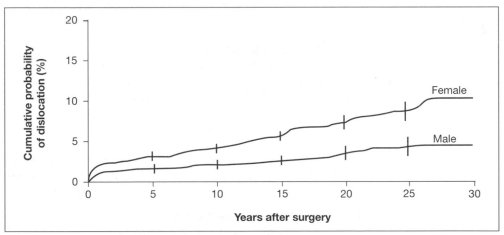

FIGURE 8.1   Cumulative probability of a first-time hip dislocation for female and male patients

From Berry DJ, von Knoch M, Schleck CD, Harmsen WS, The cumulative long-term risk of dislocation after primary Charnley total hip arthroplasty. J Bone Joint Surg Am 2004; 86:9–14. Reprinted with permission from The Journal of Bone and Joint Surgery, Inc.

following hip replacement is presented separately for females and males. You can see that at 25 years the risk of dislocation for females was 8.9% (the authors also provide the 95% confidence interval for this, 7.7% to 10.2%), whereas the risk for males was 4.5% (95% confidence interval 3.3% to 5.8%). You can also see, by looking at the slope of the curve, that female participants had both a higher early risk of dislocation as well as a higher late risk than male participants.

Precision of the estimates of likelihood

To properly interpret a prognostic study, it is necessary to know how much uncertainty is associated with its results. Just as we saw with estimates of the effect of an intervention in Chapter 4, a 95% confidence interval indicates the precision of the estimate of prognosis. As with the confidence intervals for randomised controlled trials, the larger the size of the prognostic study, the narrower (and more precise) the confidence interval will be. Confidence intervals can often be calculated if the authors of an article have not provided them.

Calculating a confidence interval for continuous outcomes

For continuous outcomes, the 95% confidence interval provides the range of average values within which we are 95% certain that the true average value lies. The confidence interval can be calculated approximately using the formula:

$$95\% \text{ confidence interval} = \text{mean} \pm (3 \times \text{standard deviation} \div \sqrt{2n})$$

where 'n' is the number of clients. Let us assume in our example of aphasia in men after their first stroke that the mean improvement of 12.3 on the Aphasia Quotient had a standard deviation of 18 and was determined using data from 83 clients.

$$95\% \text{ confidence interval} = \text{mean} \pm (3 \times \text{standard deviation} \div \sqrt{2n})$$
$$= 12.3 \pm (3 \times 18 \div \sqrt{2 * 83})$$
$$= 12.3 \pm (4.2)$$
$$= 8.1 \text{ to } 16.5$$

Therefore, we could expect that, in men with aphasia after their first stroke, the average level of improvement would be between 8 and 16 on the Aphasia Quotient 1 year after their stroke.

Calculating a confidence interval for dichotomous outcomes

For dichotomous outcomes, which are reported as the risk of an event, the 95% confidence interval provides the range of risks within which we are 95% certain that the true risk lies. The confidence interval can be calculated approximately using the formula:

$$95\% \text{ confidence interval} = \text{risk} \pm (1 \div \sqrt{2n})$$

where 'n' is the number of clients. Let us assume, in our example of postnatal depression in women, that the 62% risk of still having depression three months later was determined using data from 24 clients.

$$95\% \text{ confidence interval} = \text{risk} \pm (1 \div \sqrt{2n})$$
$$= 62\% \pm (1 \div \sqrt{2 * 24})$$
$$= 62\% \pm 14\%$$
$$= 48\% \text{ to } 76\%$$

Therefore, we could assume that the risk of postnatal depression persisting for 3 months is between 48% and 76%.

Identification and analysis of prognostic factors

In prognostic studies, data about the likelihood of the outcome are typically presented first, and then an analysis of prognostic factors is presented if the study conducts such an analysis. This data may be presented simply by reporting the prognosis for various subgroups of participants, where each subgroup has a certain prognostic factor (or if dealing with a continuous variable, varying degrees of the factor). Data about prognostic factors may also be presented in a more complex way using multivariate predictive models which assess how each prognostic factor is associated with each other prognostic factor and the overall prognosis. Explanation about multivariate analysis techniques is beyond the scope of this book.

An example of how a prognostic factor can be reported in a way that treats it as continuous data comes from a study about risk factors for hip fracture in women.[14] In this study, increasing age was reported as a risk factor for hip fracture in women over 65 years of age. For every 5-year increment in age, the risk of a hip fracture increased 1.5 times. This study also treated other risk factors dichotomously. For example, having a maternal history of hip fracture was found to double a woman's risk of hip fracture.

Clinical scenario (continued): What are the results?

In the knee arthroplasty article, the average pattern of postoperative improvement in the Lower Extremity Functional Scale is presented in a graph— see the middle curve in Figure 8.2. Note that these data are for females only. The authors elected to analyse the data for males and females separately because gender has previously been shown to influence functional mobility after total knee arthroplasty.[15,16] Females had average scores of 27 preoperatively, 18 at 1 week, 38 at 6 weeks and 53 at 6 months. The 6-month value was then maintained until 12 months.

A similar pattern of improvement was seen on the 6-Minute Walk Test. Females achieved an average distance of 353m preoperatively, 200m at 1 week, 330m at 6 weeks, and 470m at 6 months. The 6-month value was again maintained until 12 months. For a graph of the average pattern of improvement, see the middle curve in Figure 8.3.

In addition to gender, there is another prognostic factor for functional mobility in the postoperative period: preoperative functional mobility. The higher a client's Lower Extremity Functional Scale score was preoperatively, the higher their postoperative Lower Extremity Functional Scale score was throughout the following year. For a graph of the average effect of preoperative Lower Extremity Functional Scale score on postoperative recovery, see the top and bottom curves in Figure 8.2. Similarly, a client's preoperative 6-Minute Walk Test distance influenced the postoperative value—see the top and bottom curves in Figure 8.3. For simplicity, let us assume that Mrs Wilson has average pre-operative Lower Extremity Functional Scale and 6-Minute Walk Test results.

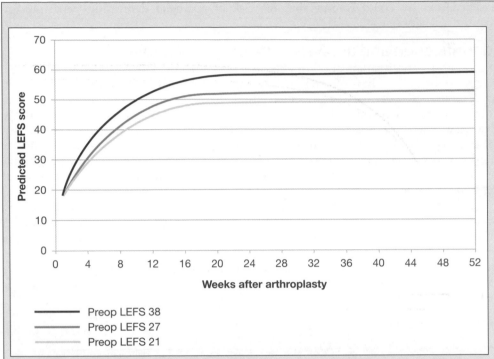

FIGURE 8.2 Change in average Lower Extremity Functional Scale (LEFS) scores for females (middle curve), with adjustment for higher (top curve) and lower (bottom curve) preoperative LEFS scores

Reproduced with permission from Kennedy D et al, Assessing recovery and establishing prognosis following total knee arthroplasty, American Physical Therapy Association, 2008[3]

It is important to remember that there is still a degree of uncertainty in using the average results for females as prognostic estimates for Mrs Wilson. For example, we have determined that her likely 6-Minute Walk Test distance at 1 year will be 470m. The article tells us that the standard deviation around this estimate was 84.7m and that this was determined with data from 44 female clients. Therefore, we can calculate a 95% confidence interval around that estimate.

$$\textbf{95\% confidence interval} = \textbf{mean} \pm (\textbf{3} \times \textbf{standard deviation} \div \sqrt{\textbf{2n}})$$
$$= 470m \pm (3 \times 84.7 \div \sqrt{2 * 44})$$
$$= 470m \pm (27)$$
$$= 443m \text{ to } 497m$$

This is a reasonably precise estimate. We can be confident when discussing our estimate with Mrs Wilson, knowing that it is a good approximation of the true value that we are seeking to estimate. However, we should acknowledge and explain to her that the true average prognosis of the 6-Minute Walk Test may be a little higher or lower than our best estimate of 470m.

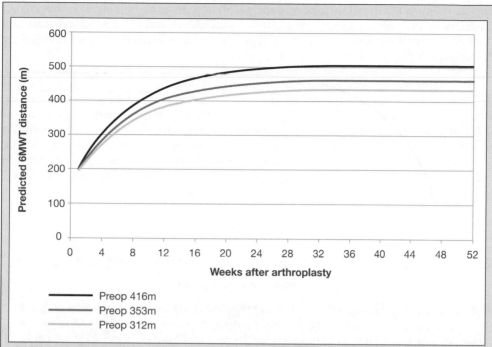

FIGURE 8.3 Change in average 6-Minute Walk Test: distances for females (middle curve), with adjustment for longer (top curve) and shorter (bottom curve) preoperative 6-Minute Walk Test distances

Reproduced with permission from Kennedy D et al, Assessing recovery and establishing prognosis following total knee arthroplasty; American Physical Therapy Association 2008[3]

How can we use this evidence to inform practice?

As we saw in Chapter 4 in the section on using evidence about interventions, before applying the evidence about interventions from a study, you need to consider whether your client is similar to the participants in the study. The same consideration needs to occur before applying the results from a prognostic study to your client.

Prognostic information has several uses in clinical practice. Having information about the likely clinical course of a condition can help you to determine whether intervention needs to be considered for the condition. If the prognosis for natural recovery is very good, there may be little point in starting any intervention. Similarly, if the prognosis for a cohort treated with a particular intervention is very good, then alternative or additional interventions may not need to be considered for clients who can be managed successfully with that intervention. In such cases, using the information to counsel clients and provide them with explanation and reassurance may be all that is necessary.

However, if the prognosis for the condition may be able to be improved by intervention and there are available interventions that are likely to make a clinically important difference, the information that you have about prognosis can form the starting point for a discussion with your client. In addition to explaining what is likely to occur in the future with respect to the condition, you also need to discuss the various intervention options (if there are more than one) with your client and engage them in the decision-making process. Shared decision making is an important component of evidence-based practice (and indeed, clinical practice in general) and further information about this and strategies to facilitate shared decision making are discussed in Chapter 14.

Central to facilitating client involvement in decision making is communicating with clients effectively. Again, Chapter 14 provides you with a number of practical strategies that you can use to ensure that you are communicating effectively with your clients. When explaining prognostic information to a client, it is important to do so in a manner that the client can understand and make it relevant to the client's goals and priorities. It is therefore good to focus on the outcomes and time frames that matter most to the client. In addition, if the client has prognostic factors that affect the prognosis, it is reasonable to consider explaining their influence, especially if any of them are modifiable (for example, being overweight).

Clinical scenario (continued): Using the evidence to inform practice

After reading about the characteristics of the study participants you decide that Mrs Wilson is similar enough to the study participants that the results could apply to her. To explain Mrs Wilson's prognosis for the return of functional mobility, we could begin by explaining her predicted status at some key time points: immediately after surgery, 6 weeks after surgery (when her support people are due to leave) and 6 months after surgery (when her maximum function is likely to be achieved). Remember that one purpose of generating this prognostic information was to help Mrs Wilson decide on arrangements for her husband's care after her surgery. Simply telling her the predicted Lower Extremity Functional Scale score and 6-Minute Walk Test distance at 6 weeks may not be very helpful in determining whether she will need assistance to care for her husband. Let us look at ways we can help Mrs Wilson to interpret these predicted results.

Mrs Wilson's Lower Extremity Functional Scale score is predicted to be 38 at 6 weeks. To link this overall score of 38 to ratings of difficulty with functional activities we can draw upon further prognostic research[17] that provides data for 20 activities. For each activity, the average total Lower Extremity Functional Scale score is scored by participants who report the difficulty that they have doing the activity as: 0 (extreme difficulty), 1 (quite a bit of difficulty), 2 (moderate difficulty), 3 (a little bit of difficulty) or 4 (no difficulty). For the activity of walking between rooms, participants who had extreme difficulty had an average overall Lower Extremity Functional Scale score of 4; those who had quite a bit of difficulty had an average score of 15; those who had moderate difficulty had an average score of 22; those who had a little bit of difficulty had an average score of 36; and those who had no difficulty had an average score of 57. With her predicted score of 38 at 6 weeks after surgery, Mrs Wilson could expect to have little difficulty walking to her husband in another room by the time her support people are due to leave.

The meaning of the 6-Minute Walk Test result that Mrs Wilson is predicted to have at 6 weeks is much easier to understand. The distance that an individual is likely to be able to walk in 6 minutes is a simple concept. However, we can still help

Mrs Wilson to interpret the distance. One way would be to compare it to normative data from healthy participants. Normative data[18] shows that healthy 60- to 69-year-old women walk an average of 505m in 6 minutes. Her 330m prognosis at 6 weeks represents 65% of the distance predicted for a healthy woman of her age (330m/505m = 65%). Viewed as a fraction of normative data, this percentage may be discouragingly low. Given that she is currently able to care for her husband, we could encourage her to compare it to her preoperative 6-Minute Walk Test distance instead. Her predicted result, 330m, represents less than a 7% reduction in her current ability, 353m, on the test.

Another approach is to compare it to distances that she must tackle in one session of walking, for example:

- Back room of the house to the front door: 40m
- Kitchen to the letterbox and return: 60m
- Front door to neighbour's house and return: 180m
- Front door to nearby convenience store: 320m

She should be able to manage all of these distances in 6 minutes. It is worth remembering that the 6-Minute Walk Test allows the participant to sit and rest as required. If she currently rests at all during her 6-Minute Walk Test and if there are no seats between her home and the nearby convenience store, she may have to consider organising assistance with shopping. She should also consider how quickly she recovered from her 6-Minute Walk Test and whether she could continue with shopping and then walk home again carrying it.

Summary points of this chapter

- Evidence about prognosis is often found in prospective cohort studies, although it may also be present in control group data from a randomised controlled trial or in a systematic review of prognostic data from several studies.
- When searching for prognostic studies, include terms for the client's problem, the intervention they receive (unless you are interested in the prognosis of the untreated condition) and the outcomes that are most important to the client.
- The most valid prognostic evidence comes from studies in which the participants were identified at an early and uniform point in their disease (known as an 'inception cohort'). The participants included in the study should be representative of the population from which they were sampled and their condition should have been accurately diagnosed. Their outcomes should have been accurately measured with an appropriate and valid tool. Follow-up of the participants in the study needed to be sufficiently long and complete.
- The two main questions that you need to ask when determining if the results of a prognostic study are important are: 1) how likely are the outcomes over time? and 2) how precise are the estimates of likelihood?
- The average prognostic estimate for clients in the study can often be tailored to your particular client by adjusting for the effect of certain characteristics which are known as prognostic factors.
- Most clients will require help to interpret prognostic estimates. This can sometimes be done by relating predicted values to threshold values, such as the client's current value, the average value for healthy people and the values required for functional activities.

References

1. Liou T, Adler S, FitzSimmons B et al. Predictive 5-year survivorship model of cystic fibrosis. Am J Epidemiol 2001; 153:345–352.
2. Roseribloom M, Pfefferbaum A, Sullivan E. Recovery of short-term memory and psychomotor speed but not postural stability with long-term sobriety in alcoholic women. Neuropsychology 2004; 18:589–597.
3. Kennedy D, Stratford P, Riddle D et al. Assessing recovery and establishing prognosis following total knee arthroplasty. Phys Ther 2008; 88:22–32.
4. Segawa H, Tsukayama D, Kyle R et al. Infection after total knee arthroplasty. A retrospective study of the treatment of eighty-one infections. J Bone Joint Surg Am 1999; 81:1434–1445.
5. Roos H, Adalberth T, Dahlberg L et al. Osteoarthritis of the knee after injury to the anterior cruciate ligament or meniscus: the influence of time and age. Osteoarthritis Cartilage 1995; 3:261–267.
6. Gelber A, Hochberg M, Mead L et al. Joint injury in young adults and risk for subsequent knee and hip osteoarthritis. Ann Intern Med 2000; 133:321–328.
7. Bullens P, van Loon C, de Waal Malefit M et al. Client satisfaction after total knee arthroplasty. J Arthroplasty 2001; 16:740–747.
8. Straus S, Richardson W, Glasziou P et al. Evidence-based medicine: how to practice and teach EBM. 3rd edn. Edinburgh: Elsevier Churchill Livingstone; 2005.
9. Robertsson O, Knutson K, Lewold S et al. The Swedish Knee Arthroplasty Register 1975–1997. Acta Orthopaedica 2001; 72:503–513.
10. White R, Romano P, Zhou H et al. Incidence and time course of thromboembolic outcomes following total hip or knee arthroplasty. Arch Intern Med 1998; 158:1525–1531.
11. Pedersen P, Vinter K, Olsen T. Aphasia after stroke: type, severity and prognosis. Cerebrovasc Dis 2004; 17:35–43.
12. Holden J, Sagovsky R, Cox J. Counselling in a general practice setting: controlled study of health visitor intervention in treatment of postnatal depression. BMJ 1989; 298:223–226.
13. Berry J, Von Knoch M, Schleck C et al. The cumulative long-term risk of dislocation after primary Charnley total hip arthroplasty. J Bone Joint Surg Am 2004; 86:9–14.
14. Cummings S, Nevitt M, Browner W et al. Risk factors for hip fracture in white women. N Engl J Med 1995; 332:767–774.
15. Kennedy D, Stratford P, Pagura S et al. Comparison of gender and group differences in self-report and physical performance measures in total hip and knee arthroplasty candidates. J Arthroplasty 2002; 17:70–77.
16. Kennedy D, Hanna S, Stratford P et al. Preoperative function and gender predict pattern of functional recovery after hip and knee arthroplasty. J Arthroplasty 2006; 21:559–566.
17. Stratford P, Hart D, Binkley J et al. Interpreting Lower Extremity Functional Status score. Physiotherapy Canada 2005; 57:154–162.
18. Bohannon R. Six-minute Walk Test: a meta-analysis of data from apparently healthy elders. Topics in Geriatric Rehabilitation 2007; 23:155–160.

CHAPTER 9

Questions about prognosis: examples of appraisals from different health professions

Tammy Hoffmann, John W Bennett, Marilyn Baird, Mark R Elkins, Craig Lockwood, Sheena Reilly and Sharon Sanders

This chapter is an accompaniment to the previous chapter (Chapter 8) where the steps involved in answering a clinical question about prognosis were explained. In order to further help you learn how to deal with prognostic clinical questions when they arise and appraise the evidence, this chapter contains a number of worked examples of questions about prognosis from a range of health professions. The worked examples in this chapter follow the same format as the examples that are in Chapter 5. In addition, as with the worked examples that were written for Chapter 5, the authors of the worked examples in this chapter were asked not to choose a systematic review (for the reason that was explained in Chapter 5), but to instead find the next best available level of evidence to answer the prognostic question that was generated from the clinical scenario.

Occupational therapy example

Clinical scenario

You are an occupational therapist who has recently rotated into the outpatient department of a brain injury rehabilitation unit. After clients are discharged as inpatients and return home to live, they return to the hospital to receive outpatient therapy. One of your clients is Mary, a 20-year-old who sustained a mild traumatic brain injury in a motor vehicle accident 8 weeks ago. Her Glasgow Coma Scale was 13 on admission to hospital. Prior to the accident Mary worked full-time as an apprentice chef. She has been working in this job for 2 years and started after finishing high school. After discharge from hospital, Mary returned home to live with her parents and has been able to do simple tasks around the home and shopping with assistance from her mother. Your initial outpatient assessment of Mary revealed that her current difficulties are poor endurance, poor standing balance and memory and planning problems. Mary is already 2 months post-injury and her employer has just advised her that he is only able to keep her position in the apprenticeship scheme reserved for her for another 4 months. Mary has asked you how likely it is that she will be able to return to her job within that time frame. As you are new to working in this area of clinical practice, you decide to search the literature to help you answer this question.

Clinical question
In adults with mild traumatic brain injury, what is the likelihood of returning to work within 6 months of the injury occurring?

Search terms and databases used to find the evidence
Database: PubMed—Clinical Queries (with 'prognosis category' and 'narrow search' selected)
Search terms: (mild traumatic brain injury) AND (return to work*)
This search retrieves eight results. After reading through the titles of these articles, only one article appears to be relevant to your clinical question. After reading its abstract, you confirm that it is relevant and you obtain the full text of it so that you can appraise it.

Article chosen
Ruffolo C, Friendland J, Dawson D et al. Mild traumatic brain injury from motor vehicle accidents: factors associated with return to work. Arch Phys Med Rehabil 1999; 80: 392–398.

Structured abstract
Study design: Inception cohort study (part of a larger case-control prospective study).
Setting: Tertiary care centre, Toronto, Canada.
Participants: 63 patients with mild traumatic brain injury who were admitted to hospital as a result of a motor vehicle accident; aged between 19 and 65 years (mean age 31.3 years, 62% male). Other eligibility criteria were: working before the accident in paid or unpaid employment; no history of head injury, neurological disease or hospitalisation for psychiatric illness; no severe disfigurement, amputation or spinal cord injury from the accident; and English-speaking.
Outcome: Return to work (at premorbid or modified level).
Prognostic factors studied: Injury severity, cognitive functioning at initial assessment and follow-up, social interaction at follow-up, discharge disposition and sociodemographic factors (age, gender, marital status, education and occupation).
Follow-up period: 6–9 months (mean = 7.4 months).
Main results: 42% of the participants who were followed up returned to work (12% to their premorbid employment and 30% to modified employment). Between the participants who returned to work and those who did not, there were statistically significant differences in levels of social interaction, premorbid occupation and discharge disposition.
Conclusion: Prognostic factors that were found to be positively related to return to work in people with mild traumatic brain injury were social interaction, jobs with greater decision-making freedom and discharge home. Cognitive impairment within the first month of the injury was not found to be a reliable indicator of likelihood of return to work.

Is the evidence likely to be biased?
* *Was there a representative and well-defined sample?*
  Yes (well-defined population); cannot tell (representative sampling). The article does not specifically state that 'all' or 'consecutive' eligible participants who were admitted to the hospital were recruited into the study. The article mentions that this study was part of a larger case-control prospective study but no further details about it or its methodology are provided. However, the target population is well-defined as clear inclusion and exclusion criteria are provided.
* *Was there an inception cohort?*
  Yes. Participants were recruited at a similar well-described point, namely after they were admitted to hospital after the traumatic brain injury occurred.
* *Was exposure determined accurately?*
  Yes. In this study, it would have been very unlikely that an error was made in recruiting participants who had suffered a traumatic brain injury as a result of a motor vehicle accident as this exposure (or in this case, eligibility criteria) can be easily determined. The authors of the article also explain how the severity of participants' traumatic brain injury was determined (mild traumatic brain injury was defined as having a Glascow Coma Scale admission score of 13 or more and/or a loss of consciousness of less than 1 hour).

- *Were the outcomes measured accurately?*
  Yes. The main outcome was clearly defined as return to work and this was further categorised into return to premorbid employment or premorbid employment under modified conditions (which were also defined). The information about this outcome measure was gathered from components of three different questionnaires. It was not possible to measure this outcome in a blind fashion as it was based on participant self-report. It was not possible to blind assessors about participants' status on each of these prognostic factors as these factors were either difficult to conceal from an assessor (for example, age, gender) or were based on participant self-report where the participant was technically the assessor.
- *Were important prognostic factors considered?*
  Yes. The authors appear to have identified the major factors that could influence the outcome of return to work. The study examined five main categories of possible prognostic factors (refer to the structured abstract).
- *Was the follow-up of participants sufficiently long and complete?*
  No, not sufficiently complete. The study recruited 63 participants and was able to follow up 50 of them (79% follow-up rate). Reasons were provided for why participants were lost to follow-up and participants who left the study were compared to those who remained in the study. Compared with participants in the group that were followed up, more participants in the group that were lost to follow-up experienced loss of consciousness at the time of injury and had jobs that had little independence and opportunity for decision making. With regards to length, the mean length of follow-up time was 6 to 9 months (mean of 7.4 months), which matches our clinical question. However, many studies that look at return to work after head injury follow participants for 12 months. Although only participants with mild traumatic brain injury were included in this study, they may have experienced impairments (either physical and/or cognitive impairments) that could continue to impact on their ability to return to work beyond 6 to 9 months post-injury.

What are the main results?

Return to work: Of the 50 participants who were able to be followed up, 21 (42%) had returned to work by the time of the follow-up assessment (12% to their premorbid employment and 30% to modified employment). You calculate the 95% confidence interval to be 32% to 52% (using the formula that was provided in Chapter 8, where 95% confidence interval = risk $\pm$ [1 $\div$ $\sqrt{2n}$]). In other words, the likelihood of having returned to work by approximately 7 months post-traumatic brain injury could be as low as 32% or as high as 52%.

Prognostic factors related to return to work: Social interaction scores were significantly higher (p values 0.01 and 0.02) in the return to work group of participants compared to the group of participants who did not return to work. Significantly more (p <0.05) of the participants who were discharged to a rehabilitation facility, as opposed to being discharged home, had not returned to work by the time of the follow-up assessment. Participants were also significantly more likely to return to work if their job involved higher levels of independence/decision-making latitude. There were no significant differences between the two groups for any of the other factors that were analysed as potential prognostic factors.

How might we use this evidence to inform practice?

As you have determined the internal validity of this study to be reasonably strong (although you keep in mind the potential bias from the incomplete follow-up) and the results useful, you proceed to assessing the applicability of the evidence by comparing your client with the participants in the study, before deciding if you can use the evidence to help inform your practice. Mary's mechanism and severity of injury is the same as participants in the study. She is younger than the mean age of study participants but meets the eligibility criterion for age and all of the other eligibility criteria of the study. In terms of the prognostic factors that were identified in this study, Mary was discharged home which, in the study, was found to be positively related to return to work, so this may increase the likelihood of her returning to work. However, you do not have much information about the other prognostic factors that were identified as being related to return to work, so you decide that you will assess her social interaction (using the measures used in the study) and find out about the extent of decision-making latitude/ independence of her job.

After you obtain this information, you will use the results of this study to inform your discussion with Mary about the likelihood of her being able to return to work within the next 4 months. As a large proportion of the study participants who returned to work returned to modified work, there is a possibility that this may also be the case for Mary. As part of your treatment planning, you will arrange a time for Mary and yourself to meet with her employer to discuss the option of her returning to work in a modified capacity (such as shorter hours, different duties, graded return to work etc) if this is necessary. During this meeting, you also plan to obtain more detailed information about Mary's duties at work and then use this, in conjunction with Mary, to set her rehabilitation program and goals.

Physiotherapy example

Clinical scenario

While working in your private physiotherapy practice, a 32-year-old baker presents 2 days after the onset of his first episode of acute low back pain. His pain is localised to his lumbar spine and is not accompanied by signs of more serious pathology such as weight loss, weakness or paraesthesia. However, it is currently preventing him from working and he urgently needs to arrange a replacement until he is able to work again. He is therefore primarily interested in any advice you can give him with regard to when he can expect to improve enough to return to work. He is also interested to know how quickly his pain is likely to improve with usual intervention.

Clinical question
In adults with acute low back pain, what is the average time to return to work and to resolution of pain?

Search terms and databases used to find the evidence
Database: PubMed—Clinical Queries (with 'prognosis category' and 'narrow search' selected)
Search terms: (acute OR recent) AND (low back pain) AND (return to work*)

The search returns 31 records. You scan the titles of the articles and read the abstracts of three studies that seem like they could be relevant. Of these, one is highly relevant as it is an inception cohort study of acute low back pain, it was conducted in the same healthcare setting as your work, it followed a large cohort and it measured the outcomes that are of primary concern to your client.

Article chosen
Henschke N, Maher C, Refshauge K et al. Prognosis in patients with recent onset low back pain in Australian primary care: inception cohort study. BMJ 2008; 377:a171. doi: 10.1136/bmj.a171.

Structured abstract
Study design: Inception cohort study.
Setting: Medical, physiotherapy and chiropractic practices in Sydney, Australia.
Participants: 973 participants (mean age 43.3 years; 54.8% male) aged at least 14 years with non-specific low back pain of less than 2 weeks' duration. Exclusion criteria included radiculopathy, cancer, spinal fracture, spinal infection and inflammatory arthritis.
Outcomes: Time to return to work (determined by self-report of returning to previous work status), time to complete resolution of pain and return to function.
Prognostic factors studied: Age, gender, intensity of low back pain and level of interference with function at baseline plus individual variables grouped into seven factors—current history, past history, features of serious spinal pathology, sociodemographics, general health, psychological health and work.
Follow-up period: 1 year (with assessments also at baseline, 6 weeks and 3 months).
Main results: Median time to return to work was 14 days (95% confidence interval [CI] 11 to 17 days). Resolution of pain was much slower, at a median of 58 days (95% CI 52 to 63 days). A reasonable proportion of patients still had unresolved problems at 1 year. The cumulative probability of having returned to previous work status at 1 year was 89% and the cumulative probability of being pain-free at 1 year was 72%.
Conclusion: Prognosis of participants was not as favourable as is claimed in clinical guidelines. Most participants experienced slow recovery and almost one-third had not recovered from the presenting episode by the 12-month follow-up.

Is the evidence likely to be biased?
*   *Was there a representative and well-defined sample?*
    Yes. The article states that consecutive participants who presented to primary care with recent onset low back pain were invited to participate. Also, the target population is well-defined as clear inclusion and exclusion criteria are provided.
*   *Was there an inception cohort?*
    Yes. Participants were recruited within 2 weeks of onset of their condition, which minimises possible bias due to variable disease duration within the cohort.
*   *Was exposure determined accurately?*
    Yes. Eligibility was determined by doctors, physiotherapists and chiropractors, so misclassification is unlikely unless participants misreported their symptoms.
*   *Were the outcomes measured accurately?*
    Cannot tell. The outcomes (pain intensity, disability and work status) were based on participant self-report. Therefore, it was not possible to measure the outcomes in a blind fashion. Also, there is little indication of psychometric validation of any of the outcome measures, which may be one source of potential bias.
*   *Were important prognostic factors considered?*
    Yes. The researchers identified an extensive range of prognostic factors (refer to the structured abstract).

- *Was the follow-up of participants sufficiently long and complete?*
  Yes. The follow-up rate was excellent (97%) and the length of follow-up appears to have been sufficient for the outcomes that were measured.

What are the results?

Return to work: The median time to return to work (to previous work hours and duties) was 14 days (95% CI 11 to 17 days). The cumulative probability of having returned to previous work status was 74.6% at 6 weeks, 83.2% at 12 weeks and 89.5% at 1 year.

Resolution of pain: The median time to resolution of pain was 58 days (95% CI 53 to 63 days). The cumulative probability of being pain-free was 39.9% at 6 weeks, 58.2% at 12 weeks and 72.5% at 1 year.

Complete recovery: This was measured by recovery on all three dimensions (return to work, no disability and no pain). The cumulative probability of being fully recovered was 39.0% at 6 weeks, 57.4% at 12 weeks and 71.8% at 1 year.

Prognostic factors: Factors associated with a longer time to recovery included older age, compensation cases, higher pain intensity, longer duration of low back pain before consultation, more days of reduced activity because of lower back pain before consultation, feelings of depression and a perceived risk of persistence.

How might we use this evidence to inform practice?

You compare your client's characteristics to those of the participants in the sample and decide that he is similar enough that you can apply this evidence to him and his situation. As this prognostic evidence has little risk of potential bias and the confidence interval extends only a few days either side of the estimate of median time to return to work, you can confidently reassure your client that about 50% of people with acute low back pain return to work at about 2 weeks. Resolution of his pain is likely to take substantially longer, with 50% of people being pain-free by about 8 weeks. However, you also explain to your client that there is a small risk that the condition will not have fully resolved by 1 year, with 28% of the study participants not considered as fully recovered by 1 year. Because he is young, self-employed and has only had the pain for 2 days, however, he does not have several of the prognostic factors that were found to predict a longer time to recovery. Therefore, it is likely that he may have a better than average prognosis for recovery. You clearly explain all of these findings to your client.

Podiatry example

Clinical scenario

You are a podiatry student on clinical placement in a hospital podiatry department. You have just seen a 62-year-old man who attended with his wife. He has been referred by the diabetes educator for foot screening, education and management. He has had type 2 diabetes for approximately 10 years and, according to the client,

(continued)

his control has been good. Your examination indicates that neuropathy is present, vascular assessment is satisfactory, there is some foot deformity and there are active pressure lesions present plantar to the first metatarsal head bilaterally. Debridement of the callosity on the right foot reveals an ulcer. Together with your supervisor, you conduct a detailed ulcer assessment. The ulceration has white, macerated margins, the base is clean and pink to red and there is no exudate. The ulcer is round, 6mm across and 4mm deep. There do not appear to be any sinuses and you cannot probe to bone. While discussing an intervention plan with your client, his wife, who appears visibly worried, asks if he will end up losing his leg. You know that this is a possibility but are not sure of the actual risk, so your supervisor suggests you conduct a search to see if you can find some evidence to guide your answer to the question. You tell your client and his wife that you will endeavour to answer her question more accurately when you see them again in a few days time.

Clinical question

In a person with a neuropathic foot ulcer, what is the risk of amputation?

Search terms and databases used to find the evidence

Database: PubMed—Clinical Queries (with 'prognosis category' selected)
Search terms: ulcer* AND (diabetic OR neuropathic) AND amputat*
This search returns 90 results and you quickly scan the titles. There are several articles which, on the basis of the title and abstract, look as though they will answer your question. They are all cohort studies that followed up participants with neuropathic ulcers. It is difficult to compare the studies in terms of the methods used by reading only the abstract, but one article stands out because it appears to include participants very similar to your client. You obtain the full text of the following cohort study of clients with diabetes who have their first foot ulcer.

Article chosen

Winkley K, Stahl D, Chalder T et al. Risk factors associated with adverse outcomes in a population-based prospective cohort study of people with their first diabetic foot ulcer. J Diabetes Complications 2007; 21:341–349.

Structured abstract

Study design: Prospective cohort study.
Setting: Community and hospital foot clinics in London, UK.
Participants: 253 people (mean age 62.0 years; 63.6% male) with diabetes (type 1 or type 2) and their first foot ulcer. Exclusion criteria included not being fluent in English, a current independent comorbid medical condition, severe mental illness (such as psychosis or dementia), duration of foot ulcer greater than 1 year, or severely ischaemic feet (ankle brachial pressure index <0.5).
Outcomes: Death, amputation and recurrence of ulceration and the time taken for each outcome to occur.
Prognostic factors studied: Age, sex, smoking status, ulcer site (dorsal or plantar), size and severity of ulcer, severity of neuropathy, ischaemia, glycosylated haemoglobin, presence of micro- and macrovascular complications and depression.

Follow-up period: 18 months (with assessments also at baseline, 6 months and 12 months).

Main results: At 18 months, 15.5% of participants had had an amputation, 15.8% had died and 43.2% had experienced ulcer recurrence. The severity of the ulcer at baseline was significantly associated with amputation (hazard ratio [HR] 3.18, 95% CI 1.53 to 6.59). Being older, having lower glycosylated haemoglobin, moderate ischaemia and depression were associated with mortality. Microvascular complications were associated with recurrent ulceration.

Is the evidence likely to be biased?

- *Was there a representative and well-defined sample?*
  Yes. It is likely that the sample was representative as the article states that the records of each participating clinic were checked fortnightly so that eligible clients could be identified (using a standardised checklist of case definition and exclusion criteria) from all of the current and new clients that were being seen by the clinics. Also, there was a very high proportion of eligible clients that were recruited into the study (of the 260 people who were eligible, 253 were recruited), which helps to ensure the representativeness of the sample. The target population is well-defined, with clear inclusion and exclusion criteria described in the article.
- *Was there an inception cohort?*
  No. Though the range of time over which the ulcers had been present is not reported (mean duration was 3.1 months with a standard deviation of 3.6 months), it appears that the participants may have had the ulcers for as little as a few weeks or for as long as a year, and only participants with an ulcer duration of greater than 1 year were excluded. As participants were not recruited at a similar point in the course of this condition, possible bias due to variable disease duration within the cohort may have been introduced into the study.
- *Was exposure determined accurately?*
  Yes. The article states that a clinically significant case definition of diabetic foot ulcer was used and go on to provide details about what this definition was. Also, participants were assessed by podiatrists at community and hospital foot clinics. Therefore it is likely that it was accurately determined whether participants had a foot ulcer or not.
- *Were the outcomes measured accurately?*
  Yes. The outcomes of death and amputation are valid and objective and specific criteria were established to define the outcome of ulcer recurrence. The methods used to identify the occurrence of the outcomes of interest appear reliable. It is not clear if the outcome assessors were blind to clinical characteristics or prognostic factors, though it does state in the discussion that they were blind to depression status. Given the objectivity of the outcome measures, the issue of blinding is not likely to be of great importance.
- *Were important prognostic factors considered?*
  Yes. The researchers identified an extensive range of factors that could have potential prognostic value.
- *Was the follow-up of participants sufficiently long and complete?*
  Yes. Follow-up was both sufficiently long and complete. Eighteen months is an adequate length of time to observe amputation and ulcer recurrence. You wonder if it is long enough to observe mortality, but notice that quite a number of participants (15%) had experienced this outcome during the follow-up period. The rate of follow-up was 100% for the death outcome, 92% for the amputation

outcome and 90.5% for the recurrence outcome. While the loss to follow-up in this study is reasonably small (that is, <10%), there were some differences in baseline characteristics between the participants who were lost to follow-up and those that remained in the cohort. Participants with missing information had a shorter duration of diabetes and fewer microvascular problems. It is unclear if this constitutes a certain type of participant who was selectively lost to follow-up.

What are the main results?

Amputation: By 18 months, 15.5% (n = 36) of the study population had undergone an amputation. Of the amputations, 10 of them were considered a major amputation (above the ankle) and the remainder were below the ankle (mainly of the toes). Using the data provided in the article, you calculate the 95% confidence interval for this 15.5% estimated risk of having an amputation to be 11.5% to 19.5%. In other words, the risk of amputation for a diabetic foot ulcer (at approximately 18 months after first seeking medical attention for the ulcer) is between 11.5% and 19.5%.

In a multivariate analysis, the severity of the ulcer was significantly associated with amputation (HR 3.34; 95% CI 1.53 to 6.59). The presence of an ulcer categorised as 'deep' according to the University of Texas Diabetic Wound Classification System increased the risk of amputation threefold. As the confidence interval for the ratio does not contain 1 (the 'no effect' value), this result is statistically significant.

Recurrence of ulcer: By 18 months, 43% of participants developed another ulcer at the same or different site to the first ulcer. Microvascular complications (such as neuropathy) were associated with recurrent ulceration (HR 3.34; 95% CI 1.53 to 6.59).

Death: Being older (HR 1.07; 95% CI 1.04 to 1.11) and having moderate ischaemia (HR 2.74; 95% CI 1.46 to 5.14) and depression (HR 2.51; 95% CI 1.33 to 4.73) increased the risk of mortality. Better glycaemic control reduced mortality risk (HR 0.73; 95% CI 0.56 to 0.96).

How might we use this evidence to inform practice?

You consider the results of the study to be relatively free of bias and your client appears to be similar to the study participants in many respects including age, type and duration of diabetes and other clinical characteristics. You have not previously seen the wound classification system used in this study to assess the severity of the ulcers. The reference provided in the study report indicates that it is a validated instrument. In the study, the ulcers were categorised as either superficial (wound extended through the epidermis or dermis only) or deep (wound penetrates tendon, joint capsule, bone or joint.) Using this categorisation, your client's ulcer would be considered superficial. Given this, you feel that you can reassure the client and his wife that he is at a lower risk of amputation than if the ulcer had penetrated to tendon, bone or joint. You will emphasise the importance of continued good control of his diabetes, as this may reduce the risk of death. However, due to the presence of peripheral neuropathy (a microvascular complication), your client is at increased risk of recurrent ulceration. In conjunction with your supervisor, you discuss the findings of the study with your client and his wife and also suggest that they schedule regular follow-up assessments to check frequently for ulcer recurrence and initiate prompt intervention if/when they recur to prevent them from progressing to deep ulcers.

Speech pathology example

Clinical scenario

You are a speech pathologist who works in a community child health centre. Mrs Overato brings her daughter Martha, aged 23 months, to see you. She is concerned that Martha has recently begun to stutter. Martha has a twin brother, Steve, who does not stutter. There is no family history of stuttering. Mrs Overato reported that Martha first started to stutter when she was about 18 months old, but this only lasted a few weeks and then stopped. The most recent bout of stuttering commenced after Martha was frightened by their neighbour's dog.

Martha repeats words and initial sounds but there is no blocking or prolongation occurring. She is reported to be as chatty as ever and appears unconcerned about her stuttering. There are no other concerns about Martha's development; she has a large vocabulary and she speaks in phrases and short sentences. There are no concerns about her speech development and she is able to articulate words very clearly for her age. Mrs Overato is very anxious as Martha and Steve will soon be beginning day care and, on a recent visit, the care staff remarked on her stuttering. She wonders if she should be seeking any intervention for Martha's stuttering. She has also heard that Martha is likely to grow out of her stuttering anyway. You decide to search the literature to obtain information about this issue.

Clinical question

When stuttering develops in infancy and early childhood in a twin, how likely is it that recovery will occur naturally and are there any indications about which children are most likely to recover?

Search terms and databases used to find the evidence

Database: PubMed
Search terms: (stutter* OR stammer*) AND (child*) AND (twin*) AND (recover*)
This search retrieves three articles, one of which is relevant to your clinical question. You also conduct a search, using the same terms, in CINAHL and this retrieves two articles. Again, only one article is relevant and it is the same article as was already located.

Article chosen

Dworzynski K, Remington A, Rijsdijk F et al. Genetic etiology in cases of recovered and persistent stuttering in an unselected, longitudinal sample of young twins. Am J Speech Lang Pathol 2007; 16:169–178.

Structured abstract

Study design: Prospective, longitudinal twin study (in the UK).
Study question: What is the recovery rate from developmental stuttering in childhood and are there factors which predict recovery and persistence?
Participants: Participants were 12,892 twins recruited at 18 months of age.
Outcomes: Recovery of stuttering.

Follow-up period: Parent reports of the children's stuttering were obtained at 2, 3, 4 and 7 years of age.

Main results: Of the 12,892 children with at least two ratings, 950 children had recovered and 135 had a persistent stutter. Ratings of stuttering at 2 years of age were not predictive of later stuttering (at 7 years), but ratings at 3 and 4 years of age were. At 3, 4 and 7 years, the liability to stuttering was highly heritable.

Conclusion: Stuttering is a disorder that appears to have high heritability and little shared environment effect in early childhood and for recovered and persistent groups of children up to 7 years of age.

Is this evidence likely to be biased?

- *Was there a representative and well-defined sample?*
  Yes. This is one of the largest and most methodologically rigorous twin studies about stuttering that has been undertaken. Its strength lies in the fact that the study of stuttering was embedded within a large study of twin development. The prospective and longitudinal nature of the study was ideal for addressing the research question. The families of all twins that were born in the UK between 1994 and 1996 were invited to participate in the larger study about twin development. Appropriate exclusion criteria were applied in participant selection, namely that children with a specific medical condition (such as a chromosomal anomaly) were excluded, as were cases where zygosity data were unavailable.

- *Was there an inception cohort?*
  No. Although the children in this study were recruited at a similar age (18 months), it is unlikely that they would have all been at a similar point with respect to the development/onset of stuttering.

- *Was exposure determined accurately?*
  No. Stuttering at ages 2, 3 and 4 years was used to predict stuttering at age 7 years. A parent questionnaire pack was sent to parents at each assessment point. Each questionnaire contained at least one question that specifically asked about stuttering/stammering. A weakness is that the study relies on parental report of the presence of stuttering and there was no clinical verification of the report. The authors argue that, in their studies of child language, clinical face-to-face assessments have verified parental report. However this has not been tested in stuttering to date.

- *Were the outcomes measured accurately?*
  No. A parent questionnaire pack was sent to parents at age 7 years (as was done for the measurement of exposure at ages 2, 3 and 4 years). The same issues that were discussed above with respect to the determination/measurement of exposure (that is, early stuttering) apply to the measurement of the outcome (that is, stuttering at 7 years).

- *Were important prognostic factors considered?*
  Yes. The researchers considered the effect of gender and genetic and environmental influences on stuttering outcomes.

- *Was the follow-up of participants sufficiently long and complete?*
  In terms of the length and completeness of follow-up, the overall length of follow-up (until children were 7 years old) is appropriate. However as the assessments were conducted when the participants were 2, 3, 4 and 7 years old, there were lengthy gaps (for example, 12 months) between the reports, so many short-lived bursts of stuttering may have been missed and data about onset prior to 2 years of age were not captured. The follow-up rate was 59% at 2 years of age, 64.8% at 3 years of age, 65% at 4 years of age and 62.4% at 7 years of age.

What are the main results?

Incidence of stuttering: The incidence was 1.1% (82/7164) at 2 years of age, 2.4% (180/7616) at 3 years and 2.5% (262/10,514) at 4 years of age. At 2 and 3 years for every girl who stuttered, there were 1.6 boys who stuttered, whereas at 4 and 7 years there were 1.8 boys for every girl who stuttered.

Recovery and persistence rates: Of the children whose parents had provided at least two ratings across the ages, 970 (7%) were classified as recovered (comprised of 429 girls (45%) and 521 boys (55%)). In the 135 (1%) children in which stuttering persisted, 35 (26%) were girls and 100 (74%) were boys. These figures can be expressed as: for every girl who continued to stutter, there were 2.9 boys who continued to stutter. Of the 82 children who were reported to be stuttering at 2 years of age, 81 had recovered by 7 years of age. Recovery rates at 3 and 4 years were reported to be 79% and 53%, respectively. Not only are fewer girls than boys affected by stuttering but this holds for each age as well as for the recovered and persistent groups.

Prediction of later stuttering: Using logistic regression, the authors explored whether reports of stuttering at early ages were predictive of stuttering at 7 years. Ratings of stuttering at 2 years of age were not predictive of later stuttering, but ratings at 3 and 4 years of age were.

Twin analyses: Monozygotic concordance rates were higher than dizygotic rates which suggest that there is substantial genetic influence operating and little evidence of shared environmental influence. This was verified in formal statistical twin modelling. The authors examined recovery and persistence patterns where one child had been affected by stuttering and the other had not. Most often the other twin was not affected, with this pattern being more apparent in dizygotic pairs compared to monozygotic pairs. The data presented did not suggest gender differences in pairs where both twins stuttered, nor were there different recovery and persistence rates. They concluded that the factors that increase liability to stuttering do not seem to be different for male or female children.

How might we use this evidence to inform practice?

In the case of Martha we can draw a number of conclusions based on the results of this study. Firstly, reports of stuttering obtained close to 2 years are not predictive of stuttering later in childhood, for example at 7 years. In this study 81 of the 82 children who were reported to be stuttering at 2 years did not stutter at 7 years. Secondly, Martha's mother can be reassured that the factors that increase liability to stuttering do not seem to be different for male or female children. Thirdly, because there is a large genetic component to stuttering and little evidence of shared environmental influences it is unlikely that the traumatic incident that Martha experienced with the neighbour's dog is implicated in the onset of stuttering, especially as this was the second bout of stuttering. Fourthly, Martha's mother can also be reassured of the likelihood of a favourable outcome as there is no family history of stuttering.

Based on the evidence from this well-conducted study we can infer that Martha's stuttering is less likely to persist because there is no family history of stuttering. Intervention therefore can be delayed and her stuttering observed and monitored over the coming 12 months. Her twin brother will not necessarily start to stutter. It is unlikely that the stuttering onset can be linked to environmental influences such as Martha's experience with the neighbour's dog.

Medicine example

Clinical scenario

As a general practitioner you regularly see a 48-year-old man who smokes about 25 cigarettes per day but is otherwise well. He is resistant to public health messages about smoking cessation partly because he feels no immediate negative consequences from smoking. You thought it may be useful to provide him with current information about the effect of smoking on mortality and quality of life.

Clinical question

In people who are heavy smokers, what is the long-term effect on their quality of life and survival?

Search terms and databases used to find the evidence

Database: PubMed—Clinical Queries (with 'prognosis category' and 'narrow search' selected)

Search terms: smok* AND (quality of life) AND (mortality OR survival)

This search returned 96 studies. The first article listed in this search was the most current, most relevant and appeared from the abstract to have sound methods, so you obtained the full text of it so that you could appraise it in detail.

Article chosen

Strandberg A, Strandberg T, Pitkälä K et al. The effect of smoking in midlife on health-related quality of life in old age: a 26-year prospective study. Arch Intern Med 2008; 168:1968–1974.

Structured abstract

Study design: Prospective cohort study.

Setting: Helsinki, Finland.

Participants: 1658 white men (born 1919–1934) of similar socioeconomic status who were participating in the Helsinki Businessmen Study. All were healthy at baseline (year 1974), when cardiovascular risk factors and smoking habits were assessed.

Outcomes: Health-related quality of life was measured with the RAND 36-Item Health Survey. Total mortality up to the year 2000 was determined from Finnish national registers.

Prognostic factors studied: Baseline smoking status.

Follow-up period: 26-year follow-up (from 1974 to 2000).

Main results: Those who had never smoked (n = 614) lived a mean of 10 years longer than heavy smokers (>20 cigarettes daily; n = 188). Those who had never smoked also had the best scores on all the RAND 36-Item Health Survey scales of survivors in 2000 (n = 1131). The largest differences were found between never-smokers and heavy smokers, ranging from 4 points on the scale of social functioning to 14 points on the physical functioning scale. The physical component summary score of the RAND decreased as the number of cigarettes that were smoked daily increased ($p = 0.01$).

Conclusion: Health-related quality of life deteriorated with an increase in daily cigarettes smoked in a dose-dependent manner. Never-smokers survived longer than heavy smokers and they had better quality of life.

Is the evidence likely to be biased?

- *Was there a representative and well-defined sample?*
  Yes. This was a well-defined sample with clear inclusion and exclusion criteria. Participants were healthy, professionally active in positions of responsibility and did not take regular medication or have signs of chronic diseases (including diabetes mellitus, cardiovascular disease, malignant neoplasms, psychiatric disorders or alcoholism). The participants were aged between 40 and 55 years at baseline. At baseline in 1974, data about detailed smoking status were available for 2464 men. However, only the data for 1658 men who were healthy were included. While these data are relevant for the particular client that you are seeing (a 48-year-old, otherwise healthy male), extrapolation of the results of this study to the general population and to women must be done cautiously.
- *Was there an inception cohort?*
  No. 'Inception' cohort refers to cohorts that are assembled at a similar well-described point in the course of a *disease*. The participants in this particular study were all healthy at baseline, showed no signs of cardiovascular disease or other serious diseases, were taking no medications permanently and were professionally active.
- *Was exposure determined accurately?*
  No. Smoking status was assessed with a questionnaire. Participants were classified into five groups according to their self-reported smoking status in 1974: 1) never-smoked (n = 614), defined as men who had never smoked regularly and were not currently smoking; 2) ex-smokers (n = 650), defined as those who had previously been smokers but had quit smoking by 1974; and participants who smoked 3) 1 to 10 cigarettes per day (n = 87), 4) 11 to 20 cigarettes per day (n = 119) or 5) over 20 cigarettes per day (n = 188). Information about the duration of the smoking habit during the study period was not available. Misclassification is possible as participants may have misreported their smoking status. However, as people who smoke may be more likely to under-report rather than over-report smoking, this would only strengthen the association if the people who smoked did not correctly identify their smoking status.
- *Were the outcomes measured accurately?*
  Partially. Health-related quality of life was measured using the RAND 36-Item Health Survey questionnaire—that is, it used participant self-report. Therefore, it was not possible to measure this outcome in a blind fashion. Total mortality of the study population was retrieved from the National Population Information System of the Finnish Population Register Centre, which includes data from all Finnish citizens. It is unclear whether the assessors who extracted this data were blind to participants' clinical characteristics or prognostic factors.
- *Were important prognostic factors considered?*
  Data about a range of factors such as alcohol consumption and cardiovascular risk factors were available from baseline to enable important prognostic factors to be adjusted for with respect to the mortality outcome. However, limited data were available for important prognostic factors for health-related quality of life at baseline. Only participants' self-rating of health and physical fitness on a 5-point scale (very good, good, fair, poor or very poor) was available as the RAND 36-Item Health Survey 1.0 questionnaire did not exist in 1974 (at baseline).

- *Was the follow-up of participants sufficiently long and complete?*
  Yes. The length of follow-up is the strength of this study. Mortality information was available for all participants. The total follow-up time was as long as 26 years, which generated 40,261 person-years of follow-up. Smoking status and health-related quality of life data were measured with a questionnaire that was mailed in the year 2000 to 1286 survivors and 1131 (87.9%) responded.

What are the results?

Mortality: Participants who had never smoked (n = 614) lived a mean of 10 years longer than heavy smokers (>20 cigarettes daily; n = 188).

Health-related quality of life: Among survivors in 2000 (n = 1131), the never-smokers had the best scores on all of the RAND 36-Item Health Survey scales. The largest differences were found between never-smokers and heavy smokers, ranging from 4 points on the scale of social functioning to 14 points on the physical functioning scale. The physical component summary score of the RAND decreased as the number of cigarettes that were smoked daily ($p = 0.01$) increased.

How might we use this evidence to inform practice?

This article clearly demonstrates that people who are heavy smokers are not only likely to live 10 years less than people who are non-smokers but that the more they smoke, the worse their physical functioning is likely to be in later years. The data provide further support for the already substantial evidence that warns about the negative risks of smoking. You consider the results of the study to be relatively free of bias. The data are directly relevant to your client (a 48-year-old, otherwise healthy male). The editorial comment about this article from the same journal issue suggests that:

> It is not just that the heavy smoker loses 10 years of life expectancy but rather that at any given age, the functional capacities of the heavy smoker are equivalent to those of non-smokers who are 10 years older. The clear message is that smoking makes you old before your time, and this reality may be far less attractive to younger smokers than the macho image of dying young while still strong and active.[1]

You discuss the findings of the study with your client and discuss methods that may support him as he quits smoking. As a starting point, you make a time to follow up with him about one of these methods, specifically nicotine replacement therapy.

Nursing example

Clinical scenario

As a nurse in an endocrine unit, you frequently provide education and support to clients and their families, particularly clients who have been newly diagnosed with diabetes. Newly diagnosed clients have many information needs and it is important these are met in order to assist their understanding of the disease, its management and potential risk factors and complications that can arise if blood glucose control is not managed well. One of your current clients is a 56-year-old woman who has just been diagnosed with type 2 non-insulin-dependent diabetes. She is the main carer for her husband who has mobility limitations as a result of a previous stroke. Your client asks you whether being diagnosed with type 2 diabetes has increased her risk of stroke. You suspect that the answer is yes, but want to be able to provide her with as clear and accurate an answer as possible, so you offer to search the evidence for information and talk with them the following day.

Clinical question

Among middle-aged women with a recent diagnosis of type 2 diabetes, what is the risk of stroke compared with women of a similar age without type 2 diabetes?

Search terms and databases used to find the evidence

Database: PubMed—Clinical Queries (with 'prognosis category' and 'narrow search' selected)

Search terms: (stroke OR CVA) AND (type 2 diabetes) AND (risk)

This search returns 145 results. As you consider this to be too many results to look through, you decide to apply four limits to the search—female, middle-aged (45–64 years), English language and humans. This search returns 80 results and you scan the titles of these articles. The title of one article seems to be a good fit with the question you constructed. You read the abstract and, as the study design is appropriate for your question and the description of the study sample population appears to be a good fit to your client, you retrieve the full text of the article.

Article chosen

Janghorbani M, Hu F, Willett W et al. Prospective study of type 1 and type 2 diabetes and risk of stroke subtypes: the Nurses' Health Study. Diabetes Care 2007; 30:1730–1735.

Structured abstract

Study design: Prospective cohort study.

Setting: Part of a larger longitudinal study in the USA (Nurses' Health Study) that ran from 1976 to 2002.

Participants: A cohort of 116,316 women, who were aged 30–55 years and were registered nurses, completed a mailed questionnaire about their health status and various lifestyle and behavioural risk factors.

Outcome: Incidence of stroke (total stroke and stroke subtypes).

Follow-up period: Follow-up questionnaires were sent every 2 years.

Main results: The incidence of total stroke was found to be four times higher in women with type 1 diabetes (relative risk [RR] 4.7; 95% CI 3.3 to 6.6) and twice as high in women with type 2 diabetes (RR 1.8; 95% CI 1.7 to 2.0) than in women without a diagnosis of diabetes.

Conclusion: Type 1 and type 2 diabetes are associated with a significantly increased risk of stroke.

Is the evidence likely to be biased?

- *Was there a representative and well-defined sample?*

    Yes. This study analyses data from the Nurses' Health Study which is the largest long-term epidemiological women's health study that has been conducted. The inclusion criteria of the Nurses' Health Study are broadly defined as married women aged between

30 and 55 years who were registered nurses. This particular article on the incidence of stroke related to diabetes reports data about a wide range of socio-demographic and clinical factors at baseline. It also detailed the characteristics of those who were excluded from analysis (for example, participants with cancer or stroke at baseline), resulting in a sample which included 116,316 women with a mean age of 54.0 years (standard deviation = 10.2 years). Although the sample is likely to be representative of women with similar characteristics to this sample, extrapolation of the results of this study to the general population and to men must be done cautiously.

- *Was there an inception cohort?*
  No. 'Inception' cohort refers to a cohort that was assembled at a similar well-described point in the course of a *disease*. Although cases of diabetes were identified from baseline in this study, the participants who had diabetes were not at a similar point in the disease.
- *Was exposure determined accurately?*
  No. A weakness of the study is that cases of diabetes were identified by participant self-report. When participants reported a diagnosis of diabetes in a biennial follow-up questionnaire, they were sent a supplementary questionnaire to gather information about diagnostic tests, treatment and complications. It is possible that some misclassification occurred as some participants may have had undiagnosed type 2 diabetes and some of the participants classified as having type 1 diabetes may have had type 2 diabetes and vice versa. However, the authors report that, in another substudy, the diagnosis of type 2 diabetes was confirmed (by medical records) in 98.4% of the participants who reported having diabetes, so the extent of any misclassification is likely to be small.
- *Were the outcomes measured accurately?*
  Yes. For all participants who reported a stroke, the researchers asked for permission to access their medical records to confirm the stroke. The review of medical records was completed by a doctor who was blind to participants' exposure status. If medical records were not available or permission to access them was refused, the cases of stroke in these participants were classed as probable if supporting information was provided. The researchers do not elaborate as to what was considered supporting information. Of the total strokes (3463) reported in this cohort, 68% were confirmed and 32% were considered as probable. For total stroke analyses, confirmed and probable cases were used, whereas only confirmed cases were used when analysing stroke subtypes.
- *Were important prognostic factors considered?*
  Yes. The researchers considered a range of possible stroke risk factors in their analyses, such as body mass index, menopausal status, use of post-menopausal hormones, smoking, physical activity, history of hypertension and hypercholesterolaemia, ischaemic heart disease and the use of aspirin and alcohol.
- *Was the follow-up of participants sufficiently long and complete?*
  Yes. The article states that the biennial follow-up rate for the larger Nurses' Health Study exceeds 90%, but no other details about this are provided. The length of follow-up in this study (24 years) is appropriate for the objective of this study.

What are the main results?

In a multivariate analysis that adjusted for age and hypertension, the relative risk of having a stroke was higher in women with type 1 diabetes (RR 4.7; 95% CI 3.3 to 6.6) and type 2 diabetes (RR 1.8; 95% CI 1.7 to 2.0) than in women without diabetes. As evidenced by the higher relative risk and narrow confidence interval, the association between diabetes and stroke was stronger with type 1 diabetes than type 2 diabetes.

How might we use this evidence to inform practice?

You consider the results of this study to be valid and appropriate to the information needs of your client. Many of the characteristics of the sample are a good match with your client's characteristics. When you next meet with her, you are able to explain the main results of the study to her and explain that she is at higher risk of stroke than someone who does not have diabetes. Your discussion with her initially focuses on blood glucose management and the importance of this, but you also provide her with verbal and written information about the risk factors for stroke. You explain the modifiable risk factors of stroke (such as hypertension, hypercholesterolaemia, smoking, obesity and physical inactivity), explain how to control or reduce these risk factors and emphasise the importance of having a regular health assessment.

Medical imaging example

Clinical scenario

You are a radiographer with 5 years post-qualification experience. The large public teaching hospital where you have just started a new job has women's health as one of its specialities. In the course of your rotation through the breast unit you become aware of the role played by the nurses in supporting the women who attend for the various breast imaging examinations. It becomes clear to you that the women rely very much upon these nurses for information about the efficacy of the various imaging modalities in diagnosing cancer of the breast. One nurse in particular is keen to know if it is possible for any of the imaging modalities (such as magnetic resonance [MR] imaging) to accurately predict which clients might survive breast cancer. She recently had some very anxious clients who asked her about their long-term chances of survival. You offer to do some searching and let the nurse know the answer later that week.

Clinical question

Can MR imaging be used to predict survival in women with breast cancer?

Search terms and databases used to find the evidence

Database: PubMed—Clinical Queries (with prognosis category and narrow, specific search filter selected)

Search terms: (MR imaging) AND (breast cancer) and (survival)

This search results in nine articles and you scan the titles, but none are relevant to your question. You return to the searching page, select the 'broad, sensitive' search filter instead and repeat your search. This produces 21 results, one of which is an article that is relevant to your clinical question.

Article chosen

Bone B, Szabo B, Perbeck L et al. Can contrast enhanced MR imaging predict survival in breast cancer? Acta Radiol 2003; 44:373–378.

Structured abstract

Study design: A longitudinal cohort study. This study followed up a cohort of participants who had previously been recruited for an earlier study that examined MR imaging in women with breast cancer.

Setting: Hospital in Sweden.

Participants: The initial study consisted of 50 consecutive breast cancer patients (mean age at diagnosis = 59 years) who had undergone a preoperative contrast-enhanced MR imaging (CE-MRI) examination between September 1992 and December 1993. Inclusion criteria for the initial study were a histopathologically verified primary breast malignancy and a detectable abnormality at MR imaging (lesion visible on at least three consecutive images).

Outcomes: Disease-free survival and overall survival.

Prognostic factors studied: A range of established classical and molecular prognostic markers were analysed, such as age, lymph node status, tumour size and proliferating cell nuclear antigen index.

Follow-up period: Median follow-up was 95 months (range 23–111 months).

Main results: The cumulative 5-year and 7-year survival rates for the whole cohort were 63% and 59% for disease-free and 81% and 77% for overall survival, respectively. Local recurrence or metastasis of the primary disease developed in 20 (40%) patients. Independent and significant predictors of disease-free survival were tumour size and the signal enhancement ratio. Independent and significant predictors of overall survival were age, lymph node status, tumour size and proliferating cell nuclear antigen index.

Conclusion: CE-MRI is useful in predicting the disease-free survival of women with breast cancer.

Is the evidence likely to be biased?

- *Was there a representative and well-defined sample?*
  Cannot tell. When the cohort was gathered for the initial study, the article states that participants were consecutively investigated breast cancer patients, which may indicate that the cohort was likely to be representative. However, it is not clear what is meant by 'investigated' as this could imply that only patients who had undergone a CE-MRI investigation were included and, if this was the situation, it is possible that these patients may have systematically differed in some way to the patients who did not undergo this investigation. The sample was reasonably well-defined as clear inclusion criteria are provided, however no exclusion criteria are stated.

- *Was there an inception cohort?*
  Cannot tell. The article does not provide any clear details about whether participants were in a similar stage in the disease process when they were recruited. Although it is likely that participants were recruited shortly after the time of diagnosis as they were patients who had undergone a CE-MRI examination preoperatively, no further details about this are provided.

- *Was the exposure determined accurately?*
  Yes. One of the inclusion criteria was that participants needed to have a histopathologically verified primary breast malignancy. In addition, all imaging and other clinical predictive markers were correlated and confirmed with the histopathological description of the biopsied tumour samples.

- *Were the outcomes measured accurately?*
  Yes. Data about the outcomes of overall survival and disease-free survival were obtained from the hospital medical records. Disease-free survival and overall survival

are objective outcomes that were defined and the articles states that participants who died from causes other than breast cancer were censored.

* *Were important prognostic factors considered?*
No. The researchers identified some prognostic factors, but not all potentially important ones. For example, there was a mix of tumour types in this cohort and this may have affected the results, especially in such a small group. Ideally, results should have been stratified according to tumour type and grade but this would require a much larger cohort.

* *Was the follow-up of participants sufficiently long and complete?*
No. A major weakness of the study is that the follow-up was conducted retrospectively via hospital medical records. This implied that participants continued to be cared for by the same hospital throughout the study period, which may not have been the case. No information is provided as to whether all participants were able to be followed up (in this case, if current medical records were available for all participants from the initial study). A prospective follow-up of patients would have strengthened the study. Additionally, the follow-up of participants was not long enough. Although the median follow-up time was appropriate at 95 months, the range was very large (23 to 111 months) and the reason for this large variation in the follow-up period is not explained.

What are the main results?

Predictors of disease-free survival: In a multivariate analysis, only the signal enhancement ratio obtained during the CE-MRI ($p = 0.014$) and tumour size at excision ($p = 0.001$) were significant and independent prognostic factors for disease-free survival.

Predictors of overall survival: In a multivariate analysis, age ($p = 0.003$), lymph node status ($p = 0.014$), tumour size ($p = 0.039$) and the proliferating cell nuclear antigen index ($p = 0.053$) were found to be significant and independent prognostic factors for overall survival.

How might we use this evidence to inform practice?

Because the study had a number of flaws which cast doubt on the validity of the results, you decide that the results should be treated with caution. You decide to tell the nurse that, although the results of this study seem to indicate a possible role for CE-MRI in predicting survival in breast cancer, the evidence is currently not adequate for it to be used to replace biological markers as predictors of survival in women with breast cancer.

References

1. Burns D. Live fast, die young, leave a good-looking corpse. Arch Intern Med 2008; 168:1946–1947.

CHAPTER 10

Evidence about clients' experiences and concerns

Alan Pearson

LEARNING OBJECTIVES

After reading this chapter, you should be able to:
- Appreciate the role of qualitative research in providing information about clients' experiences and concerns
- Develop a qualitative clinical question
- Describe the basic assumptions that underpin the common qualitative research methodologies of phenomenology, grounded theory, ethnography, action research, feminist research and discourse analysis
- Critically appraise qualitative research articles
- Interpret the findings of qualitative research articles
- Discuss how the findings of qualitative research may be used in practice

Clinical scenario

A team of general practitioners, nurses, physiotherapists, occupational therapists, dieticians and medical receptionists working in a government-funded health centre have invested a great deal of energy and resources to develop a team-based approach to client care. Overall, they are pleased with the progress made and are anxious to consider the degree to which their efforts relate to improving clients' experiences. They have agreed that, given the growing size of the team and the increase in the number of different members of the team interacting with clients with chronic illnesses, their most urgent need is to find out what, from the clients' perspective, continuity really means.

This chapter focuses on questions that relate to the experiences of clients and health professionals and the meaning that clients and health professionals associate with these experiences. In general terms, evidence-based health care has tended to focus on the search for objective evidence to establish the degree to which a particular intervention or activity results in defined outcomes. The importance of basing practice on the best available evidence is now well accepted and ways of finding, appraising and applying evidence related to diagnosis, prognosis or the effects of an intervention are becoming increasingly well understood. Thus, evidence-based practice is generally conceptualised as searching for, appraising and synthesising the results of experimental or quantitative research and transferring the findings to practice and policy domains to improve health outcomes.

Health professionals, however, seek evidence to substantiate the worth of a very wide range of activities and interventions and thus the type of evidence needed depends on the nature of the activity and its purpose. Pearson and colleagues[1] have described a model of evidence-based health care in which they assert that, if evidence is needed to address the multiple questions, concerns or interests of health professionals or the users of health services, it must come from a wide range of research traditions. Evidence that arises out of qualitative inquiry is frequently sought and utilised in clinical practice.[2] Qualitative research seeks to make sense of phenomena in terms of the meanings that people bring to them.[3] Evidence from qualitative studies that explore the experience of clients and health professionals has an important role in ensuring that the particularities associated with individual clients, families and communities are just as important as information that arises out of quantitative research.

Qualitative researchers attempt to increase our understandings of:
- how individuals and communities perceive health, manage their own health, and make decisions related to health service usage
- the culture of communities and of organisations in relation to implementing change and overcoming barriers to the use of new knowledge and techniques
- how clients experience health and illness and the health system
- the usefulness, or otherwise, of components and activities of health services that cannot be measured in quantitative outcomes (such as health promotion and community development)
- the behaviours/experiences of health professionals and the contexts of health care.

Qualitative research generates evidence that informs clinical decision making on matters related to feasibility, appropriateness or meaningfulness. Pearson et al[2] describe feasibility as the extent to which an activity is practical and practicable. Clinical feasibility is about whether or not an activity or intervention is physically, culturally or financially practical or possible within a given context. They define appropriateness as the extent to which an intervention or activity fits with or is apt in a situation. Clinical appropriateness is about how an activity or intervention relates to the context in which care is given. Meaningfulness refers to how an intervention or activity is experienced by the client. Meaningfulness relates to the personal experience, opinions, values, thoughts, beliefs and interpretations of clients. Evidence-based practice in its fullest sense is about making decisions about feasibility, appropriateness, meaningfulness and effectiveness—and quantitative and qualitative evidence are of equal importance in this endeavour.

This chapter explores the development of qualitative clinical questions and the role and methods of qualitative research. It will also explain how to appraise and apply qualitative evidence. Throughout the chapter, a clinical scenario and relevant qualitative article will be referred to as an example as we consider how to appraise a qualitative article and how the findings of qualitative research can be applied in practice.

Qualitative research: its role in researching clients' experiences and concerns

Qualitative research that focuses on clients' (and health professionals') experiences and concerns assists people to tell their stories about what it is like to be a certain person, living in a particular time and place, in relation to a set of circumstances, and analyses the data generated to describe human experience and meaning. The 'data' that are collected and analysed in qualitative research are words because they are the media through which people express themselves and their relationships to other people and their world. This means that, if researchers want to know what the experience of care is like, they will ask the people receiving that care to describe their experience in order to capture the rich meaning.

Through these approaches the enduring realities of people's experiences are not over-simplified and subsumed into a number or a statistic. Because qualitative researchers draw relationships between sets of data and interpret the material, qualitative research is flexible in design and adaptive. For example, it is possible to use multiple methods for any one study. Qualitative approaches in health services research represent a relatively new disciplinary approach and there is still much debate concerning the rigour of analysis[4-6] and the benefits of one method over another: for instance, the benefits of an ethnographic approach over a phenomenological or a grounded theory approach. Each of these approaches is briefly explained later in this chapter. Different qualitative research approaches set out to achieve different things and, when differing perspectives are put together, they provide a multifaceted view of the subject of inquiry that deepens our understanding of it. In this sense they are not substitutes for each other due to some essential superiority of one method over another, but rather they represent a theoretical 'tool kit' of devices. Depending on the task at hand, one methodology on one occasion may be a more useful tool than another.

How to structure a qualitative question

The team that was described in the clinical scenario at the beginning of this chapter want to find out what receiving care from a large primary healthcare team is like for people who have a chronic illness. The PICO format that was described in Chapter 2 can be used to structure a qualitative question, but generally there is no 'comparison' in a qualitative question and the 'I' refers to 'interest' or 'issue' rather than intervention.

> ## Clinical scenario (continued): Structuring the question
>
> From this scenario, a suitable qualitative question would be: In adults with any chronic condition that requires frequent primary health care (Population), what is their experience of continuity and of receiving that care from different members of the primary healthcare team (Issue) and how does this experience help or hinder their daily lives (Outcomes)?

Because the question for our clinical scenario explicitly seeks *qualitative* information, clearly, the team will need to search for qualitative research articles. Using the term 'qualitative research' is, however, in itself problematic. The word 'qualitative' is frequently used to describe a singular, specific methodology (for example '... in this study a qualitative methodology was pursued') when in its broadest sense it is an umbrella term that encompasses a wide range of methodologies stemming from a number of diverse traditions.

Although we can be clear in saying that there are easy-to-describe qualitative data (that is, data that consist of words and the meaning they convey) and that there are easy-to describe ways to approach qualitative data analysis (that is, manual and electronic approaches to analysing words and their meanings), to design and conduct qualitative research requires the identification of a well understood methodology that is appropriate to the question and the use of methods of data collection and analysis that are congruent with the chosen methodology. There are many different qualitative methodologies and we will outline six commonly used approaches in the following section. Although they are discussed separately, qualitative researchers often combine elements from different methodologies when undertaking their research.

Qualitative methodologies used in health research

Phenomenology

A phenomenological research approach values human perception and subjectivity and seeks to explore what an experience is like for the individual concerned.[7] The basis of this approach is a concept called 'lived experience', which means that people who are living presently, or have lived an experience previously, are in the best position to speak of it, to inform others of what the experience is like or what it means to them. Phenomenology is concerned with discovering the 'essence' of experience. It asks the question: 'What was it like to have that experience?'

Data are collected using a focussed, but non-structured, interview technique to elicit descriptions of the participant's experiences. This style of interview supports the role of the researcher as one who does not presume to know what the important aspects of the experience to be revealed are. Several steps are involved in thematic data analysis.[7] The interviews are transcribed verbatim and are then read by researchers who attempt to totally submerge themselves in the text in order to identify the implicit or essential themes of the experience, thus seeking the fundamental meaning of the experience.

The strength of the phenomenological method is that it seeks to derive meaning and knowledge from the phenomena themselves and, although it is generally conceded that unmediated access to a phenomenon is never a possibility (that is, the exclusion of all prior perceptions and research bias), the emphasis on the experience of the participants ensures that this model represents as closely as possible the participants' perspective.[5,6] In this sense the perspectives that arise from the phenomenological approach help to shape the categories of concern in terms of the issues that the participants themselves identify. Through the phenomenological method, participants contribute substantially to informing and describing the field of inquiry that future policy needs to address.

Clinical scenario (continued): Potential contribution of evidence from phenomenological research

The findings of phenomenological research studies could usefully provide evidence to the primary healthcare team related to the lived experience of being a patient/client and the meanings that clients associate with this experience.

Grounded theory

Grounded theory is a term chosen by sociologists Glaser and Strauss[8] to express their ideas of generating theory from the 'ground' using an 'iterative' (or cyclical/circular) approach whereby data are gathered using an ongoing collection process from a variety of sources. They developed this approach in their ground-breaking work on death and dying in hospitals.[8] Strauss and Corbin[9] have developed an approach that begins with open coding of data that requires the researcher to take the data apart and ask, 'What is going on here?'

Clinical scenario (continued): Potential contribution of evidence from grounded theory research

The findings of grounded theory research studies could usefully provide evidence to the primary healthcare team related to the development of a new, theoretical understanding of what being a person receiving primary health care means, grounded or based on the experience of clients themselves.

Ethnography

The term ethnography was used originally to describe a research technique that was used to study groups of people who: shared social and cultural characteristics; thought of themselves as a group; and shared common language, geographic locale and identity. Classic ethnographies portray cultures, providing 'a portrait of the people' (the literal meaning of the term ethnography) and move beyond descriptions of what is said and done in order to understand 'shared systems of meanings that we call culture'.[10]

An ethnographer comes to understand the social world of the group in an attempt to develop an inside view while recognising that it will emerge from an outside perspective. In this sense the researcher attempts to experience the world of the 'other' (euphemistically referred to as 'going native'), while appreciating that the experience emerges through the 'self' of the researcher. Ethnography involves participant observation, the recording of field notes and interviewing key informants. The identifying feature of participant observation is the attempt to reconstruct a representation of a culture that closely reflects 'the native's point of view'.

Clinical scenario (continued): Potential contribution of evidence from ethnography

The findings of ethnographic research studies could usefully provide evidence to the primary healthcare team related to the norms, patterns and group meanings of clients who are receiving primary health care, based on observation and the accounts of members of the group.

Action research

Phenomenology, grounded theory and ethnography are described as 'interpretive' approaches to research because they all aim to describe and understand phenomena. Some approaches to qualitative research take a more 'critical' approach—asking not just what is happening, but why. Critical researchers seek to question why things are as they are and to generate change by bringing problems or injustices forward for conscious debate and consideration. Critical approaches involve working with people collaboratively to analyse and seek out understandings of the real situation and to search out alternative ways of seeing the situation.

Action research is the pursuit of knowledge through working collaboratively on describing the social world and acting on it in order to change it. Through acting on the world this way, critical theory and understandings are generated. Action research asks the question, 'What is happening here and how could it be different?' It involves reflecting on the world in order to change it and then entering into a cyclical process of reflection, change and evaluation.

Data collected in action research include transcripts of group discussions as well as quantitative and qualitative data suggested by the participative group. Both of these types of data are analysed concurrently. Themes, issues and concerns are extracted and discussed by both the research team and the participative group. Action research provides a potential means for overcoming the frequent failure of externally generated research to be embraced by research consumers, who often regard this form of research as unrelated to and not associated with their practice.

Clinical scenario (continued): Potential contribution of evidence from action research studies

The findings of action research studies could usefully provide evidence to the primary healthcare team related to outcomes of involving clients themselves in critiquing the care they receive and in developing and implementing action to change those things that they identify as inappropriate or as barriers to optimal living.

Feminist research

Feminist research grew in the 1960s[11] from the premise that existing research and theory was biased to a male perspective that had not been challenged and that it overshadowed female and feminine experiences, contributions and perspectives. Science (including social and human sciences) and research were, and still are, largely carried out in academic departments which, it was argued, were male domains with a masculine driven agenda. It is argued that this agenda steered research towards the quantitative or experimental type of research. Feminist researchers sought to challenge this domination. Feminist research must therefore be considered political, critical and constructivist in orientation.

In terms of the methods used in research, feminist researchers seek to remove the hierarchical relationship that exists between the researcher and the participant. Rogers,[12] from an ethical perspective, indicates that 'a feminist approach leads us to examine not only the connections between gender, disadvantage and health, but also the distribution of power in the processes of public health, from policy making through to programme delivery'. It could therefore be argued that a feminist approach, one which uses appropriate methods, could help, in public health terms, to illuminate the experience and perspective of 'hidden' or difficult to reach groups and enhance practice and policy.

Feminist research that is undertaken within the broad umbrella of health research has often been linked to women's health research and as such has probably had an over-focus on women's reproductive related issues (such as fertility, menstruation, menopause and breast and gynaecological cancers). In addition, it might also be considered it has sought to address broader areas of women's health such as family roles, sexual exploitation, areas of mental health (for example, eating disorders) and inequality. While the latter areas might not be related to biological health, they are clearly related to an overall holistic view of health and as such are appropriate areas to research.

Clinical scenario (continued): Potential contribution of evidence from feminist research

The findings of feminist studies could provide evidence to the primary healthcare team related to the role of gender and gender relations in the care that female clients receive and in developing and implementing action to change those things that they identify as inappropriate or as barriers to optimal living.

Discourse analysis

Postmodernism and relativism

Postmodernist thought emerged in a number of academic disciplines in the last two or so decades of the 20th century and has played an important role in creating new ways of developing ideas in the arts, science and culture. At its simplest (and it is far from simple!) postmodernism is a response to modernity—the period when science was trusted and represented progress—and essentially focuses on questioning the centrality of both science and established principles, disciplines and institutions to achieving progress. The nature of 'truth' is a recurring concern to postmodernists, who generally claim that there are no truths but instead that there are multiple realities and that understandings of the human condition are dynamic and diverse. The notion that no one view, theory or understanding should be privileged over another is a belief of postmodernist critique and analysis. The scrutiny and breakdown of ideas that are associated with postmodernism is most frequently applied through the discursive analysis of texts. The most popular application of this in health services research is discourse analysis.

Discourse analysis

Discourse is defined as to '… talk, converse; hold forth in speech or writing on a subject; give forth'.[13] Thus, discourse analysis essentially refers to the capturing of public, professional, political and even private discourses and deconstructing these 'messages'. Discursive analysis aims at revealing what is being said, thought and done in relation to a specific topic or issue. Discursive analysis is applicable to every situation and subject. Although the discursive analysis of health policy, service delivery priorities, systems and methods or the practices of health professionals will not result in definitive answers to questions, it can be useful in uncovering dominant and marginalised discourses and in locating inconsistencies that require explanation.

> ## Clinical scenario (continued): Potential contribution of evidence from discursive studies
>
> **The findings of discursive studies could usefully provide evidence to the primary healthcare team that arises out of deconstructing what clients and health professionals say; the origins of existing, dominant views; and the way in which strongly held, powerful discourses may 'silence' or 'marginalise' the voices of clients/ patients.**

Hopefully by now you will have realised that qualitative research evidence is an important source of knowledge related to the 'culture, practices, and discourses of health and illness'.[14,15] The value of such research and its methodologies lies in its ability to systematically examine questions about issues such as experiences, opinions and reasons for behaviours that are unable to be answered by means of quantitative research that often uses frequencies and associations.

Searching for qualitative evidence

Finding qualitative research papers through database searches is often difficult.[16] It has been claimed that finding quantitative studies is much easier because the progress that has been made in indexing specific quantitative designs has not been paralleled in the qualitative domain. In Chapter 3, we provided you with some search strategies for locating qualitative research in MEDLINE, CINAHL, Embase and PsycINFO (refer to Table 3.1 in Chapter 3). For example, you may remember that, in MEDLINE, the best multiple term strategy that minimised the difference between a sensitive and specific search[17] was to combine the content terms with the following methodological terms: interview:.mp. OR experience:.mp. OR qualitative.tw. However, if you wish to look for a particular method, relevant terms such as phenomenology or grounded theory will need to be used.

Clinical scenario (continued): Finding the evidence to answer the question

One possible search strategy that the primary healthcare team could use is to search in PubMed, with the following search terms: (primary health care) AND (chronic illness) AND (patient experience) AND continuity.

This search resulted in 53 articles. One of these articles seemed to directly address patient experiences of continuity of care in a chronic illness. It specifically explores continuity of care in a group of people with diabetes.

Clinical scenario (continued): Structured abstract of the chosen article

Citation: Naithani S, Gulliford M, Morgan M. Patients' perceptions and experiences of 'continuity of care' in diabetes. Health Expect 2006; 9:118–129.[18]

Study design: This is a 'qualitative' study.

Study question: The study explored patients' experiences and values with respect to continuity in diabetes care.

Context: Participants lived in relatively deprived inner city areas of London that have young, mobile and ethnically diverse populations.

Participants: Participants were 25 people with type 2 diabetes from 14 general practices in two inner London boroughs. Participants were purposively sampled to include main ethnic minority groups.

Data collection method: In-depth semi-structured interviews.

Analysis: Analysis initially involved coding segments of transcripts that described patients' views and experiences of their diabetes care. These were then mapped to the dimensions of continuity of Freeman et al, which are further described in the article. This model was selected as forming the product of a synthesis of previous approaches to continuity of care and emphasising the primary–secondary interface.

Key findings: Patients' accounts identified four dimensions of experienced continuity of care. These were: 1) receiving regular reviews with clinical testing and provision of advice over time (longitudinal continuity); 2) having a relationship with a usual care provider who knew and understood them (relational continuity); 3) flexibility of service provision in response to changing needs or situations (flexible continuity); 4) consistency and coordination between different members of staff and settings (team and cross-boundary continuity). Lack of continuity occurred largely at transitions between sites of care, between providers or with significant changes in patients' needs.

Conclusion: The study offers a patient-based framework for determining continuity of care in chronic disease management. It also identifies problematic aspects of continuity related to key transition points. The authors suggest that it is important that service design for chronic disease management take patients' experience of continuity of care into account.

Is the evidence likely to be biased? Appraising qualitative evidence: rigour and reporting

Dixon-Woods, Agarwal and Smith[19] suggest that 'there are now over 100 sets of proposals on quality in qualitative research' and assert that:

> Some means of appraising qualitative research is needed if it is to contribute appropriately to systematic reviews. Proposals for criteria that might define high quality qualitative research have proliferated, but sometimes do not overlap or are difficult to operationalise.

The major aim in critically appraising experimental or quantifiable data is to limit bias and thus establish the validity of a study. As you have seen in earlier chapters of this book, from a quantitative perspective, sources of bias include selection bias, performance bias and attrition bias. Validity is assessed by establishing the extent to which the design and conduct of a study address potential sources of bias. This focus on limiting bias to establish validity does not fit with the philosophical foundations of qualitative approaches to inquiry. The focus of critical appraisal of qualitative evidence is on the rigour of the research design and quality of reporting. Qualitative approaches are located in diverse understandings of knowledge; they do not distance the researcher from the researched; and the data analysis is legitimately influenced by the researcher when they interpret the data. Critical appraisal therefore focuses on:

1. congruity between philosophical position adopted in the study, study methodology, study methods, representation of the data and the interpretation of the results
2. the degree to which the biases of the researcher are made explicit
3. the relationship between what the participants are reported to have said and the conclusions drawn in analysis.

Drawing from the literature and input from a panel of experts, a critical appraisal instrument is described by Pearson.[20] This instrument has been extensively piloted and refined and is referred to as the QARI (Qualitative Assessment and Review Instrument). It consists of ten appraisal criteria which we will now explore.

1 Is there congruity between the stated philosophical perspective and the research methodology?

In responding to this question, consider whether the article clearly states the philosophical or theoretical premises on which the study is based. Does the article clearly state the methodological approach on which the study is based? Is there congruence between the two?

For example, an article may state that the study adopted a critical perspective and a participatory action research methodology was followed. There is congruence between a critical view (focussing on knowledge arising out of critique, action and reflection) and action research (an approach that focuses on working with groups to reflect on issues or practices and to consider how they could be different, on acting to change and on identifying new knowledge arising out of the action taken). However, consider another example in which an article states that the study adopted an interpretive perspective and that a survey methodology was followed. In this example, there is incongruence between an interpretive view (focussing on knowledge arising out of studying what phenomena mean to individuals or groups) and surveys (an approach that focuses on asking standard questions to a defined study population). Sometimes an article may state that the study was qualitative or used qualitative methodology (such statements do not demonstrate rigour in design) or make no statement about the philosophical orientation or methodology.

Clinical scenario (continued): Critical appraisal of the chosen article

1 Congruity between the stated philosophical perspective and the research methodology

The study sought to understand patients' experience (interpretation) and used what it describes as '… a qualitative …' approach. This is a somewhat meaningless description that offers little when trying to address this criterion. However, it appears that the researchers were taking an interpretive position and used a constructivist methodology, but they do not explicitly describe the methodology. Thus, when evaluating this criterion, it appears that there is insufficient information to make a judgement.

2 Is there congruity between the research methodology and the research question or objectives?

This question seeks to establish if the study methodology is appropriate for addressing the research question. For example, an article may state that the research question was to seek understandings of the meaning of pain in a group of people with rheumatoid arthritis and that a phenomenological approach was taken. Here, there is congruity between this question and the methodology. Consider another example in which an article states that the research question was to establish the effects of counselling on the severity of pain experience and that an ethnographic approach was pursued. A question that tries to establish cause-and-effect cannot be addressed by using an ethnographic approach (as ethnography sets out to develop understandings of cultural practices) and, therefore, this would be incongruent.

Clinical scenario (continued): Critical appraisal of the chosen article

2 Congruity between the research methodology and the research question or objectives

Given that the aim was to understand patient/client experiences, this criterion appears to be met.

3 Is there congruity between the research methodology and the methods used to collect data?

This question guides reviewers to consider whether the data collection methods are appropriate to the stated methodology. For example, an article may state that the study pursued a phenomenological approach and that data were collected through phenomenological interviews. In this instance there is congruence between the methodology and data collection. However if an article stated that the study pursued a phenomenological approach and that data were collected through a postal questionnaire, this would indicate incongruence between the methodology and data collection. This is because phenomenology seeks to elicit rich descriptions of the experience of a phenomenon that cannot be achieved through seeking written responses to standardised questions.

Clinical scenario (continued): Critical appraisal of the chosen article

3 **Congruity between the research methodology and the methods used to collect data**
The method used was in-depth semi-structured interviews with 25 people with type 2 diabetes. This method is consistent with the overall design of the study.

---

4 Is there congruity between the research methodology and the representation and analysis of data?

Are the data analysed and represented in ways that are congruent with the stated methodological position? For example, an article may state that the study pursued a phenomenological approach to explore people's experience of grief by asking participants to describe their experiences of grief. If the text generated from asking these questions is searched to establish the meaning of grief to participants and the meanings of all participants are included in the report findings, then this represents congruity. However if the same article focussed only on the meanings that were common to all participants and discarded single reported meanings, this would not be appropriate in phenomenological work.

Clinical scenario (continued): Critical appraisal of the chosen article

4 **Congruity between the research methodology and the representation and analysis of data**
Interviews were transcribed and responses analysed thematically and grouped into dimensions of continuity of care. This is congruous with the overall approach.

---

5 Is there congruence between the research methodology and the interpretation of results?

Are the results interpreted in ways that are appropriate to the methodology? For example, an article may state that a study pursued a phenomenological approach to explore people's experience of facial disfigurement and these results are used to inform health professionals about accommodating individual differences in care. In this example, there is congruence between the methodology and this approach to interpretation. However, consider the example of an article that states that the study pursued a phenomenological approach to explore people's experience of facial disfigurement and the results are used to generate practice checklists for assessment. In this case, there is incongruence between the methodology and this approach to interpretation as phenomenology seeks to understand the meaning of a phenomenon for the study participants and cannot be interpreted to suggest that this can be generalised to total populations to a degree where standardised assessments will have relevance across a population.

Clinical scenario (continued): Critical appraisal of the chosen article

5 Congruence between the research methodology and the interpretation of results

The results were interpreted as clients valuing four dimensions of continuity of care. These were: receiving regular reviews with clinical testing and provision of advice over time (longitudinal continuity); having a relationship with a usual care provider who knew and understood them, was concerned and interested and took time to listen and explain (relational continuity); flexibility of service provision in response to changing needs or situations (flexible continuity); and consistency and coordination between different members of staff and between hospital and general practice or community settings (team and cross-boundary continuity). Problems of a lack of experience of continuity mainly occurred at transitions between sites of care, between providers or with major changes in clients' needs.

---

6 Is the researcher located culturally or theoretically?

Are the beliefs and values and their potential influences on the study declared? The researcher plays a substantial role in the qualitative research process and it is important when appraising evidence that is generated in this way to know the researcher's cultural and theoretical orientation. A high quality report will include a statement that clarifies this.

Clinical scenario (continued): Critical appraisal of the chosen article

6 Locating the researcher culturally or theoretically

The researchers do not describe this.

---

7 Is the influence of the researcher on the research, and vice versa, addressed?

Are the potential for the researcher to influence the study and the potential of the research process itself to influence the researcher and the interpretations acknowledged and addressed? For example:

- Is the relationship between the researcher and the study participants addressed?
- Does the researcher critically examine their own role and potential influence during data collection?
- Is it reported how the researcher responded to events that arose during the study?

> ## Clinical scenario (continued): Critical appraisal of the chosen article
>
> **7 Influence of the researcher on the research, and vice versa, is addressed**
> The researchers do not describe this.

8 Is there representation of participants and their voices?

Generally, articles should provide illustrations from the data (such as quotes from participants) to show the basis of their conclusions and to ensure that participants are represented in the article.

> ## Clinical scenario (continued): Critical appraisal of the chosen article
>
> **8 Representation of participants and their voices**
> The article illustrates each of the themes by presenting excerpts from the patient interview transcripts and therefore demonstrates compliance with this criterion.

9 Was ethical approval provided by an appropriate body?

A statement on the ethical approval process that was followed should be provided in the article.

> ## Clinical scenario (continued): Critical appraisal of the chosen article
>
> **9 Ethical approval by an appropriate body**
> An ethics committee approved the project proposal.

10 Do conclusions drawn in the research article appear to flow from the analysis or interpretation of the data?

This criterion concerns the relationship between the findings reported and the views or words of study participants. In appraising an article, appraisers seek to satisfy themselves that the conclusions drawn by the research are based on the data collected—the data being the text that is generated through observation, interviews or other processes.

How then do we make sense of the appraisal as a whole? Pearson[20] offers the following categorisation of judgement about a qualitative article. Overall the article may be considered:

• *Unequivocal:* The evidence is beyond reasonable doubt and includes findings that are factual, directly reported/observed and not open to challenge.

- *Credible:* The evidence, while interpretative, is plausible in light of the data and theoretical framework. Conclusions can be logically inferred from the data but because the findings are essentially interpretative, these conclusions are open to challenge.
- *Unsupported:* Findings are not supported by the data and none of the other level descriptors apply.

While the QARI tool has been the focus of this chapter, there are many different approaches to determining the quality of qualitative research. For example, the Critical Appraisal Skills Programme (CASP) that was used in the earlier chapters of this book in relation to the appraisal of quantitative evidence also has a checklist that is widely used. It also addresses the issues of rigour, credibility and relevance of qualitative research. Regardless of which approach is used, it is important to remain aware of the specific qualitative methodology that is being used.

Clinical scenario (continued): Critical appraisal of the chosen article

10 Relationship of conclusions to analysis or interpretation of the data
The study develops a patient-based framework for assessing continuity of care in chronic disease management and identifies key transition points with problems of lack of continuity. It concludes that it is important that service redesign and developments in vertically integrated services for chronic disease management take account of impacts on the patient's experience of continuity of care.

Applying qualitative evidence

Research from qualitative studies can inform health professionals' thinking about similar situations/populations that they are working with. However, the way in which findings from qualitative evidence might be used in practice differs from quantitative research. Quantitative research findings are reported in terms of the probability (for example) of an outcome occurring when a particular intervention is implemented, in the same way, for a defined client group and therefore require health professionals to accept a generalisation that the research findings can be applied to most clients. In quantitative research, this concept is referred to as generalisability.

There are objections to the application of qualitative findings in practice because of the theoretical underpinnings of many qualitative methodologies. Principally this relates to the idea that 'truth' is contextual, or 'in the moment', and therefore only representative of a particular person or group at *that* time and within *that* context. Therefore it is argued that the findings of a qualitative study of one group of people in a single study cannot be extrapolated to other people, groups or contexts. Researchers who follow this line of argument claim that the pooling and/or application of qualitative findings is, in effect, an attempt to formulate a result that can be generalised across a population and, as such, is an inappropriate use of qualitative findings. Other researchers have developed a strong opposing view and suggest that the term *generalisability* is being misinterpreted. Sandelowski and colleagues have put forward that the argument against the pooling or application of qualitative findings is founded on a 'narrowly conceived' view of what constitutes generalisability—that is, a view that sees it in relation to the representativeness (in terms of size and randomisation) of a sample and of statistical significance. They argue that qualitative research has the capacity to produce generalisations—but they are suggestive or naturalistic (or realistic) in nature rather than generalisations that are predictive as is the case in quantitative research.[21]

Clinical scenario (continued): Applying qualitative evidence to the clinical scenario

A strategy for applying the findings of qualitative research within the primary healthcare team could include:
- Raising awareness of the client's experiences within the team in relation to longitudinal continuity, relational continuity, flexible continuity and team and cross-boundary continuity
- Conducting a clinical audit of care giving to people with a chronic illness and assessing the degree to which these four areas of continuity are achieved
- Involving the multidisciplinary team in reviewing the way in which people with a chronic disease are cared for in relation to longitudinal continuity, relational continuity, flexible continuity and team and cross-boundary continuity
- Engaging the multidisciplinary team in service redesign and the development of services for chronic disease management that include:
  - offering clients regular reviews
  - identifying a 'usual care provider' for all clients with a chronic condition
  - a degree of flexibility of service provision in response to changing needs or situations
  - consistency and coordination between different members of staff and between hospital and general practice or community settings
- Evaluating the effects of the changes implemented on the client experience by eliciting client feedback and analysing this feedback.

Summary points of this chapter
- The experiences of clients are a rich source of evidence for practice and can increase our understandings of how individuals and communities perceive health, manage their own health and make decisions related to health service usage.
- Qualitative research uses rigorous processes to elicit and analyse data related to client experience.
- There are a number of well established qualitative research methodologies including (but not limited to) phenomenology, grounded theory, ethnography, action research, feminist research and discourse analysis. These methods are adaptive and may be used in conjunction with each other.
- Appraising qualitative evidence requires an assessment of the quality of the research in relation to the research methodology, methods and analyses used and the interpretation of data. Critical appraisal focuses on the congruity between the philosophical position adopted in the study, study methodology, study methods, representation of the data and the interpretation of the results; the degree to which the biases of the researcher are made explicit; and the relationship between what the participants are reported to have said and the conclusions that have been drawn in the analysis.

References

1. Pearson A, Wiechula R, Court A et al. The JBI model of evidence-based healthcare. Int J Evidence-based Healthcare 2005; 3:207–215.
2. Pearson A, Field J, Jordan Z. Evidence-based clinical practice in nursing and health care. Oxford: Blackwell Publishing; 2007.
3. Denzin NK. The art and politics of interpretation. In: Denzin N, Lincoln Y eds. Handbook of qualitative research. Thousand Oaks, CA: Sage; 1994:500–515.
4. Gubrium JF. Qualitative research comes of age in gerontology. Gerontologist 1992; 32:581–582.
5. Koch T. Establishing rigour in qualitative research: the decision trail. J Adv Nurs 1993; 19: 976–986.
6. Koch T. Implementation of a hermeneutic inquiry in nursing: philosophy, rigour and representation. J Adv Nurs 1996; 24:174–184.
7. van Manen M. Researching lived experience: human science for an action sensitive pedagogy. Toronto: Althouse Press; 1997.
8. Glaser B, Strauss AL. The discovery of grounded theory: strategies for qualitative research. New York: Aldine de Gruyter; 1967.
9. Strauss A, Corbin J. Basics of qualitative research: grounded theory procedures and techniques. London: Sage; 1990.
10. Boyle JS. Styles of ethnography. In: Morse J (ed). Critical issues in qualitative research methods. Thousand Oaks CA: Sage; 1994:159–185.
11. Green J, Thorogood N. Qualitative methods for health research. London: Sage Publications; 2004.
12. Rogers W. Feminism and public health ethics. J Med Ethics 2006; 32:351–354.
13. Concise Oxford English Dictionary. Oxford: Oxford University Press; 1964.
14. McCormick J, Rodney P, Varcoe C. Reinterpretations across studies: an approach to meta-analysis. Qual Health Res 2003; 13:933–944.
15. Green J, Britten N. Qualitative research and evidence based medicine. BMJ 1998; 316:1230–1232.
16. Shaw R, Booth A, Sutton A et al. Finding qualitative research: an evaluation of search strategies. BMC Med Res Methodol 2004; 4:5.
17. Wong S, Wilczynski N, Haynes RB et al. Developing optimal search strategies for detecting clinically relevant qualitative studies in MEDLINE. Medinfo 2004; 11:311–316.
18. Naithani S, Gulliford M, Morgan M. Patients' perceptions and experiences of 'continuity of care' in diabetes. Health Expect 2006; 9:118–129.
19. Dixon-Woods M, Shaw R, Agarwal S et al. The problem of appraising qualitative research. Qual Saf Health Care 2004; 13:223–225.
20. Pearson A. Balancing the evidence: incorporating the synthesis of qualitative data into systematic reviews. JBI Reports 2004; 2:45–64.
21. Sandelowski M, Docherty S, Emden C. Focus on qualitative methods. Qualitative metasynthesis: issues and techniques. Res Nurs Health 1997; 20:365–371.

CHAPTER 11

Questions about clients' experiences and concerns: examples of appraisals from different health professions

Sally Bennett, John W Bennett, Craig Lockwood, Sharon Sanders
Jemma and Skeat

This chapter is an accompaniment to the previous chapter (Chapter 10) where the steps involved in answering a clinical question about clients' experiences and concerns were explained. In order to further help you learn how to appraise the evidence for this type of question, this chapter contains a number of worked examples of questions about clients' experiences and concerns that are relevant to health professions such as the therapies, nursing, medicine and complementary and alternative medicine. The QARI tool for appraising qualitative research that was outlined in Chapter 10 has been used for these examples. Although there are other checklists available for appraising qualitative evidence that have a slightly different focus, there is no consensus about the ideal approach that should be used when appraising qualitative research. The QARI tool has been tested and used extensively. Chapter 1 explained how to access the QARI tool.

As was explained in Chapter 10, when the QARI tool is used, critical appraisal focuses on:
- congruity between philosophical position adopted in the study, study methodology, study methods, representation of the data and the interpretation of the results
- the degree to which the biases of the researcher are made explicit
- the relationship between what the participants are reported to have said and the conclusions drawn in analysis.

Occupational therapy and physiotherapy example

Clinical scenario

You have been working as a therapist in a multidisciplinary stroke rehabilitation unit and want to understand why some clients seem more motivated to participate in rehabilitation than others.

Clinical question
What factors might motivate people who have had a stroke to participate in stroke rehabilitation?

Search terms and databases used to find the evidence
Database: PubMed
Search terms: A simple search using the following text words was used: (stroke rehabilitation) AND motivation AND qualitative.

This search strategy retrieved 16 articles, two of which focussed on stroke rehabilitation and motivation. One article considered motivation from the health professionals' perspective and the other considered motivation from the perspective of clients. This is the article that you choose to appraise.

Article chosen
Maclean N, Pound P, Wolfe C et al. Qualitative analysis of stroke patients' motivation for rehabilitation. BMJ 2000; 321:1051–1054.

Structured abstract

Study design: 'Qualitative study with semi-structured interviews' is the design stated in the article. However, it is likely to have used a phenomenological approach.

Study question: To explore the attitudes and beliefs of stroke patients identified by professionals as having either 'high' or 'low' motivation for rehabilitation.

Context: The stroke unit of an inner city teaching hospital.

Participants: 22 patients with stroke who were undergoing rehabilitation—14 with high motivation for rehabilitation and 8 with low motivation.

Data collection method: Semi-structured interviews were used covering the following topics: confidence about making a good recovery, views about relationships with professionals, ideas about important factors in recovery, ideas about the patient's role in rehabilitation, ideas about the nature and purpose of rehabilitation and feelings about what sort of life is desired after the stroke. Participants were free to structure the conversation within each topic. New topics brought up by the participants were discussed as and when they arose.

Analysis: Transcribed interviews were coded for themes and constant comparison was used. The codes in each interview were then compared with those in each other interview to create broader categories that linked codes across interviews.

Key findings: People with stroke who were identified as having high motivation for rehabilitation were more likely to understand the purpose of rehabilitation than those who were identified as having low motivation. Positive determinants of motivation included: being given information about rehabilitation, positive comparisons with other people with stroke and wanting to leave hospital. Negative determinants of motivation included: overprotection from family members and professionals, lack of information and the provision of mixed messages about rehabilitation to patients and less favourable comparisons with others.

Conclusion: Differences in beliefs were evident between stroke patients who were identified as having low or high motivation for rehabilitation. Environmental factors (behaviour of health professionals, information available, hospital environment and so on) appear to influence motivation in addition to the individual's personality. Health professionals need to be aware of the ways in which their behaviour affects motivation.

Is the evidence rigorous and sufficiently reported?

1. *Is there congruity between the stated philosophical perspective and the research methodology?*

   The study does not clearly state the philosophical or theoretical premises on which it is based but clearly takes an interpretive perspective in trying to understand motivations for rehabilitation among people with stroke. The methodology is not clearly stated either. The article simply states that it was a qualitative study using semi-structured interviews. It can be seen from reading the methods, however, that a phenomenological perspective has been taken to understand the attitudes and beliefs of people with stroke. Phenomenology seeks to uncover lived experience through spoken and unspoken communication to establish meaning associated with lived experiences as perceived by people and this was clearly undertaken in this study.

2. *Is there congruity between the research methodology and the research question or objectives?*

   The objective of the research was to explore the attitudes and beliefs of stroke patients who were identified by professionals as having either 'high' or 'low' motivation for rehabilitation. Therefore the objectives are congruent with the phenomenogical methodology.

3. *Is there congruity between the research methodology and the methods used to collect data?*
   Data collection relied upon health professionals identifying 'high' and 'low' motivation patients and therefore used purposeful sampling. Semi-structured interviews were employed and these were then transcribed. This is appropriate to the methodology of a phenomenological approach.

4. *Is there congruity between the research methodology and the representation and analysis of data?*
   Analysis of the data was conducted using a process of constant comparison. Data were first coded and care taken to ensure that the codes captured the respondents' meanings. The codes in each interview were then compared with those in each other interview to create broader categories that linked codes across interviews (constant comparison). These methods of analysis are congruent with the methodology (phenomenology). The study did not involve any reflective validation by the research participants. The representation of the data is also congruent with the methodology. It draws on quotes from participants to validate the identified themes.

5. *Is there congruity between the research methodology and the interpretation of results?*
   The results have been interpreted appropriately as they have been used to inform the researchers of the experiences and perceptions of people who have had a stroke. The focus on establishing meaning based on experience is appropriate for a phenomenological study.

6. *Is there a statement locating the researcher culturally or theoretically?*
   The beliefs and values of the researchers are not described.

7. *Is the influence of the researcher on the research, and vice versa, addressed?*
   The influence of the researcher was not clearly addressed. The primary author interviewed all participants but there was no indication in the report that the researcher had reflected on the influence that their role, position, values or beliefs might have had on the interview process with the participants.

8. *Are participants and their voices adequately represented?*
   Quotes were used to illustrate most themes; however, a few themes were not validated through the use of quotes. Further it was clear that different participants' voices were represented (indicated by participant number for each quote used).

9. *Is the research ethical according to current criteria or, for recent studies, is there evidence of ethical approval by an appropriate body?*
   No specific statement about obtaining ethical approval is evident in the report; however, it does state that participants agreed to participate.

10. *Do conclusions drawn in the research article appear to flow from the analysis, or interpretation, of the data?*
    The researcher's conclusions are clearly drawn from the key themes identified and inform the strategies for interacting with stroke patients that may increase motivation for rehabilitation.

What are the main findings?

People with stroke who were identified as having high motivation for rehabilitation were more likely to understand the purpose of rehabilitation than those who were identified as having low motivation. Positive determinants of motivation included: information about rehabilitation, positive comparisons with other people with stroke and wanting to leave hospital. Negative determinants of motivation included: overprotection from family members and professionals, lack of information and the provision of mixed messages about rehabilitation to patients and less favourable comparisons with others.

How might we use this evidence to inform practice?

This study emphasises the need for health professionals to look past an individual client's personality to environmental factors and health professional behaviours that may influence the motivation of people who have had a stroke to participate in rehabilitation. In particular, overprotection from family members and professionals and providing clients with insufficient information and/or mixed messages about rehabilitation may contribute to a reduced level of motivation. There are aspects of the methods and reporting of this study that could have been improved and this, in turn, would have strengthened your confidence in the findings of the study.

Podiatry example

Clinical scenario

You are a member of a recently established multidisciplinary team of health professionals who are involved in the management of clients who have diabetic foot complications. During a case conference, you begin a discussion about a client who has developed a new ulcer on the plantar surface of her foot after a recent digital amputation. The client has a pair of therapeutic shoes but refuses to wear them. Though you have spoken to her about the importance of appropriate footwear, she does not regularly wear any type of footwear that can accommodate pressure deflective devices or that provides sufficient protection to her feet. Recognising that many of the clients who are seen by the team seem not to wear their prescribed footwear or to follow footwear advice, the endocrinologist asks if you have any suggestions about how to tackle this problem. Before coming up with any strategies, you say that first you would like to gain an understanding of people's attitudes to, beliefs about and experiences with prescribed footwear. You think this understanding may help you come up with strategies that may improve clients' concordance with footwear advice. You agree to present your findings at the next case conference.

Clinical question

What are people's experience with prescribed footwear and what factors determine whether they will follow footwear advice?

Search terms and databases used to find the evidence

Database: You know that this question is best answered by a qualitative study. Your hospital librarian suggested that CINAHL is a probably a good database for you to start your search in.

Search terms: (footwear OR shoes) AND (complian* OR adheren* OR concordan*)

This search retrieves 50 titles. There are three studies that have examined people's experiences with prescribed footwear or investigated factors associated with a person's decision to follow footwear advice. You think that it will be important that you review them all for your presentation. To begin with, you select the following study which gives client and health professional views on the use of therapeutic footwear.

Article chosen

Johnson M, Newton P, Goyder E. Patient and professional perspectives on prescribed therapeutic footwear for people with diabetes: a vignette study. Pat Educ Couns 2006; 64:167–172.

Structured abstract

Study design: Qualitative analysis of semi-structured interviews using the framework approach.

Study question: The purpose of the study was to explore the experiences and views of people involved in prescribing and wearing footwear designed to reduce diabetes-related complications.

Context: Diabetes foot clinics, North Sheffield, UK.

Participants: 15 health professionals with experience in delivering care to people with diabetes-related foot complications and 15 clients from two diabetes foot clinics who had been prescribed footwear designed to reduce diabetes-related complications.

Data collection method: Participants were interviewed using a vignette depicting the experiences of a fictitious client with diabetes-related foot complications. Prompts were used after each vignette section to explore participant views.

Analysis: Interviews were taped and analysed using the framework approach.

Key findings: There was incongruence between clients and health professionals in terms of the expectations and reality of preventive behaviour. Health professionals, while advocating preventive measures in order to limit morbidity, are aware of how difficult this can be for clients. For clients, the reality of wearing prescribed footwear conflicted with personal and social norms. Both clients and health professionals expressed concerns about shoe fit when foot shape, size and structure are constantly changing.

Is the evidence rigorous and sufficiently reported?

1. *Is there congruity between the stated philosophical perspective and the research methodology?*
   The study does not clearly state the philosophical or theoretical premises on which it is based but clearly takes an interpretive perspective in trying to understand the experiences and views of people involved in prescribing and wearing footwear that is designed to reduce diabetes-related complications. The methodology is not clearly stated either. It simply states that it was a qualitative study that used semi-structured interviews and vignettes. One can see from reading the methods, however, that a phenomenological perspective has been taken. Phenomenology seeks to uncover lived experience through spoken and unspoken communication to establish meaning associated with lived experiences as perceived by people and this was clearly undertaken in this study.

2. *Is there congruity between the research methodology and the research question or objectives?*
   The purpose of the study was to explore the experiences and views of people who are involved in prescribing and wearing footwear designed to reduce diabetes-related complications. Therefore the objectives are congruent with the phenomenological methodology.

3. *Is there congruity between the research methodology and the methods used to collect data?*

Purposive sampling was used to identify health professionals and clients. Different types of health professionals (consultants, general practitioners, nurses, orthotists, podiatrists and a dietitian) with experience in delivering care to people with diabetes-related foot complications were interviewed. The clients who agreed to participate had long-term experience with foot care services and were from diverse socio-economic circumstances. The researchers believed these clients would provide a broad spectrum of beliefs and attitudes to prescribed footwear.

In this study, one-on-one interviews with health professionals and clients were conducted using vignettes. A piloted vignette which depicts the experiences of a fictitious client with diabetes-related foot complications was used. Prompts were used after each vignette section to explore participant views. Responses were then followed up as necessary to increase the clarity and depth of information. The researchers discuss why vignettes were used and why face-to-face interviews were conducted (as opposed to focus groups) with participants. These are appropriate to the methodology of a phenomenological approach.

4. *Is there congruity between the research methodology and the representation and analysis of data?*

The interviews were taped and analysed using the framework approach. In this method, after becoming familiar with the data, investigators classified the data according to key themes and concepts. In this study, two researchers carried out this process with a sample of transcripts before applying the framework to the remaining data. The validity of the interpretations does not appear to have been examined. These methods of analysis are congruent with the methodology (phenomenology). The representation of the data is also congruent with the methodology. It draws on quotes from different participants to validate the identified themes.

5. *Is there congruity between the research methodology and the interpretation of results?*

The results have been interpreted appropriately as they have been used to inform the researchers of the experiences and perceptions of people prescribing and wearing footwear designed to reduce diabetes-related complications. The focus on establishing meaning based on experience is appropriate for a phenomenological study.

6. *Is there a statement locating the researcher culturally or theoretically?*

The beliefs and values of the researchers are not described.

7. *Is the influence of the researcher on the research, and vice versa, addressed?*

The potential for the researchers' values and expectations to influence the conduct and conclusions of the study have not been discussed.

8. *Are participants and their voices adequately represented?*

Quotes were used to illustrate themes. It was clear that different participants' voices were represented (indicated by participant gender and number or letter for each quote used).

9. *Is the research ethical according to current criteria or, for recent studies, is there evidence of ethical approval by an appropriate body?*

The article states that ethical approval was obtained from the local research ethics committee. Issues of informed consent and confidentiality were not discussed.

10. *Do conclusions drawn in the research report appear to flow from the analysis, or interpretation, of the data?*

The study concluded that client perspectives need to be taken into account in shoe provision. The researchers' conclusions are clearly drawn from the key themes they identified and inform the people prescribing footwear designed to reduce diabetes-related complications.

What are the main findings?

The researchers present two themes which summarise issues relating to prescribed footwear that are important to clients and health professionals. The first theme relates to prescribed versus routine behaviour. There is incongruence between health professional recommendations regarding footwear and clients' behaviour, with clients finding it difficult to carry out advice that does not fit in with usual behaviour or that of others. The second theme explores issues related to the fitting of footwear when foot shape, size and structure may be constantly changing. This was problematic for prescribers and clients. The researchers conclude that the insensitiveness of prescribed shoes to the varying contexts in which they are to be used, or the varying shapes of the client's foot, may be the reason for low levels of use of prescribed footwear.

How might we use this evidence to inform practice?

The researchers discuss how the results of this study may be used in practice and suggest that negotiating the extent of use of prescribed footwear, providing varied styles of therapeutic footwear for different contexts and more detailed evaluation of shoe fit may improve the acceptance of prescribed footwear. Furthermore, involving clients in footwear design and obtaining views about the acceptability of the recommendations may help in developing more realistic aims that are relevant to the client. The researchers do mention transferability of the findings, suggesting that the small sample in this study prevents generalisation to a larger population of people with foot complications but that the issues raised are transferable to similar settings.

There is limited information provided by which you can compare your setting with the study setting. However, the demographic details of the study sample seem similar to your clients in terms of their age, duration of diabetes and the type of intervention being received. There is no further detail on the types of footwear that participants in this study had been prescribed or were prescribing.

You reflect on discussions that you have had with clients about their footwear. Some of the experiences described in the study seem consistent with your clients. Many clients prescribed therapeutic shoes (shoes that have features such as extra depth, broad sole, deep toe box) comment negatively on the appearance and many complain that the shoes are not suitable for the hot climate in which they live. They also report difficulty being able to put the shoes on. Before moving on to the next study, you draw up a table which you will use to summarise the methods and results of the studies that you have found. You plan to present this at the next case conference, using it to stimulate discussion on possible strategies to improve concordance with footwear advice.

Speech pathology example

Clinical scenario

Mr Fallon, a 34-year-old man with a moderate–severe stutter, has previously attended your speech pathology clinic and has returned today for advice. He has previously received individual speech therapy for 6 months but was disappointed when this did not 'cure' his fluency difficulties. He would like to discuss some other options for therapy, particularly a 'prolonged speech'/'smooth speech' group program which he has heard about. From this program, he wants to see a difference in himself and is concerned at being able to maintain and transfer the techniques to everyday life after the program and to 'sound normal'. You wonder whether there is evidence about how clients perceive prolonged speech approaches to therapy for dysfluency.

Clinical question

How do adults with moderate–severe chronic dysfluency experience the outcomes of prolonged speech approaches?

Search terms and databases used to find the evidence

Database: Given that this clinical question is about client experiences, qualitative methods are considered the most appropriate research design to locate. For the topic of focus in this question, MEDLINE/PubMed, CINAHL or Embase would be appropriate to search in.

Search terms: The terms that could be used include 'stuttering' or 'fluency disorders'; 'prolonged speech' or 'smooth speech'; 'easy speech' or 'rate control'; 'treatment outcome' or 'patient satisfaction' or 'consumer satisfaction' or 'experiences'. In this instance, a free text search of PubMed using the terms 'stutter*' AND (prolonged speech) AND 'experience*' returned three articles, one of which was relevant to the question.

Article chosen

Cream A, Onslow M, Packman A et al. Protection from harm: the experience of adults after therapy with prolonged-speech. Int J Lang Commun Disord 2003; 38:379–395.

Structured abstract

Study design: Qualitative investigation using phenomenology as the method of inquiry.

Study question: What are the experiences of adults who use prolonged speech to control stuttering?

Context: Sydney, Australia. Therapy based on prolonged speech had been available through the speech pathology departments of public hospitals in Sydney for some time.

Participants: 10 adults (aged 24–54 years; 9 male, 1 female) who had received prolonged speech treatment. Participants were purposively sampled, on the basis of representing different viewpoints or experience. However, all had objectively experienced success with the prolonged speech treatment as a criterion for inclusion was 'they had experienced zero stuttering at the end of treatment'.

Data collection method: Face-to-face interviews and informal discussions (face-to-face or over the telephone) were held with participants over a 2-year period. At the end of the study, participants attended group interviews for further discussion. Interviews were 'conversational' in nature, with an open-ended rather than structured format. A total of 34 interviews/discussions were included in the data.

Analysis: Content analysis was used to determine emerging themes. Transcripts were analysed using consecutively a line-by-line approach (to identify all emergent themes), a holistic approach (to understand the overall meaning of the interviews/discussions) and a selective approach (aiming to discover the primary themes). Additional data were sought and analysed to gain further understanding of experiences of people who have undertaken prolonged speech treatment. Analysis occurred concurrently to data collection, and emerging themes were discussed with participants.

Key findings and conclusion: Even after prolonged speech treatment, there is an ongoing risk of stuttering occurring. Although clients may have experience of being able to control stuttering, they also continue to feel different from people who do not stutter and these feelings may be exacerbated after treatment. The maximum benefits of prolonged speech are achieved when clients use a strategic approach to control stuttering and everyday communication.

Is the evidence rigorous and sufficiently reported?

When considering these features of qualitative research methodology we can see that the authors have used phenomenology, which is both a philosophy and a methodology for qualitative research. Phenomenology is appropriate to discovering what makes up others' experiences and attempting to get to the 'essence' of these experiences. Underpinning this approach, the authors have used a constructivist paradigm for their research, a theoretical standpoint where reality and truth are understood to be 'constructed' differently by every individual, rather than something 'objective' that can be described or understood (and generalised). Summarising from the QARI tool, the research aims, methodology, data collection and analysis are all congruent with this approach and theoretical context. Additionally, the rigour of this study has been enhanced through the following methods:

- The researchers have stated their position within the research and procedures to address the trustworthiness of the research, including member checking/discussion of interpretations with participants and triangulation of data, were employed.
- The participants' voices are represented through quotes that exemplify the discovered themes.
- Ethical procedures have been followed.
- The conclusions flow clearly from the themes identified and presented by the authors.

What are the main findings?

The themes that emerged describe interwoven experiences of adults after prolonged speech therapy. As prolonged speech therapy does not 'cure' stuttering, participants reported that their feelings about their stuttering and the need to 'protect themselves' from the negative consequences that they associate with stuttering do not diminish even after success with prolonged speech therapy. Being fluent speakers 'has a price' for participants, as prolonged speech feels unnatural to produce and may also sound unnatural. Thus, participants were bound to be 'different' whether they used prolonged speech or stuttered. Prolonged speech became a 'tool' that participants could apply, along with their own existing resources, to protect themselves from harm.

The authors concluded that successful use of prolonged speech from a client's perspective is the strategic application of the technique in order to reduce harm from stuttering. In some situations, clients may choose the risk of sounding different by stuttering, rather than the risk of sounding different through prolonged speech. The findings suggest that practising the technique (either in therapy or in booster/maintenance programs) is not likely to increase the long-term use of the technique. Clinical programs to teach prolonged speech should focus not just on the behavioural changes, but the integration of the technique alongside existing resources that the client has for reducing harm. Speech pathologists should consider whether clients have the resources to benefit from prolonged speech—for example, clients who are already considerably anxious about being different may not be suitable for this type of treatment.

How might we use this evidence to inform practice?

In the case of Mr Fallon, caution should be used in recommending a prolonged speech therapy course to him, given his existing anxiety about 'sounding normal' and his emphasis on maintaining any therapy technique that he tries. Mr Fallon could be counselled about the realistic benefits that he might perceive from using prolonged speech—for example, although he might be able to use the technique well, he may find it unnatural and will have to weigh up the benefits of applying the technique versus stuttering. It should be emphasised that prolonged speech is not a 'cure' for stuttering. If Mr Fallon does choose to begin prolonged speech therapy, he should be directed towards groups/therapists who emphasise the integration of prolonged speech in everyday life, rather than simply 'teaching' clients how to be good users of the technique.

Medicine example

Clinical scenario

As a general practitioner you are involved in the care of a number of clients who have breast cancer. A few of them regularly ask you about various vitamins and strategies such as relaxation that they have heard might improve their health. To increase the confidence that you have in your role in providing information about complementary and alternative medicine alongside maintaining the treatment regimens that are outlined by their oncologists, you look to the literature for reassurance about the role that general practitioners play in providing support for both complementary and alternative medicine and traditional medicine.

Clinical question

What role do general practitioners play in providing support for both complementary and alternative medicine and traditional medicine for people with cancer?

Search terms and databases used to find the evidence

Database: PubMed—Health Services Research Queries screen
Search terms: (CAM or complementary and alternative medicine) AND cancer
This search retrieved 46 articles and the second article appeared to be the most relevant to the question under consideration.

Article chosen

Brazier A, Balneaves L, Seely D et al. Integrative practices of Canadian oncology health professionals. Curr Oncol 2008; 15:s110.es87–91.

Structured abstract

Study design: This study used an interpretive description qualitative methodology (phenomenological approach).
Study question: To explore the practices of health professionals integrating complementary medicine and traditional medicine (integrative care) for people with breast cancer and to understand their perspectives about what this involves.

Context: This study was part of a larger qualitative study of integrative care delivered by 'conventional' oncology health professionals for people in Canada who have breast cancer.
Participants: Using purposive sampling, 16 oncology health professionals including medical and radiation oncologists, nurses and pharmacists were recruited from cancer agencies, hospitals, integrative clinics and private practice settings in four Canadian cities.
Data collection method: A series of in-depth interviews were used to understand the integrative practices used, how they discussed complementary and alternative medicine with their patients, referrals made to complementary health professionals and which complementary services were available within their practice setting.
Data analysis: Data analysis used the constant comparative approach.
Key findings and conclusion: None of the health professionals interviewed provided both complementary and traditional medicine themselves but acted as integrative care guides and collaborated with other health professionals. They were, however, open to complementary and alternative medicine. Some health professionals took on integrative care roles with women with breast cancer to support their decisions about complementary and alternative medicine. Openness to integrative practices provides much needed support for women with breast cancer.

Is the evidence rigorous and sufficiently reported?

1. *Is there congruity between the stated philosophical perspective and the research methodology?*
   The study describes an interest in the perspectives and experiences of oncology health professionals and situates itself in the interpretive paradigm. Specifically, the article described a primary interest in examining the practices of health professionals for integrating complementary and traditional medicine within the context of decisions being made by women with breast cancer. It uses the interpretive description method.[1] The interpretive description method differs from phenomenology in that it incorporates prior knowledge in the design, analysis and interpretation of data. The interpretive description method is congruent with the interpretive paradigm as it aims to 'describe the experience of the participant, while simultaneously capturing the meaning that the participant attributes to the experience' (p S88).[2]

2. *Is there congruity between the research methodology and the research question or objectives?*
   The aims of this study were to explore the practices of health professionals integrating complementary medicine and traditional medicine (integrative care) for people with breast cancer and to understand their perspectives about what this involves. The objectives are congruent with the interpretive description methodology.

3. *Is there congruity between the research methodology and the methods used to collect data?*
   The data collection relied upon purposive sampling, in-depth interviews and verbatim transcripts. These are appropriate to the methodology of interpretive description.

4. *Is there congruity between the research methodology and the representation and analysis of data?*
   Data analysis was conducted using constant comparative approaches in which pieces of data are compared to locate similarities and understand relationships among the data. These methods of analysis are well suited to the interpretive description methodology. The findings used quotes from participants to validate and illuminate the two main practices that were identified.

5. *Is there congruity between the research methodology and the interpretation of results?*
   The two main findings were that health professionals acted as integrative care guides and collaborated with other health professionals as a means of supporting women

with breast cancer making decisions about complementary and alternative medicine. The results have been interpreted appropriately as they have been used to inform the researchers of the experiences and perceptions of health professionals faced with integrating complementary and traditional medicine and are consistent with the aims of interpretive description methodology.

6. *Is there a statement locating the researcher culturally or theoretically?*
Although the beliefs and values of the researchers are not explicitly described, the introduction provided by the authors clearly indicates a positive stance towards complementary and alternative medicine. The subsequent aim of the study was not just to understand integrative practices that were being undertaken but to provide suggestions for oncology health professionals wanting to provide integrative care in their practice. Again this indicates a positive stance towards complementary and alternative medicine and integrative practices.

7. *Is the influence of the researcher on the research, and vice versa, addressed?*
The influence of the researcher was not clearly addressed in this study even though it is recommended as part of interpretive description methodology.

8. *Are participants and their voices adequately represented?*
The participants were adequately quoted in the article, indicating reasonable representation.

9. *Is the research ethical according to current criteria or, for recent studies, is there evidence of ethical approval by an appropriate body?*
No specific statement about obtaining ethical approval is evident in the report; however, as this study was part of a larger qualitative study, ethical considerations may have been detailed in another article.

10. *Do conclusions drawn in the research report appear to flow from the analysis, or interpretation, of the data?*
The researchers' conclusions are clearly drawn from the two types of integrative practices that were identified and use the participants' views to inform the strategies recommended for supporting health professionals in the use of integrative practices.

What are the main findings?

Depending on the interest, knowledge and skills that different health professionals had in supporting clients with decisions about complementary and alternative medicine, two main integrative practices were evident. Firstly, oncology health professionals described acting as integrative care guides by using practices such as interpreting complementary and alternative medicine information for clients, supporting them in working out further questions to ask or supporting clients' exploration of complementary and alternative medicine. Secondly, oncology health professionals described liaising and collaborating with other health professionals.

How might we use this evidence to inform practice?

This study suggested that health professionals can support clients' exploration of complementary and alternative medicine at the same time as delivering traditional treatments, even if they do not actively participate in providing complementary and alternative medicine. This can be done by acting as a guide to complementary and alternative medicine and traditional medicine or by collaborating with complementary and alternative medicine health professionals or services. Although this information is based on interviews with oncology health professionals, this same information might help you, as a general practitioner, to decide to what extent and perhaps how you might want to be involved in supporting your clients with their decisions about complementary and alternative medicine.

Nursing example

Clinical scenario

As the quality manager in a residential care facility you have booked a meeting with a family of three daughters whose aged mother (a frail 84-year-old woman) is being admitted later that week for placement. She has mild dementia and has been living with her youngest daughter who is no longer able to cope with her mother's increasingly complex needs. This is the family's first experience of a residential care facility as their father has already passed away. Your past experience suggests that their mother's ability to settle in to the new environment will be complicated, partly due to the family's lack of experience with the aged care sector and because it does represent a significant life transition for older adults.

With excellent systems in place (validated by recent accreditation approval), it is not the process of admission that troubles you. Rather, you want to have a better understanding of what the experience of being admitted to a residential care environment means to older adults. How older adults perceive their sense of belonging might just be the key to a smoother transition from home to residential services for all involved. The nature of this information need is one that is best addressed by qualitative research as you are concerned about concepts such as experiences and perspectives.

Clinical question

How does the lived experience of older adults who are transitioning to residential aged care facilities influence their ability to integrate and find a sense of identity?

Search terms and databases used to find the evidence

Database: CINAHL

Search terms: transition AND (care facilit*) AND resident*

This search returns 14 articles. Four of these were broadly relevant to the issue at hand, but only one was directly relevant to your clinical question.

Article chosen

Heliker D, Scholler-Jaquish A. Transition of new residents to long-term care: basing practice on residents' perspective. J Gerontol Nurs 2006; 32:34–42.

The abstract confirms that this article focuses on the experience (a qualitative concept) of new residents related to settling in to what is initially an unfamiliar environment. The article uses the descriptor 'long-term' in place of the term 'residential', although these terms mean the same thing in the literature.

Structured abstract

Study design: The methods used in the paper were from the interpretive perspective, using in-depth interviews to ascertain the views and experiences of recently admitted older adults.

Study question: The study sought to understand the perspectives and experiences of newly admitted residents to assist in better anticipation of individual residents' needs on admission.

Participants: The participants were a convenience sample of 10 older adults who had recently been admitted to a residential aged care facility.

Data collection methods: Participants were interviewed within 1 week of admission and then at intervals over the next 3 months.

Analysis: The interviews were analysed using hermeneutical phenomenology.

Context: A large, multi-level facility in Texas, USA where senior nursing staff were keen to establish a better understanding of residents' experiences and to use that information to develop new strategies that would help older adults transition to aged care from their home environments.

Key findings: Three key themes emerged from the data related to patterns of transition from home to residential care: 1) becoming homeless; 2) getting settled and learning the ropes; and 3) creating a place. Becoming homeless was associated with leaving one's home and moving to a new environment where a sense of identity has yet to be created. Homelessness also occurred as the familiar life, its memories, self, friends and neighbourhoods were lost to older adults following admission to residential care. Getting settled and learning the ropes began to emerge as a theme for people who had been in the facility for 1 to 2 months. This was a process of negotiation to learn the new layout, routines and people. It followed a time of isolation and was characterised by spending less time in one's room or less time alone. Creating a place occurred over time—between 2 and 3 months for most people interviewed. It related to developing new memories and neighbours and friends. Importantly, room ownership developed and facilitated a safe sense of perspective for the residents' sense of identity and neighbourhood. It gave them a base from which to reach out and relate to their new world.

Conclusion: Residential care facilities which can create opportunities for residents to share stories and lived experiences are facilitating the development of identity for new residents. Staff in residential care facilities who share their stories create a sense of neighbourhood which new residents can relate to, enhancing their ability to understand their new environment.

Is the evidence rigorous and sufficiently reported?

1. *Is there congruity between the stated philosophical perspective and the research methodology?*

   The study describes an interest in the perspectives and experiences of residents and situates itself in the critical and interpretive paradigm. Therefore the methodology is congruent with the philosophical perspectives. Specifically, the article described a primary interest in examining the lived experience within the context of transition to residential care. This situates the article within the interpretive paradigm and is congruent with the choice of hermeneutical phenomenology as the research methodology. Hermeneutic phenomenology seeks to uncover lived experience through spoken and unspoken (such as facial expression and body posture) communication to establish the meaning that is associated with lived experiences as perceived by people.

2. *Is there congruity between the research methodology and the research question or objectives?*

   The objective of the research was to uncover the meaning of transition by examining the perspectives and experiences of new residents. Therefore the objectives are congruent with the methodology.

3. *Is there congruity between the research methodology and the methods used to collect data?*
   The data collection relied upon convenience sampling, in-depth interviews and verbatim transcripts. These are appropriate to the methodology of hermeneutic phenomenology.
4. *Is there congruity between the research methodology and the representation and analysis of data?*
   Data analysis was conducted using a process of reading and re-reading to understand the whole of the text leading to the identification of themes, metaphors and meanings. The researchers continued reading and re-reading to establish a higher order hermeneutical analysis of the emerging relationships between themes, followed by a period of reflective validation by the research participants. These methods of analysis are congruent with the methodology (hermeneutic phenomenology). The representation of the data is also congruent with the methodology. It draws on quotes from participants to validate and illuminate the identified themes and includes voices from many participants.
5. *Is there congruity between the research methodology and the interpretation of results?*
   The results have been interpreted appropriately as they have been used to inform the researchers of the experiences and perceptions of new residents. The focus on establishing meaning based on experience is appropriate for a phenomenological study.
6. *Is there a statement locating the researcher culturally or theoretically?*
   The article describes the researchers as desiring to understand the residents' experiences to better inform supportive strategies following admission. The researchers are clearly located within the critical and interpretive paradigm. The beliefs and values of the researchers are not described.
7. *Is the influence of the researcher on the research, and vice versa, addressed?*
   The methods describe how each researcher kept a record of reflections and comments on the developing thematic analysis, including group discussions of the transcripts, summaries and emerging themes. There was explicit mention of engagement of the researchers (as actual instruments in the research) and this was recorded in the researchers' diaries. Therefore the influence of the researchers was clearly addressed.
8. *Are participants and their voices adequately represented?*
   The participants were frequently quoted in the article which indicates adequate representation.
9. *Is the research ethical according to current criteria or, for recent studies, is there evidence of ethical approval by an appropriate body?*
   Ethical approval was sought and obtained from all organisations involved in the research.
10. *Do conclusions drawn in the research report appear to flow from the analysis, or interpretation, of the data?*
    The researchers' conclusions are clearly drawn from the three key themes they identified and participants' stories are used to inform the strategies that they recommended to assist new residents in making the transition to a residential care facility.

What are the main findings?

Three key themes emerged from the data related to patterns of transition from home to residential care: 1) becoming homeless; 2) getting settled and learning the ropes; and 3) creating a place. The implications for practice arising from this study were that staff who listen to a new resident's stories are better able to plan care appropriately for that individual. Further to this, the study found that listening and respecting the elderly, while sharing stories and experiences, facilitates the process of transition to the new facility. Creating commonalities enables new residents to seek assistance and integrate their concept of belonging with the facility. Minimising the perceived rift between a resident's sense of 'home' and the new environment is the central goal in facilitating transition.

How might we use this evidence to inform practice?

The evidence from this study shows that admission is characterised by a period of disorganisation and adaptation. The learning of new rules and relationships is part of the adaptation (transition) process. Transitioning their sense of belonging or home can be facilitated. Facilities which base care planning not only upon assessment, but also on engagement with new residents and through listening to their stories, are better equipped to help individuals find their place in the new environment. Having learnt this from the research, you convene a staff meeting to discuss integrating story seeking questions into the admission assessments and care plan. These questions now guide staff in facilitating the development of care plans which consider an individual's experiences and perceptions.

References

1. Thorne S, Kirkham SR, MacDonald–Emes J. Interpretive description: a noncategorical qualitative alternative for developing nursing knowledge. Res Nurs Health 1997; 20:169–177.
2. Brazier A, Balneaves L, Seely D et al. Integrative practices of Canadian oncology health professionals. Curr Oncol 2008; 15:s110.es87–91.

CHAPTER 12

Appraising and understanding systematic reviews and meta-analyses

Sally Bennett, Sue Leicht Doyle and Denise O'Connor

LEARNING OBJECTIVES

After reading this chapter, you should be able to:
- Understand what systematic reviews and meta-analyses are
- Know where to look for systematic reviews
- Understand how systematic reviews are carried out
- Critically appraise a systematic review
- Understand how to interpret the results from systematic reviews and meta-analyses
- Understand how systematic reviews can be used to inform practice

A systematic review is a method for systematically locating, appraising and synthesising research from primary studies and is an important means of condensing the research evidence from many primary studies. This chapter will describe systematic reviews and meta-analyses, discuss their advantages and disadvantages and briefly illustrate the use of systematic reviews for different types of clinical questions. The methods for carrying out systematic reviews will be described and key factors that can introduce bias into reviews will be explained. Using a worked example, we will also demonstrate how to critically appraise a systematic review and how it can be used to guide decision making in practice.

What are systematic reviews?

Due to the massive increase in the volume of health research over the last 50 years or so, it was recognised that some system of synthesising this information was essential. The health literature has a long tradition of using literature or narrative reviews to help readers grasp the breadth of a particular topic. These literature reviews typically provide a reasonably thorough description of a particular topic and refer to many articles that have been published in that particular area. Nearly all students are required to do at least one literature review as part of their studies so you probably know what literature reviews are all about.

More recently, **systematic reviews** have been embraced as a more comprehensive means of synthesising the literature.[1] While literature reviews provide an overview of the research findings for a given topic they often address a broad range of issues, whereas systematic reviews address specific clinical questions in depth.[2] Systematic reviews also differ from literature reviews in that they are prepared using transparent, explicit and pre-defined strategies that are designed to limit bias.[2] In contrast to literature reviews, systematic reviews involve a clear definition of eligibility criteria; incorporate a comprehensive search of *all* potentially relevant studies; use explicit, reproducible and uniformly applied criteria in the selection of articles for the review; rigorously appraise the risk of bias within individual studies; and systematically synthesise the results of included studies.[2]

Where possible, a systematic review uses statistical methods to combine the results of two or more individual studies, and this type of review is then referred to as a **meta-analysis**. Meta-analyses generally provide a better overall estimate of a clinical effect than the results from individual studies. Often it is not possible to combine the results of individual studies because the interventions or outcomes used in the different studies are just too diverse, so results from these studies are synthesised narratively. It may help you to think about these different types of reviews visually. As you can see in Figure 12.1, literature reviews make up the vast majority of reviews that are found in the overall health literature. Systematic reviews can be considered a subset of reviews, and meta-analyses are a smaller set again. Note that the circle representing meta-analyses overlaps both systematic and literature reviews. This is because not all meta-analyses are carried out systematically. For example, it is technically possible for someone to take a collection of articles that report randomised controlled trials from their desk and undertake a meta-analysis of these articles. This would not be considered systematic as methods were not used to ensure that a systematic search for all relevant articles was conducted. Sometimes the terms systematic review and meta-analysis are used interchangeably, but in this chapter they are conceptualised as different entities. A systematic review does not need to incorporate a meta-analysis, but a meta-analysis should only be done within the context of a systematic review (although occasionally it is not).

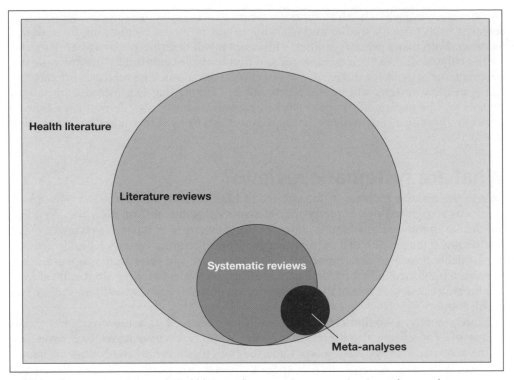

FIGURE 12.1 The relationships between the health literature, literature reviews, systematic reviews and meta-analyses

Advantages and disadvantages of systematic reviews

By combining the results of similar studies, a properly conducted systematic review can improve the dissemination of evidence,[2] hasten the assimilation of research into practice,[3] assist in clarifying the heterogeneity of conflicting results between studies[3] and establish generalisability of the overall findings.[2] Systematic reviews are important for health professionals who are seeking answers to clinical questions, for researchers who are identifying gaps in research and defining future research agendas and for administrators and purchasers who are developing policies and guidelines.[2]

Although systematic reviews have many advantages, as with any other study type, they may be subject to bias. Limitations of systematic reviews include:

• Publication bias. This relates to a researcher's tendency to only submit interesting and positive results for publication or the tendency of journal editors to only accept articles with such results for publication. Researchers often feel that there is no point in submitting for publication the results of a trial that showed that an intervention had no effect as they believe that no journal will want to publish it. The consequence of this is that studies sourced from the published health literature may not be representative of all the studies that have been conducted about a particular intervention or issue.

• Inclusion of low quality primary data in their synthesis.

In addition to these problems, it may be possible for researchers to design a review that is based upon their retrospective knowledge of the relevant trials, which could influence the criteria used to select studies for inclusion in the review, assess the quality of those studies and extract data.[4] A further problem of meta-analyses in particular is that, as they combine data from many individual studies, unfortunately they can also magnify the effect of the bias that may be in these individual studies if they are of low quality (or high risk of bias).

Systematic reviews for different types of clinical questions

Systematic reviews synthesise different study methodologies depending on the research question of interest.[5] As we saw in Chapter 2 when we examined the hierarchies of evidence for various question types, systematic reviews are at the top of the hierarchy of evidence for questions about the effects of intervention, diagnosis and prognosis. For example, a properly conducted systematic review of randomised controlled trials is generally considered to be the best study design for assessing the effectiveness of an intervention because it identifies and examines all of the evidence about the intervention from randomised controlled trials that meet pre-determined inclusion criteria.[6] This type of systematic review is by far the most common type of systematic review available. However, systematic reviews may be carried out to address other types of questions such as questions about diagnosis, prognosis and client experiences.

Systematic reviews that focus on questions of prognosis or prediction often undertake a synthesis of cohort studies. Consider the following example in which a systematic review of cohort studies of clients in the subacute phase of ischaemic or haemorrhagic stroke was conducted with the aim of identifying prognostic factors for future place of residence at 6 to 12 months post-stroke.[7] The authors searched MEDLINE, EMBASE, CINAHL, Current Contents, Cochrane Database of Systematic Reviews, PsycLIT and Sociological Abstracts as well as reference lists, personal archives and consultations of experts in the field and guidelines to locate relevant cohort studies. They then assessed the internal, statistical and external validity of the 10 studies that they had selected for inclusion. Although the review found many factors that were predictive of a client's future place of residence (for example, low initial functioning in activities of daily living, advanced age, cognitive disturbance, paresis of arm and leg), the authors concluded that there was insufficient evidence concerning possible predictors in the subacute stage of stroke with respect to place of future residence.

Systematic reviews of diagnostic test studies are carried out to determine estimates of test performance and consider variation between studies. This type of systematic review uses different methods to assess study quality and combine results than those used for systematic reviews of randomised controlled trials.[8] An example of this type of review is one that used meta-analytic procedures in a review of the accuracy of the Mini-Mental State Examination in the detection of dementia and mild cognitive impairment.[9] Thirty-four dementia studies and five mild cognitive impairment studies were included in the meta-analysis. It was concluded that the Mini-Mental State Examination offers modest accuracy with best value for ruling-out a diagnosis of dementia in community and primary care.

There have recently been advances in the methodology for undertaking systematic reviews of qualitative research, allowing us to have a more comprehensive understanding of clients' experience in relation to a particular issue and to understand the acceptability of interventions to clients or the reasons why an intervention is not readily implemented. Some work has also been done to develop methods for combining results from both quantitative and qualitative research within a single review. However, discussion among researchers about how systematic reviews of qualitative research should best be conducted continues.[10] There is still significant debate about whether a synthesis of qualitative studies is appropriate and whether it is acceptable to combine studies that use a variety of different methods.[11]

An interesting example of a review that combines qualitative and quantitative methods can be seen in a systematic review that examined older people's views, perceptions and experiences of falls prevention interventions.[12] The authors of the review searched eight databases using a broad search strategy in order to locate relevant qualitative and quantitative studies. The systematic review contained 24 studies, which consisted of 10 qualitative studies, one systematic review, three narrative reviews, three randomised controlled trials, three before/after studies and four cross-sectional observational studies. Synthesis of the *quantitative* studies in this review identified factors that encouraged older people's participation in falls prevention interventions, while the findings from the 10 *qualitative* studies demonstrated the importance of considering older people's views about falls interventions to ensure that these interventions are properly targeted.

So, contrary to common misconception, systematic reviews are not just limited to syntheses of randomised controlled trials. They are a methodology that can be used for many different study types and research questions. Having pointed this out, the remainder of this chapter will, however, focus on systematic reviews for questions about the effects of interventions. As we mentioned earlier, this type of systematic review is by far the most common type and we want you to gain a deeper understanding of the methods and appraisal of this type of systematic review.

Locating systematic reviews

It has been mentioned a number of times already in this book that a significant difficulty in locating research evidence is the overwhelming quantity of information that is available and the diverse range of journals in which information is published. Unfortunately, systematic reviews are not immune to this problem. As you saw in Chapter 3, the premier source for systematic reviews is the Cochrane Database of Systematic Reviews. These reviews are written by volunteer researchers who work with one of many review groups that are coordinated by The Cochrane Collaboration (www. cochrane.org). Each review group has an editorial team which oversees the preparation and maintenance of the reviews, as well as the application of rigorous quality standards. This is why Cochrane reviews are so highly regarded. Those of you who are particularly interested in methodology issues may like to know that The Cochrane Collaboration has Method Groups who continue to refine methods for various types of reviews such as ones about effectiveness, diagnostic tests and prognostic information, as well as methods for qualitative reviews.

Another source of reliable information contained within the Cochrane Library is the Database of Abstracts of Reviews (DARE). It contains abstracts of systematic reviews that have been quality assessed. Each abstract includes a summary of the review together with a critical commentary about the overall quality. Chapter 3 provided the details of other resources that can be used to locate systematic reviews. These include the Joanna Briggs Institute, PEDro, OTseeker, PsycBITE, speechBITE and the large biomedical databases such as CINAHL and MEDLINE/PubMed (the latter contains a search strategy specifically for locating systematic reviews on the PubMed Clinical Queries screen).

How are systematic reviews conducted?

We believe that it is easier to learn how to appraise a systematic review if you first have an understanding of what is involved in performing a systematic review. Undertaking a systematic review requires a significant time commitment, with estimates varying depending on the number of citations/abstracts involved. Obviously, for some topics there is very little research that has been done whereas, for other topics, there is a huge amount of research to find and sort through. To give you an idea, one estimation is that it takes approximately 1139 hours or the equivalent of 6 months full-time work to complete a systematic review.[13]

We will now explain the basic steps involved in undertaking a systematic review, which are:
1. Define the research question.
2. Determine the types of studies to be included.
3. Search for potentially eligible studies.
4. Apply eligibility criteria to select studies.
5. Assess the risk of bias in individual studies.
6. Extract data from the included studies.
7. Synthesise the data.
8. Interpret and report the results.
9. Update the review at an appropriate time point in the future.

Plan and define the research question for a systematic review

As with any research study, when conducting a systematic review, the first place to start is planning the overall project. Planning also ensures that all aspects important to the scientific rigour of a review are undertaken to reduce the risk of bias. Each stage of the review needs to be thoroughly understood prior to moving on to plan the next stage. The question needs to be clearly focussed as too broad a question will not produce a useful review. The question should also make sense clinically. Involving consumers, at both the health professional and client level, may also be helpful when developing a plan, as this will ensure that areas of concern such as interventions or outcomes that might not otherwise be considered are addressed.[14] Planning a review also requires decisions to be made about the methods for searching, screening, appraisal and synthesis. These decisions should be made before commencing the review itself as this will help to make the whole process systematic and more transparent for all involved.

Determine the types of studies to be included in the review

Review authors must decide: 1) which studies to include in the review; 2) how to locate the studies to include in the review; 3) how to assess the quality of the studies included; and 4) what data to extract from the studies. The type of studies to include will depend on the type of review question (for example, whether the review is about effects of intervention or about diagnostic tests). Within each type of review question there is then a further choice about study methods to include. Traditionally, inclusion criteria for systematic reviews about the effects of interventions, for instance, have focussed on including randomised controlled trials or quasi-randomised controlled trials. However, the frequency of inclusion of non-randomised studies and qualitative studies in effectiveness reviews may increase as methods for their synthesis become further developed.

Search for potentially eligible studies

The search methodology needs to be developed prior to commencing the review and to be clearly explained and reproducible. All components of the question of the review (such as the participants, interventions, comparisons and outcomes) need to be considered when developing the search strategy of the review. Each of the synonyms for each of the components also needs to be included in the search.[15] The search strategy should be planned to include both English and non-English publications where possible and no date exclusions should be used. Searching should occur across multiple databases as it has been found that search strategies that are limited to one database do not identify all of the relevant studies.[15] The review authors should also contact authors in the field in an attempt to locate other studies that have not already been identified and ongoing or planned studies in the area, and to ask about and obtain written copies of unpublished studies.[16] The reason for doing this is to limit a problem called 'publication bias' that was explained earlier in the chapter and can occur due to study authors being more likely to submit studies with statistically significant results and journals being more likely to publish studies with positive results than those with negative outcomes.

As an illustration of how important it is that review authors use a comprehensive search strategy, one study found that 35% of all appropriate randomised controlled trials were not located by computerised searching[17] and another reported that 10% of suitable trials for systematic reviews were missed when only electronic searching was conducted.[18] Hand searching journals has been identified as vitally important to conducting a high quality systematic review[19] as not all journals are indexed in electronic databases or may be missed by the search strategy used. It is highly recommended[20] that authors of systematic reviews perform hand searching of the major journals that publish in the area relevant to the review question to increase the comprehensiveness of their search strategy. Citation tracking or use of the references from the studies found may help the reviewer to locate further studies on the topic and increase comprehensiveness of the search. Attempts should also be made to obtain unpublished studies (including masters and doctoral research and conference presentations) by searching the CENTRAL database in the Cochrane library and other trial registries.

Apply eligibility criteria to select studies

Once the search has been completed and potentially relevant studies identified, the next task is to decide which of the studies should be included in the systematic review. Not all articles that are located during the search will be directly relevant to the review question. Eligibility criteria are established to guide the selection of studies to be included in the review. The criteria specify the type of research methodologies that are to be included, the population and outcomes of interest and the interventions that will be considered. The selection process should then be carried out by two or more authors independently to minimise bias. Titles and abstracts are screened for relevance and eligibility. The full text of potentially relevant studies is retrieved so that a more detailed evaluation can be done. Studies that are not eligible (and this decision can be made on the basis of title and abstract information) are excluded at this point. A final evaluation by at least two authors is conducted on the full text articles and a decision is made whether to include or exclude the studies. If the review authors are conducting a Cochrane systematic review, studies that are excluded at this stage of the review process are listed in the review along with the reason why they were excluded.[20]

Assess the risk of bias in individual studies

The next step is to evaluate the quality of the studies that have been included in the review. Assessing the quality of the individual studies is vital to conducting a quality systematic review. Including poor quality trials would raise doubts about the reliability of the systematic review's results and conclusions.[21] To guard against errors and increase the reliability of the quality assessment, it is recommended that two or more review authors independently assess the quality of the included studies.[20] Determining the potential for bias in individual studies can be done in a number of different ways, such as using the approach to appraising randomised controlled trials that was explained in Chapter 4 of this book. From the beginning of 2008, systematic reviews that are carried out through The Cochrane Collaboration have to use the 'Risk of Bias' tool.[22] The risk of bias tool includes six different domains which are shown in Table 12.1, along with a definition of each of these criteria. Implementation of this tool requires two steps: 1) extracting information from the original study report about each criterion (see description column in Table 12.1); and then 2) making a judgement about the likely risk of bias in relation to each criterion (scored as 'yes', 'no' or 'unclear') (see Review authors' judgement column in Table 12.1).

Extract data from the included studies

Generally the data that are collected concern participant details, intervention details, outcome measures used, results of the study and the study methodology.[20] A standardised data collection tool or process is typically established so that the data are collected in a consistent manner and relevant to the research question.

Synthesise the data

Before we explain what review authors do at this stage of the process, you first need to understand the principles of meta-analysis in more detail. As we mentioned at the beginning of this chapter, a meta-analysis pools the data obtained from all the studies included in a systematic review and re-analyses it using statistical procedures. The rationale behind a meta-analysis is that, as you are combining the samples of individual studies, the overall sample size is increased, which improves the power of the analysis as well as the precision of the estimates of the effects of the intervention.[15]

When review authors plan a systematic review, the process by which they will conduct the meta-analysis should be clearly outlined. It has been suggested that the process should include the following steps:[23]

1. The analysis strategy should clearly match the goals of the review.
2. Decide what types of study designs should be included in the meta-analysis.
3. Establish the criteria that would be used to decide whether or not to complete a meta-analysis (see when not to complete a meta-analysis below).
4. Identify what types of outcome data are likely to be found in the studies and outline how each will be managed.
5. Identify in advance what effects measures will be used.
6. Decide the type of meta-analysis that will be used (random effects or fixed effects).
7. Decide how clinical and methodological diversity will be managed, what characteristics would define the heterogeneity and if and how this will be incorporated into the analysis.
8. Decide on how missing data will be managed.
9. Decide how publication and reporting bias will be investigated and addressed.

Domain	Description	Review authors' judgement
Sequence generation	Describe the method used to generate the allocation sequence in sufficient detail to allow an assessment of whether it should produce comparable groups.	Was the allocation sequence adequately generated?
Allocation concealment	Describe the method used to conceal the allocation sequence in sufficient detail to determine whether intervention allocations could have been foreseen in advance of, or during, enrolment.	Was allocation adequately concealed?
Blinding of participants, personnel and outcome assessors Assessments should be made for each main outcome (or class of outcomes)	Describe all measures used, if any, to blind study participants and personnel from knowledge of which intervention a participant received. Provide any information relating to whether the intended blinding was effective.	Was knowledge of the allocated intervention adequately prevented during the study?
Incomplete outcome data Assessments should be made for each main outcome (or class of outcomes)	Describe the completeness of outcome data for each main outcome, including attrition and exclusions from the analysis. State whether attrition and exclusions were reported, the numbers in each intervention group (compared with total randomised participants), reasons for attrition/exclusions where reported and any re-inclusions in analyses performed by the review authors.	Were incomplete outcome data adequately addressed?
Selective outcome reporting	State how the possibility of selective outcome reporting was examined by the review authors and what was found.	Are reports of the study free of suggestion of selective outcome reporting?
Other sources of bias	State any important concerns about bias not addressed in the other domains in the tool.	Was the study apparently free of other problems that could put it at a high risk of bias?

TABLE 12.1   The Cochrane Collaboration's tool for assessing risk of bias in individual studies [22]

There are two stages to doing a meta-analysis. Firstly, the intervention effect, including the confidence intervals, for each of the studies is calculated. The statistics used will depend on the type of outcome data found in the studies, with commonly used statistics including odds ratios, relative risks and mean differences.[15] As we saw in Chapter 4 when learning how to interpret the results of randomised controlled trials, if the outcome is dichotomous, odds ratios or relative risks may be used. For continuous outcomes, mean differences may be used.

Table 12.2 lists some of the statistical measures of intervention effect that can be used in a meta-analysis based on the outcome data type as outlined in the *Cochrane Handbook for Systematic Reviews of Interventions*.[23]

Type of outcome data	Measures of intervention effect
Dichotomous or binary (one of two categories)	Risk ratio (RR) Odds ratio (OR) Risk difference (RD) Number needed to treat (NNT)
Continuous (numeric)	Mean difference
Ordinal (including measurement scales)	Proportional odds ratio Recalculated as binary data
Counts and rates (for example, number of events)	Rate ratio
Time to event (survival data)	Hazard ratio

TABLE 12.2   Examples of statistical measures of intervention effect that can be used in a meta-analysis

The second stage in a meta-analysis is calculating the overall intervention effect. This is generally a weighted average of the summary statistics from the individual studies, with the weighting being determined by a function of the sample size and variance of each study. This is illustrated later in this chapter.

Interpret and report the results

While the results of the review are discussed in the text of the review, the results of a meta-analysis are typically displayed visually using a forest plot. Forest plots are like a series of tree plots (which were explained in Chapter 4) that are represented in one figure. In meta-analyses, forest plots generally display both the information (such as the intervention effect and the associated confidence interval) from the individual studies that were included in the review *and* an estimate of the overall effect (see Figure 12.2). In systematic reviews where data are not statistically combined, forest plots may still be presented but do not include an overall estimate. Forest plots are useful as they allow readers to visually assess the amount of variation among the studies that are included in the review.[15] How do you interpret a forest plot? There was a previous convention that risk ratios and odds ratios less than one indicated that the experimental intervention was more effective than the control. When looking at the forest plot, this would mean that effect estimates to the left of the vertical line (the line of no effect) implied that the intervention was beneficial. This convention is no longer used as the position of the effect estimates on the forest plot is influenced by the nature of the outcome (that is, outcome of benefit or harm). Instead, when interpreting a forest plot, you should look for clear markings on the horizontal axis of the plot to indicate which side of the line of no effect is associated with benefit from the intervention.[24] We will take a closer look at interpreting a forest plot towards the end of this chapter when we look at the results from a specific systematic review.

Not all systematic reviews can undertake a meta-analysis, particularly when substantial heterogeneity exists. This might be due to large variations among studies in terms of the interventions or outcomes that they used. For example, in a systematic review of family therapy for depression, three trials were found but the results were not combined as the studies were very heterogeneous in terms of the interventions, participants and measurement instruments that were involved.[25] Large variations can make pooling results difficult or impossible. When this occurs (which unfortunately is often), review authors describe the results of each study separately in a narrative way.

Conclusions that are commonly reached in systematic reviews include:

1. The results from a review consistently show positive (or negative) effects of an intervention. In this case a review might state that the results (that is, the evidence) are convincing.
2. Where there are conflicting results from studies within the review, the authors might state that the evidence is inconclusive.
3. A number of reviews find only a few studies (or sometimes none) that meet their eligibility criteria and conclude that there is insufficient evidence about that particular intervention.

As a reader of systematic reviews it is important that you do not confuse the concept of 'no evidence' (or 'no evidence of an effect') with 'evidence of no effect'. When there is inconclusive evidence, it is incorrect for review authors to state that the results of the review show that an intervention has 'no effect' or is 'no different' from the control intervention.[21]

Critical appraisal of systematic reviews

Now that you have an understanding of just what is involved in undertaking a systematic review, let us move on to looking at how to critically appraise systematic reviews. As with other types of studies, not all systematic reviews are carried out using rigorous methods and, therefore, bias may be introduced into the final results and conclusion of the review. A review of 300 systematic reviews found that not all systematic reviews were equally reliable and that their reporting could be improved by following a universally agreed upon set of standards and guidelines.[26] Just because the evidence that you have found to answer your clinical question is a systematic review, this does not mean that you can automatically trust the results of the review. It is important that you critically appraise systematic reviews and determine whether you can trust their results and conclusions.

Using the three-step critical appraisal process that we have used elsewhere in this book to appraise other types of studies, the three key elements to be considered when appraising a systematic review are: the validity of the review methodology, the magnitude and precision of the intervention effect and the applicability of the review to your specific client or client population.

There are a number of tools that can be used to critically appraise systematic reviews, many of which are based on the 'Users' guides to evidence-based medicine' article about overviews.[27] Three commonly used appraisal checklists are The Centre for Evidence Based Medicine appraisal tool (http://ssrc.tums.ac.ir/SystematicReview/CEBM.asp), the CASP checklist for appraising reviews (http://www.phru.nhs.uk/Pages/PHD/resources.htm) and the criteria proposed by Greenhalgh and Donald.[28]

Box 12.1 lists key questions that you can ask when critically appraising a systematic review. These questions are adapted from the appraisal criteria suggested by Greenhalgh and Donald.[28]

Critical appraisal of systematic reviews—a worked example

To help you further understand how to critically appraise and use systematic reviews to inform clinical decisions, we will consider a clinical scenario, formulate a clinical question, locate a systematic review that might address that question and critically appraise the review. The text box describes the clinical scenario that we will use.

BOX 12.1 KEY QUESTIONS TO ASK WHEN CRITICALLY APPRAISING A SYSTEMATIC REVIEW

A. Were the methods used in the review valid?

1. Did the review address a clearly focussed question with clearly defined eligibility criteria? The question should be focussed in terms of the:
   a. Participants
   b. Intervention(s) and comparison(s)
   c. Outcome(s)

2. Did the review include high quality, relevant studies?
   a. Of robust study design (for example, randomised controlled trials)?
   b. That addressed relevant questions?
   c. Selected by more than one independent assessor?

3. Is it unlikely that the review missed important, relevant studies?
   a. Is the search strategy reproducible?
   b. Did the search strategy include synonyms for all terms?
   c. Is the search strategy sufficiently comprehensive? (Consider what sources were searched—for example, bibliographic databases, trial registers, unpublished literature, hand searching, reference lists, correspondence with experts, unpublished data.)

4. Did the review include an assessment of the risk of bias of included studies and was this assessment incorporated into the review findings?
   a. Is the method for assessing risk of bias reproducible?
   b. Is the method for assessing risk of bias adequate?
   c. Was the risk of bias assessment conducted by more than one independent assessor?
   d. Was the risk of bias assessment incorporated into the review findings? For example, were results analysed for different sets of studies according to level of bias evident (sometimes referred to as sensitivity analyses) where possible?

5. Did the review combine the results from studies and, if so, was it reasonable to do so?
   a. Were the results similar from study to study (was an examination of heterogeneity undertaken)? In systematic reviews this might be tested statistically using the I^2 statistic or by looking at the degree of overlap between the studies' confidence intervals.
   b. Were reasons for variations in results discussed?

B. What are the results of the review?

1. What are the overall results of the review?
2. How precise are the results?

C. How relevant are the results to me?

1. Were all important outcomes considered (from the points of view of individuals/clients, policy makers, healthcare professionals, family/carers, the wider community)?
2. Can the results be applied to my client/s? Consider how well your client(s) and practice setting compare with the review population (for example, participant characteristics and disease/impairment characteristics), intervention(s) and outcomes(s).

Clinical scenario, clinical question and finding the evidence to answer the question

James, Samantha and Louise are a physiotherapist, occupational therapist and speech language pathologist who have been working in the acute care wards of a large regional hospital. They have been involved in an ongoing debate with the administration of the hospital about stroke clients who continue to be triaged to various medical wards on admission rather than consistently admitted to the stroke unit. They are concerned that clients who are sent to regular medical wards may not receive the optimal care and therapy that is needed to achieve the best outcomes after stroke. The administrator argues that clients still have access to all of the therapies in the regular medical wards. To assist with clarifying their thoughts and developing an argument in preparation for a meeting that will be taking place next week, the therapists decide to do a search of the literature to see if there is any evidence to support their argument. They know that the hospital administration is worried about the costs involved and the decreased flexibility to manage the overall hospital and feels that the benefits do not outweigh the costs. The team formed the clinical question: For people with acute stroke who are admitted to hospital, do patients cared for in stroke units have greater improvements in independence compared with patients who are cared for in general medical wards?

They searched using the phrase 'stroke unit*' in the search box on the homepage of the Cochrane library and located a systematic review[29] in the Cochrane Database of Systematic Reviews that appears relevant to their question.

Clinical scenario (continued): Structured abstract of chosen article[29]

Citation: Stroke Unit Trialists' Collaboration. Organised inpatient (stroke unit) care for stroke. Cochrane Database of Systematic Reviews 2007, Issue 4. Art. No.: CD000197. DOI: 10.1002/14651858.CD000197.pub2.

Objectives: The aim of this systematic review was to compare the effectiveness of care received in stroke units with other types of care.

Search strategy: The authors searched the Cochrane Stroke Group trials register and the reference lists of studies found through the initial search, and contacted researchers who were working in this area. The search was not limited by date or language.

Selection criteria: Individual studies that were included in the review were randomised controlled clinical trials that compared organised inpatient stroke unit care with an alternative form of care.

Data collection and analysis: The eligibility and quality of randomised controlled trials were assessed by two reviewers.

> **Main results:** The review included 31 trials and found that more organised care was associated with improved outcomes. In 26 trials, care in general wards was compared with care in stroke units. Stroke unit care showed reductions in the odds of death at 1 year follow-up (odds ratio 0.86; 95% confidence interval [CI] 0.76 to 0.98), the odds of death or institutionalised care (odds ratio 0.82; 95% CI =0.73 to 0.92) and death or dependency (odds ratio 0.82; 95% CI 0.73 to 0.92). Organised stroke unit care did not increase the length of hospital stay.
>
> **Authors' conclusions:** People who had a stroke were more likely to have better outcomes in terms of survival, independence and avoiding institutional care when they received care in an organised inpatient stroke unit compared with those who did not receive care in a stroke unit.

Using the questions that are outlined in Box 12.1 we will now step you through a critical appraisal of the stroke unit systematic review.

A Were the methods used in the review valid?

1 Did the review address a clearly focussed question with clearly defined eligibility criteria?

Yes. The research question for this review is concisely and clearly spelt out in the abstract. 'Objective: To assess the effect of stroke unit care compared with alternative forms of care for patients following a stroke.' The question is elaborated on further in the study but is still clearly defined prior to the review being completed.

a) Participants: Yes. The review stated that 'Any patients admitted to hospital who had suffered a stroke were eligible. We recorded the delay between stroke onset and hospital admission but did not use this as an exclusion criterion. We used a clinical definition of stroke: focal neurological deficit due to cerebrovascular disease, excluding subarachnoid haemorrhage and subdural haematoma'.

b) Intervention(s) and comparison(s): Yes. The intervention under consideration in this review included stroke wards, acute stroke units which accept patients acutely but discharge early, rehabilitation stroke units and comprehensive stroke units (that is, combined acute and rehabilitation care). Each of these interventions was clearly defined in the review. The comparisons included mixed rehabilitation wards, mobile stroke teams or general medical wards.

c) Outcome(s): Yes. As stated in this review: 'The primary analysis examined death, dependency and the requirement for institutional care at the end of scheduled follow-up of the original trial (two trials subsequently extended follow-up). Dependency was categorised into two groups where "independent" was taken to mean that an individual did not require physical assistance for transfers, mobility, dressing, feeding or toileting. Individuals who failed any of these criteria were considered "dependent". The criteria for independence were approximately equivalent to a modified Rankin score of 0 to 2, a Barthel Index of more than 18 out of 20, or an Activity Index (AI) of more than 83. The requirement for long-term institutional care was taken to mean care in a residential home, nursing home, or hospital at the end of scheduled follow-up. Secondary outcome measures included patient quality of life, patient and carer satisfaction, and duration of stay in hospital or institution or both.'

2 Did the review include high quality, relevant studies?

a) Of robust study design? Yes. The review authors stated that they 'included all prospective trials that used some form of random allocation of stroke patients to an organised system of inpatient (stroke unit) care or an alternative form of inpatient care. Trials were included if treatment allocation was carried out on a strictly random basis or with a quasi-random procedure (such as bed availability or date of admission)'.

b) That addressed relevant questions? Yes. Refer to previous point.

c) Selected by more than one independent assessor? Yes. The review stated that two review authors assessed the eligibility and methodological quality of published trials.

3 Is it unlikely that the review missed important, relevant studies?

a) Is the search strategy reproducible? Yes. The full search strategy used in this review is not documented within the review itself, but the authors provide a link to the Cochrane Stroke Group methods used in reviews, which provides the full search strategy.

b) Is the search strategy sufficiently comprehensive? Yes, if you assume that all trials in most databases (such as CINAHL, EMBASE) had been located and entered into the Cochrane Stroke Group Trials Register. The review authors stated that they 'searched the Cochrane Stroke Group Trials Register, which was last searched by the Review Group Coordinator in April 2006. In an effort to identify further published, unpublished and ongoing trials, we scanned the reference lists of relevant articles, contacted colleagues and researchers and publicised our preliminary findings at stroke conferences in the UK, Scandinavia, Germany, Netherlands, Switzerland, Spain, Canada, South America, Australia, Belgium, USA, and Hong Kong. The search was not restricted by date, language or any other criteria to the best of our knowledge'.

4 Did the review include an assessment of the risk of bias of included studies and was this assessment incorporated into the review findings?

a) Is the method for assessing risk of bias reproducible? Yes. The review authors stated that they 'did not use a formal scoring system to record methodological quality but recorded the method of allocation concealment, completeness of follow-up, presence of an intention-to-treat analysis, and the presence of a blinded assessment of outcome'.

b) Is the method for assessing risk of bias adequate? Yes, as above.

c) Was the risk of bias assessment conducted by more than one independent assessor? Yes. The review stated that two review authors assessed the eligibility and methodological quality of published trials.

d) Was the risk of bias assessment incorporated into the review findings (for example, were sensitivity analyses used where possible)? Yes. The review stated: 'In view of the variety of trial methodologies described we carried out a sensitivity analysis based only on those trials with a low risk of bias: (1) secure randomisation procedures; (2) unequivocally blinded outcome assessment; (3) a fixed one-year period of follow-up. Seven trials are known to have met all of these criteria'.

5 Did the review combine the results from studies and, if so, was it reasonable to do so?

a) Were the results similar from study to study (was an examination of heterogeneity undertaken)? Yes. Tests of heterogeneity were undertaken for all pooled outcomes. For the outcomes of 'death', 'death or institutional care' and 'death or dependency', there was no evidence of statistical heterogeneity in any of the comparisons, indicating that the results were similar from study to study for these outcomes. However, the outcome of 'length of stay (days) in a hospital or institution or both' had too high a level of heterogeneity.

b) Were reasons for variations in results discussed? No. The only attempt at explaining variations in results for the outcome, 'length of stay (days) in a hospital or institution or both', comes from the following statement: 'The analysis of length of stay is complicated by the different methods of reporting results, the widely varying baseline lengths of stay, and the statistically significant heterogeneity between different trials'.

B What are the results of the review?

In the stroke unit systematic review, you can see that the authors were dealing with dichotomous outcomes and therefore used odds ratios to calculate effect measures. The review authors state that they 'analysed dichotomous outcomes as the odds ratio (OR) with 95% confidence interval (CI) of an adverse outcome' and explained the statistical models used to do so. They went on to elaborate that 'subgroup analyses involved a re-analysis stratified by patient or service subgroup using tabular subgroup data provided by the trialists. We analysed data on length of stay in a hospital or institution using standardised mean difference ...'

1 What are the overall results of the review?

When organised stroke unit care was compared to an alternative service, it was found that 'Case fatality recorded at the end of scheduled follow-up (median follow-up 12 months; range six weeks to 12 months) was lower in the organised (stroke unit) care in 22 of the 31 trial comparisons. The overall estimate gave an odds ratio of 0.82 (95% CI 0.73 to 0.92; $p = 0.001$), which was not complicated by statistically significant heterogeneity between trials'.

When reporting the second outcome, which was the odds of death or requiring institutional care at the end of scheduled follow-up, the review found a highly statistically significant result (odds ratio 0.81; 95% CI 0.74 to 0.90; $p < 0.0001$) and no statistically significant heterogeneity between the trials.

The third outcome that was analysed was the combined adverse outcome of being dead or dependent in activities of daily living at the end of the scheduled follow-up. The authors report that 'the summary odds ratio for being dead or dependent if receiving organised (stroke unit) care rather than alternative (less organised) services was 0.79 (95% CI 0.71 to 0.88; $p < 0.0001$), indicating a significant reduction in odds of death or dependency in the organised (stroke unit) care group. There was no statistically significant heterogeneity between trials'.

2 How precise are the results?

The precision of the summary effect size estimates that are reported in the previous results section is relatively high as the confidence intervals are quite narrow.

Earlier in this chapter we introduced the idea of forest plots as a way of visually representing the results from multiple studies within a systematic review. Let us look at the first forest plot from the stroke unit systematic review, shown in Figure 12.2, in a bit more detail. We find that the forest plot is labelled to show that effect measures to the *left* of the vertical line favour the intervention and those to the *right* of the line favour the control (comparison intervention).

The top of each forest plot is labelled to tell you what the *comparisons* are. The first forest plot that is included in the systematic review (and shown in Figure 12.2) is titled 'Organised stroke unit care versus alternative service' and has several subgroup analyses involved, with the first comparison being stroke ward versus general medical ward. The *outcome* of interest to each forest plot is also identified at the top of the forest plot. The outcome being reported in this forest plot is 'death by the end of scheduled follow-up'.

Each forest plot consists of a number of *horizontal lines*, with each horizontal line representing one of the individual studies that is included in the review. The length of the horizontal line represents the precision of the result or the confidence interval of the result of the study. In the forest plot in Figure 12.2, the first subgroup analysis involved 16 studies. There is a *square* on each of the lines which represents the intervention effect estimate from each of the individual studies. The *diamond* at the bottom of the plot represents the pooled quantitative result from the meta-analysis of the first subgroup.

At the bottom of the forest plot there is a line that tells you the *scale* for the intervention effect that you are measuring and at the top of the vertical line the type of effect (for example, odds ratio) is identified. In this example forest plot, it is the odds ratio. The *vertical line* in the middle of the plot is the line of no effect where the treatment and the placebo have the same effect on the risk of death in the follow-up period after stroke. To the left of the line, where the odds ratio is less than one, the interpretation is that the intervention (organised stroke unit care) made death during follow-up less likely. Results to the right of the vertical line, where the odds ratio is more than one, mean the intervention made the risk of death during the follow-up period more likely.

The second and third columns in the forest plot are headed 'Treatment n/N' and 'Control n/N'. The 'n' represents the number of deaths in the group (treatment or control) and the 'N' represents the total number of participants in the group. The weight column (the fifth column in this forest plot) is the percentage weight given to each of the individual studies in the pooled meta-analysis. The weight used is a function of the sample size and its variance. The size of the square on each of the horizontal lines is proportional to the percentage of weight that is given to the study in the meta-analysis.

If the horizontal line for a study crosses the vertical line it means that the study found no significant difference between the two groups. In our example forest plot, all of the studies except two[30,31] cross the vertical line. The study given the largest weight is the second study in the analysis (author is Athens). The squares positioned to the left of the vertical line show that those studies found that the stroke unit was beneficial compared to the general ward. The squares positioned to the right of the vertical line show that the studies found that the general ward was beneficial compared to the stroke unit.

As mentioned earlier in this chapter, the middle of the diamond is the pooled treatment effect calculated in the meta-analysis. The width of the diamond is the certainty of the result, generally the 95% confidence interval.[32] In the first subgroup analysis shown in the forest plot, the intervention effect is significant. That is, the stroke ward was more effective than the general ward in reducing the number of deaths in the follow-up period after stroke. If the confidence interval crosses the vertical line, as is the case in the second subgroup analysis in our example forest plot, this indicates that there was no significant difference between the effectiveness of a mixed rehabilitation ward versus a general medical ward.

C How relevant are the results to me?

1 Were all important outcomes considered?
(from the points of view of individuals/clients, policy makers, healthcare professionals, family/carers, the wider community)

For people who have had a stroke, the important outcomes of death, dependency, requirement of institutional care, patient satisfaction and quality of life were considered by the review authors and results for these outcomes were analysed where available. Other outcomes which may be of interest to policy makers and healthcare professionals are the costs of providing organised stroke unit care in comparison to general care. The

Analysis 1.1. Comparison 1 Organised stroke unit care versus alternative service, Outcome 1 Death by the end of scheduled follow up.

Review: Organised inpatient (stroke unit) care for stroke
Comparison: 1 Organised stroke unit care versus alternative service
Outcome: 1 Death by the end of scheduled follow up

Study or sub group	Treatment n/N	Control n/N	Peto Odds Ratio Peto.Fixed. 95% CI	Weight	Peto Odds Ratio Peto.Fixed. 95% CI
1. Stroke ward versus general medical ward					
Akershus	61/271	70/279		13.8%	0.87 [0.59, 1.28]
Athens	103/302	127/302		19.7%	0.71 [0.51, 0.99]
Beijing	12/195	19/197		4.0%	0.62 [0.30, 1.29]
Dover (GMW)	34/98	35/89		6.0%	.082 [0.45, 1.48]
Edinburgh	48/155	55/156		9.5%	0.82 [0.51, 1.32]
Goteborg-Ostra	16/215	12/202		3.6%	1.27 [0.59, 2.73]
Goteborg-Sahlgren	45/166	19/83		5.9%	1.25 [0.68, 2.27]
Joinville	9/35	12/39		2.1%	0.78 [0.29, 2.14]
Nottingham (GMW)	14/98	10/76		2.8%	1.10 [0.46, 2.61]
Orpington 1993 (GMW)	3/53	6/48		1.1%	0.43 [0.11, 1.70]
Orpington 1995	7/34	17/37		2.2%	0.33 [0.12, 0.87]
Perth	4/29	6/30		1.2%	0.65 [0.17, 2.50]
Stockholm	49/269	45/225		10.4%	089 [0.57, 1.40]
Svendborg	14/31	12/34		2.2%	1.50 [0.56, 4.02]
Trondheim	27/110	36/110		6.2%	0.67 [0.37, 1.20]
Umea	43/11/	75/183		9.2%	0.92 [0.57, 1.50]
Subtotal (95% CI)	**2171**	**2090**		**100%**	**0.83 [0.71, 0.96]**

Total events: 489 (Treatment). 556 (Control)
Heterogeneity: Chi2 = 11.47, df = 15 (p = 0.72); I2 = 0.0%
Test for overall effect: z = 2.57 (P = 0.010)

2. Mixed rehabilitation ward versus general medical ward					
Birmingham	4/29	2/23		6.9%	1.63 [0.30, 8.90]
Helsinki	26/121	27/122		54.1%	096 [0.52, 1.77]
Illinois	0/56	0/35		0.0%	0.0 [0.0, 0.0]
Kuopio	8/50	10/45		19.1%	0.84 [0.31, 2.28]
New York	0/42	0/40		0.0%	0.0 [0.0, 0.0]
Newcastle	11/34	12/33		19.9%	0.84 [0.31, 2.28]
Subtotal (95% CI)	**332**	**298**		**100%**	**10.91 [0.58, 1.42]**

Total events: 49 (Treatment), 51 (Control)
Heterogeneity: Chi2 = 0.86, df = 3 (p = 0.84); I2 = 0.0%
Test for overall effect: z = 0.43 (P = 0.67)

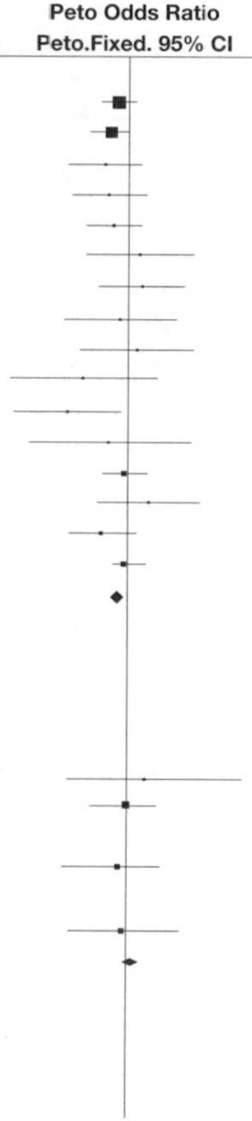

FIGURE 12.2 Example of a forest plot
Stroke Unit Trialists' Collaboration, Organised inpatient (stroke unit) care for stroke, Issue 4, 2007, Copyright The Cochrane Collaboration, reproduced with permission (cont'd)

Study	Treatment	Control	Weight	OR (95% CI)
3. Mobile stroke team versus general medical ward				
Cape Town	19/58	28/91	21.3%	1.10 [0.54, 2.22]
Manchester	45/157	35/151	41.0%	1.33 [0.80, 2.21]
Montreal	16/65	21/65	18.4%	0.69 [0.32, 1.47]
Uppsala	27/60	26/52	19.3%	0.82 [0.39, 1.72]
Subtotal (95% CI)	**340**	**359**	**100%**	**1.03 [0.74, 1.42]**

Total events: 107 (Treatment). 110 (Control)
Heterogeneity: Chi2 = 2.45, df = 3 (p = 0.48): I2 = 0.0%
Test for overall effect: z = 0.17 (P = 0.86)

Study	Treatment	Control	Weight	OR (95% CI)
4. Stroke ward versus rehabilitation ward				
Dover (MRW)	5/18	11/28	11.4%	0.61 [0.18, 2.08]
Nottingham (MRW)	11/78	16/63	24.3%	0.48 [0.21, 1.12]
Orpington 1993 (MRW)	6/71	12/73	17.7%	0.48 [0.18, 1.30]
Osaka	0/91	0/87	0.0%	0.0 [0.0, 0.0]
Tampere	30/98	27/113	46.5%	1.40 [0.76, 2.58]
Subtotal (95% CI)	**356**	**364**	**100%**	**1.82 [0.54, 1.24]**

Total events: 52 (Treatment), 66 (Control)
Heterogeneity: Chi2 = 5.83, df = 3 (p = 0.412: I2 = 49%
Test for overall effect: z = 0.96 (P = 0.34)

Study	Treatment	Control	Weight	OR (95% CI)
5. Stroke ward versus mobile stroke team				
Orpington 2000	13/152	34/152	100.0%	0.35 [0.19, 0.65]
Subtotal (95% CI)	**152**	**152**	**100%**	**0.35 [0.19, 0.65]**

Total events: 13 (Treatment), 34 (Control)
Heterogeneity: not applicable
Test for overall effect: z = 3.33 (P = 0.00088)

Study	Treatment	Control	Weight	OR (95% CI)
6. Stroke team versus stroke ward				
Groningen	1/27	7/27	34/3%	0.18 [0.04, 0.79]
Pavia	6/134	8/134	65.7%	0.74 [0.25, 2.17]
Subtotal (95% CI)	**161**	**161**	**100%**	**0.45 [0.19, 1.08]**

Total events: 7 (Treatment). 15 (Control)
Heterogeneity: Chi2 = 2.33, df = 1 (p = 0.13): I2 = 57%
Test for overall effect: z = 1.78 (P = 0.076)
Test for subgroup differences: Chi2 = 11.13 , df = 5 (p = 0.05): I2 = 55%

0.1 0.2 0.5 1.0 2.0 5.0 10.0
Favours treatment Favours control

review authors also point out that the results do not explain why stroke units may result in improved client outcomes. They suggest that this may be the result of a number of factors such as better diagnostic procedures, better nursing care, early mobilisation, the prevention of complications or more effective rehabilitation procedures. These variables may be important to measure in future trials.

2 Can the results be applied to my client(s)?

Based on the large number of trials and participants (31 trials, involving a total of 6936 participants) and the subgroup analysis findings that outcomes were independent of patient age, sex or stroke severity, it can be suggested that the results can be extrapolated from the review population to other people who have had a stroke and receive organised stroke unit care. If we go back to our clinical scenario that we raised at the beginning of this worked example, we see that the health professionals in the scenario are working in an acute hospital setting and with clients who have had a stroke. The question that they raised was: For people with acute stroke admitted to hospital, do stroke units have greater improvements in independence compared with general medical wards? This is directly addressed by this systematic review. The scenario does not provide us with details about the characteristics of the stroke clients that they see but, given that the therapists work in a general hospital setting and the studies included in the review were conducted in general hospital settings in various locations throughout the world, it is likely that the characteristics of the clients would be similar.

Resolution of clinical scenario

The systematic review that we have just appraised indicates that stroke units can result in improved outcomes in terms of survival, independence and avoiding institutional care when compared with care that is provided in alternative services. The outcome data from this review, particularly the data that compared stroke unit care with care in medical wards, could be used by the therapists in our scenario when they are discussing hospital policy with the administrator to argue that people who have had a stroke should be cared for in the stroke unit. Data about the costs involved were not provided in the review; however, the review did find that there was no increase in the length of stay for participants who received care in stroke units. This is only a proxy for cost and in future studies it would be important to ascertain full details of the costs involved. Discussions with the administrator about the feasibility of implementing a plan to ensure that all people who are admitted to hospital with a stroke are admitted to the stroke unit as soon as possible would also be needed.

Summary points of this chapter

- Systematic reviews differ from literature reviews because they are prepared using explicit, transparent and pre-specified strategies that limit bias. They involve a comprehensive search of *all* potentially relevant articles; use explicit, reproducible and uniformly applied criteria in the selection of articles for the review; rigorously appraise the risk of bias within individual studies; and systematically synthesise the results of included studies.
- Systematic reviews synthesise different study methodologies depending on the research question of interest.
- A properly conducted systematic review can improve the dissemination of evidence, hasten the assimilation of research into practice, assist in clarifying the heterogeneity of conflicting results between studies and establish generalisability of the overall findings.

- Because systematic reviews vary in quality, you should know how to appraise them and recognise the key features that introduce bias into systematic reviews. When examining whether the review used valid methods, key questions that need to be asked are whether the review: 1) addressed a clearly focussed question with clearly defined eligibility criteria; 2) included high quality, relevant studies; 3) is unlikely to have missed important, relevant studies; 4) included an assessment of the risk of bias of the included studies and incorporated this assessment into the review findings; and 5) combined the results from studies and, if so, was it reasonable to do so?
- The main questions that you need to ask when examining the results of a systematic review are: 1) What are the overall results? 2) How precise are the results? 3) Did the review consider all the important outcomes? and 4) Can the results be applied to your clients?

References

1. Mulrow C, Cook DJ, Davidoff F. Systematic reviews: critical links in the great chain of evidence. Ann Intern Med 1997; 126:389–391.
2. Cook D, Mulrow C, Haynes RB. Systematic reviews: synthesis of best evidence for clinical decisions. Ann Intern Med 1997; 126:376–380.
3. Greenhalgh T. How to read a paper: papers that summarise other papers (systematic reviews and meta-analyses). BMJ 1997; 315:672–675.
4. Herbert R, Jamtvedt G, Mead J et al. Practical evidence-based physiotherapy. Edinburgh: Elsevier; 2005.
5. Phillips B, Ball C, Sackett D et al. Oxford Centre for Evidence-based Medicine levels of evidence. Online. 2001. Available: http://www.cebm.net/index.aspx?o=1025 (11 Sept 2008).
6. National Health and Medical Research Council. How to use the evidence: assessment and application of scientific evidence. Online. 2000. Available: http://www.nhmrc.gov.au/publications/synopses/_files/cp69.pdf (12 Sept 2008).
7. Meijer R, Ihnenfeldt DS, van Limbeek J et al. Prognostic factors in the subacute phase after stroke for the future residence after six months to one year. A systematic review of the literature. Clin Rehab 2003; 17:512–520.
8. Irwig L, Tosteson AN, Gatsonis CA et al. Guidelines for meta-analyses evaluating diagnostic tests. Ann Intern Med 1994; 120:667–676.
9. Mitchell AJ. A meta-analysis of the accuracy of the mini-mental state examination in the detection of dementia and mild cognitive impairment. J Psychiatr Res 2009; 43:411–431.
10. Popay J. Qualitative research and process evaluation in systematic reviews: the methodological research agenda. The Cochrane Collaboration Methods Groups Newsletter. Online. 2000. Available: http://www.cochrane.org/newslett/mg4-1.htm (10 Oct 2008).
11. Goldsmith MR, Bankhead CR, Austoker J. Synthesising quantitative and qualitative research in evidence-based patient information. J Epidemiol Community Health 2007; 61:262–270.
12. McInnes E, Askie L. Evidence review on older people's views and experiences of falls prevention strategies. World Views on Evidence-Based Nursing 2004; 1:20–37.
13. Allen IJ, Okin I. Estimating the time to conduct a meta-analysis from number of citations retrieved. JAMA 1999; 282:634–635.
14. Jackson N, Waters E. Criteria for the systematic review of health promotion and public health interventions. Health Promot Int 2005; 20:367–374.
15. Akobeng AK. Understanding systematic reviews and meta-analysis. Arch Dis Child 2005; 90: 845–848.
16. Bhandari M, Guyatt G, Montori V et al. Current concepts review: users guide to orthopedic literature: how to use a systematic review. J Bone Joint Surg 2002; 84A:1672–1682.
17. Hopewell S, Clarke M, Lefebvre C et al. Handsearching versus electronic searching to identify reports of randomised trials. Cochrane Database of Methodological Rev 2002; 4: Art. No. MR 000001. DOI:10.1002/14651858.
18. Kennedy G, Rutherford G. Identifying randomised controlled trials in the journal. Presentation at the Eighth International Cochrane Colloquium. 2000. Cape Town, South Africa.
19. Armstrong R, Jackson N, Doyle J et al. It's in your hands: the value of handsearching in conducting systematic reviews. J Pub Health 2005; 27:388–391.

20. Higgins JP, Green S (eds). Cochrane handbook for systematic reviews of interventions. Version 5.0.0 (updated February 2008). The Cochrane Collaboration; 2008. Online. Available: http://www.cochrane-handbook.org.
21. Juni P, Altman D, Egger M. Systematic reviews in health care: assessing the quality of controlled clinical trials. BMJ 2001; 323:42–46.
22. Higgins J, Altman D (eds). Chapter 8: Assessing risk of bias in included studies. In: Higgins J, Green S (eds). Cochrane handbook for systematic reviews of interventions. Version 5.0.0 (updated February 2008). The Cochrane Collaboration; 2008. Online. Available: http://www.cochrane-handbook.org.
23. Deeks J, Higgins J, Altman D (eds). Chapter 9: Analysing data and undertaking meta-analyses. In: Higgins J, Green S (eds). Cochrane handbook for systematic reviews of interventions. Version 5.0.0 (updated February 2008). The Cochrane Collaboration; 2008. Online. Available: http://www.cochrane-handbook.org.
24. Schünemann H, Oxman A, Higgins J et al. Chapter 11: Presenting results and Summary of findings tables. In: Higgins J, Green S (eds). Cochrane handbook for systematic reviews of interventions. Version 5.0.0 (updated February 2008). The Cochrane Collaboration; 2008. Online. Available: http://www.cochrane-handbook.org.
25. Henken H, Huibers M, Churchill R et al. Family therapy for depression. Cochrane Database Syst Rev 2007; 3: Art. No.: CD006728. DOI: 10.1002/14651858.CD006728.
26. Moher D, Tetzlaff J, Tricco A, et al. Epidemiology and reporting characteristics of systematic reviews. PLoS Med 2007; 4:e78. doi:10.1371/journal.pmed.0040078.
27. Oxman A, Cook D, Guyatt G. Users' guides to the medical literature: VI. How to use an overview. JAMA 1994; 272(17):1367–1371.
28. Greenhalgh T, Donald A. Evidence-based health care workbook: understanding research: for individual and group learning. London: BMJ Publishing Group; 2000.
29. Stroke Unit Trialists' Collaboration. Organised inpatient (stroke unit) care for stroke. Cochrane Database Syst Rev 2007; 4: Art. No.: CD000197. doi: 10.1002/14651858.CD000197.pub2.
30. Kalra L, Eade J. Role of stroke rehabilitation units in managing severe disability after stroke. Stroke 1995; 26:2031–2034.
31. Vemmos K, Takis K, Madelos D et al. Stroke unit treatment versus general medical wards: long term survival. Cerebrovasc Dis 2001; 11:8.
32. Leonardi-Bee J. Presenting and interpreting meta-analyses. RLO, School of Nursing and Academic Division of Midwifery, University of Nottingham; 2007. Online. Available: http://www.nottingham.ac.uk/nursing/sonet/rlos/ebp/meta-analysis2/index.html (14 Sept 2008).

CHAPTER 13

Clinical guidelines

Rachel Yates, Jonathon Kruger, Jeff Coombes and Tammy Hoffmann

LEARNING OBJECTIVES

After reading this chapter, you should be able to:

- Describe what clinical guidelines are, their uses and their limitations
- Be aware of the major online resources for locating clinical guidelines
- Explain the major steps that are involved in the development of guidelines
- Appraise the quality of a clinical guideline to determine whether you should trust the recommendations that it contains
- Describe some of the issues related to using a clinical guideline in practice
- Be aware of the some of the legal issues associated with the use of guidelines

Put simply, the term 'clinical guideline' refers to information, compiled from various sources, that recommends ways of dealing with specified clinical conditions. Clinical guidelines (also often called clinical practice guidelines) can range from simple protocols that have been compiled by an individual health agency to quality evidence-based guidelines which have undergone a much more rigorous development and review process. The latter is the type that we are interested in and will focus on in this chapter. However, we will also discuss how to assess which category different guidelines fall into as it is likely that you will come across a variety during your clinical practice. In this chapter we will look at what clinical guidelines are, why they are used, where to search for guidelines, the steps involved in developing a guideline and how to appraise the quality of a guideline. We will also discuss some of the issues involved with using guidelines in clinical practice, including legal issues surrounding their use.

What are clinical guidelines?

An internationally accepted definition of clinical guidelines is that they are *systematically developed statements to assist health professional and client decisions about appropriate health care for specific circumstances.*[1]

A well-developed guideline contains rigorously compiled information and recommended actions to guide practice that are based on a comprehensive review of the available research evidence about a particular topic area, often combined with client input and expert opinion. Guidelines are designed to help health professionals decide how to prevent, diagnose and/or treat the client's presenting symptoms. For example, occupational therapists, physiotherapists, speech pathologists or other health professionals who work with people who are recovering from a stroke may find the National Stroke Foundation's 'Clinical Guidelines for Stroke Rehabilitation and Recovery' useful for informing practice (available from http://www.nhmrc.gov.au/publications/synopses/cp105syn.htm).

Why use guidelines?

As we saw in Chapter 2, health professionals are continually exposed to an overwhelming amount of health research and there are thousands of new studies published each year. Keeping abreast of this enormous volume of information is not possible for busy health professionals and the development of healthcare guidelines is one way in which information overload is being addressed. Guidelines are a useful tool for evidence-based practice as they help us to translate evidence into practice recommendations, which can then be applied to clinical situations.

Guidelines aim to help health professionals and clients make better decisions about health care. They aim to reduce variations in practice across health professionals for the same condition and improve client outcomes. Guidelines achieve these aims by clarifying and providing recommendations about those parts of healthcare practice that can be examined through established scientific methods.[2] The *development* of guidelines—the act of amassing and scrutinising the relevant research about a specific topic and making research accessible to health professionals and clients—is part of evidence-based practice at the organisational level. The subsequent *translation* of guidelines in the clinical setting is more about evidence-based individual decision making, as well as the implementation of evidence into practice.

Clinical guidelines are increasingly being used by health professionals. It is anticipated that their use will continue to become more common. The direct applicability to contemporary clinical practice is what makes a clinical guideline useful. As with other types of evidence, care needs to be taken to ensure that guidelines are of high quality and that they are implemented effectively. This process includes adapting them for a local setting and tailoring evidence-based implementation strategies to local settings. Guidelines will not address all the uncertainties of current clinical practice and should be seen as only one strategy that can help improve the quality of client care.[3]

Guidelines: the pros and cons

Guidelines have a number of benefits. By drawing together all of the evidence that is known about a particular clinical topic and making sense of it, a guideline can save health professionals a lot of time. Clinical guidelines typically provide an overview of the management of a condition or the use of an intervention. They usually have a broader scope than systematic reviews, which tend to focus on a single clinical question. A guideline may also provide a more coherent synthesis of research about how to manage a condition. Compared to systematic reviews, which usually draw conclusions from only the best available research evidence, the conclusions (recommendations) of guidelines are typically the result of a synthesis of the best available research evidence, expert opinion (such as clinicians and researchers) and client input. Guideline development is not easy and involves large amounts of time, money, expertise and effort. As the development process can be lengthy, there is a possibility that the evidence used in a guideline may not be the most current evidence by the time the guideline is finally published.

When considering using a guideline, the key word to remember is 'guide'. Rigorously developed guidelines are the result of a comprehensive examination of the literature by a panel of experts. This panel has drawn research findings together into a useful, practical resource that can assist in the prevention, diagnosis and treatment of health conditions. However, guideline recommendations are *not* fixed protocols that must be followed. As with evidence-based practice in general, responsible and informed clinical judgement about the management of clients remains important. You need to work together with your client to develop an individual intervention plan that is tailored to their specific needs and circumstances, and that is achievable, affordable and realistic.[4]

One of the potentially limiting factors about guidelines is that they generally tend to deal with a specific situation in isolation. However, in practice, clients often present with a range of comorbid conditions. Even when a client presents without comorbidities, translating a guideline in practice still needs to take into account factors such as:
- client preferences and desired outcomes
- the likelihood of adherence
- client's readiness to change behaviours
- the risk to the client if the guidelines are not followed
- the availability and affordability of any services, medications or other interventions that are recommended in the guidelines.

Client factors will be discussed in more detail later in this chapter when we discuss using a clinical guideline in practice.

How guidelines fit with other evidence-based practice products

As well as clinical guidelines, there are other evidence-based practice products or aids that can help health professionals and clients to make decisions about care. Examples of these products include:

- 'Handbooks', of which there are many and which differ from country to country. Some examples, primarily Australian ones, include:
  - ○ The *Australian Immunisation Handbook* (http://www.health.gov.au/internet/immunise/publishing.nsf/Content/Handbook-home)
  - ○ The Royal Australian College of General Practitioners' evidence-based guides, which include handbooks on preventative health and also care in residential aged care facilities (http://www.racgp.org.au/guidelines)
  - ○ The *Australian Medicines Handbook* (http://www.amh.net.au/index.php?page=about)
  - ○ The *Asthma Management Handbook* (http://www.nationalasthma.org.au/cms/index.php)
  - ○ Bandolier publications on evidence-based health care (http://www.medicine.ox.ac.uk/bandolier/)
- Decision support tools for health care (sometimes these are available for both clients and health professionals). More detail about decision aids is provided in Chapter 14.
- Practice software and personal digital assistants (PDAs) which incorporate, or have links to, evidence-based guidelines
- Educational modules and information packs which are sent out to health professionals by federal and state health departments

Guidelines can complement these other products, when the information contained in them is aligned and consistent. Some of these products may contain guidelines and sometimes the products may share the same evidence base as the relevant guidelines. However, there is not always consistency across products. Situations can arise where there are discrepancies in the recommendations made in various products. When discrepancies occur, you need to decide which resource to use. Later in this chapter, we discuss how to evaluate the quality of guidelines so that you can choose the one with the highest quality that will be of the most use to your particular clinical situation.

Where and how to find guidelines

It is probably clear to you by now that there are thousands of clinical guidelines across the health professions. The obvious question is: Where and how should you look for guidelines relevant to your client/clinical situation? In general, there are three main electronic sources that can be used to locate clinical guidelines:
- large bibliographic databases (such as PubMed, Embase, CINAHL)
- guideline-specific databases (such as the National Guidelines Clearinghouse, The National Library of Guidelines)
- specific organisations (such as the Heart Foundation, Diabetes Australia).

Bibliographic databases

Although the large bibliographic databases do contain some clinical guidelines, the problem is that only a small proportion of guidelines are published in journals. As a result, only a small proportion is indexed in the traditional databases. In addition, none of these bibliographic databases appraise the quality of guidelines, and it may be difficult to access more than just the abstract from their sites. However, if you decide to search the large bibliographic databases to locate guidelines, here are a few tips:
- PubMed: When searching for clinical guidelines in PubMed, you can select the limit 'practice guideline' under publication type.
- MEDLINE: Methodological search strategies for retrieving guidelines in MEDLINE (via Ovid) have been created[5] and are summarised in Table 13.1, showing strategies

that are aimed at locating all articles classified as a guideline and strategies that are aimed at locating methodologically sound guidelines. In the study that developed these search filters, all articles retrieved that met the definition of a clinical practice guideline were evaluated for methodological quality according to the following criteria if they were concerned with the development of a guideline: 1) the article contained an explicit statement that described the process of developing the guideline, including methods of evidence assembly, method of review of studies and at least one of a) the organisations and the individuals involved, b) the methods of formulating guidelines and c) the methods of reaching agreement or consensus and 2) evidence was cited in support of at least one of the recommendations contained in the guideline. If the article related to the application (as opposed to development) of a clinical guideline, the following criterion was used to evaluate the article's scientific merit: at least one of the exact guidelines was provided in a table, figure or text of the article. Combine the methodological search strategies in Table 13.1 with your content terms (such as the keywords from your clinical question) when searching for clinical guidelines in MEDLINE.

- Embase: Embase has a thesaurus term 'practice guideline' which you can use as part of your search strategy; however, be aware that the term refers to more than just clinical practice guidelines.
- CINAHL: You can select the limit 'practice guideline' under publication type when searching in CINAHL.

Chapter 3 provides further details about these databases, as well as advice about how to use search strategies such as those shown in Table 13.1 when looking for evidence to answer a clinical question.

Guideline-specific databases

One of the best ways to find a clinical guideline can be by searching a guideline-specific database. Details about some of the major guideline-specific databases in Australia, the UK and the USA are provided below and Table 13.2 lists many others.

- **National Guidelines Clearinghouse (NGC)** (http://www.guideline.gov/). This database is maintained as a public resource by the USA Department of Health and Human Services. An interesting feature is the Guideline Comparison Utility, which

Hedge	All classified guidelines	Methodologically sound guidelines
Best sensitivity	exp health services administration OR tu.xs. OR management.tw.	guideline:.tw. OR exp data collection OR recommend:.tw. guidelines.tw. OR practice guidelines.sh. OR recommend:.tw.
Best specificity	guideline:.tw.	guideline adherence.sh. OR physician's practice patterns.sh. practice guidelines.tw. OR practice guidelines.sh.
Best optimisation of sensitivity and specificity	guide:.tw. OR recommend:.tw. OR exp risk	exp "quality assurance (health care)" OR recommend:.tw. OR guideline adherence.sh.

Colon = truncation; tw = textword; exp = explosion; tu = therapeutic use; sh = subject heading; xs = exploded subheading; + = explode

TABLE 13.1 Search strategies (hedges) for locating practice guidelines in MEDLINE (via OVID) [5]

Database	Website	Scope of guidelines
EBM Guidelines: Evidence-Based Medicine	http://ebmg.wiley.com/ebmg/ltk.koti	Contains a collection of clinical guidelines for primary care combined with the best available evidence. There are approximately 1000 primary care practice guidelines.
PEDro (Physiotherapy Evidence Database)	http://www.pedro.org.au/	Contains evidence-based clinical guidelines of relevance to physiotherapy. Some guidelines are also of relevance to other health professions. PEDro was described in more detail in Chapter 3.
Evidence-Based Practice: Clinical Practice Rehabilitation Guidelines	http://www.health.uottawa.ca/rehabguidelines/en/login.php	Maintained by the School of Rehabilitation Sciences at the University of Ottawa, this database contains web-based guidelines of relevance to rehabilitation health professionals. The guidelines have been appraised using the AGREE instrument.
Canadian Medical Association Infobase: Clinical Practice Guidelines	http://www.cma.ca/index.cfm/ci_id/54316/la_id/1.htm	Contains over 1200 guidelines that were developed or endorsed by an authoritative medical or health organisation in Canada.
Scottish Intercollegiate Guidelines Network (SIGN)	http://www.sign.ac.uk	Most of the guidelines are about medical topics, but some will also be of relevance to other health professionals such as allied health and nursing.
Guidelines Advisory Committee (Ontario Medical Association, Canada)	http://www.gacguidelines.ca	Reviews existing guidelines using the AGREE instrument and creates summaries of guidelines they consider worthy of endorsing. Most of the guidelines reviewed concern medical topics.
New Zealand Guidelines Group	http://www.nzgg.org.nz/	This group oversees the development and implementation of guidelines across the health and disability sectors in New Zealand. Guidelines on a wide range of topics are available.
Medical Journal of Australia: Clinical Guidelines	http://www.mja.com.au/public/guides/guides.html	Contains guidelines on a broad range of medical topics.

TABLE 13.2   Details of other guideline-specific databases

gives users the ability to generate side-by-side comparisons of a combination of two or more guidelines. The NGC staff also prepare syntheses of selected guidelines that cover similar topic areas. In these syntheses, there is often a comparison of guidelines developed in different countries. This tool may assist health professionals by providing insight into the commonalities and differences in international health practices.

- **National Library of Guidelines** (UK) (http://www.library.nhs.uk/GuidelinesFinder/). This database contains the full text of over 2000 selected care guidelines. The focus is on guidelines that have been produced in the UK, but some guidelines from other countries are included for topics where no UK-developed ones exist. The guidelines

that it contains are those produced by the National Institute for Health and Clinical Excellence (NICE; http://www.nice.org.uk) and other national agencies.
- **National Health and Medical Research Council (NHRMC, Australia;** http://www.nhmrc.gov.au/guidelines/health_guidelines.htm). As discussed later in this chapter, the NHMRC has a rigorous process for appraising guidelines. At the time of writing this chapter (September 2008), approximately 40 guidelines were available.
- **Turning Research Into Practice (TRIP).** The TRIP database was discussed in detail in Chapter 3. The search results are grouped according to the type of evidence (for example, systematic review). For guidelines, the search can be filtered further by specifying North America, Europe or 'other'. At the time of writing, there were over 2500 clinical guidelines available via the North American filter, 1400 under Europe and 270 under 'other'.

Specific organisations

In many countries, organisations for specific conditions or diseases, such as the Heart Foundation in Australia, also provide access to clinical guidelines that are relevant to the health condition. These guidelines are often included in the bibliographic or guideline-specific databases that we have already discussed; however, it may be quicker to locate a guideline of interest by going directly to one of these organisation's websites. Some Australian examples of these are:
- Heart Foundation (http://www.heartfoundation.org.au/)
- Diabetes Australia (http://www.diabetesaustralia.com.au/For-Health-Professionals/Diabetes-National-Guidelines/)
- Kidney Health Australia (http://www.cari.org.au/guidelines.php)
- National Stroke Foundation (http://www.strokefoundation.com.au/clinical-guidelines)
- Australian Cancer Network (http://www.cancer.org.au/Healthprofessionals/clinicalguidelines.htm)
- National Breast Cancer Centre (http://www.nbcc.org.au/bestpractice/)

How are guidelines developed?

In most cases, the development of a guideline follows a process which involves:
1. Gathering the relevant evidence about the topic
2. Assessing the evidence
3. Linking the evidence to desirable clinical outcomes
4. Writing recommendations which become the draft guidelines
5. Obtaining feedback about and external review of the draft guidelines
6. Altering the draft guidelines according to the feedback to produce the finalised guidelines

What gives rise to the variable quality of guidelines is that differences occur in this development process, typically in the following areas:
- the comprehensiveness of the search used to locate evidence (it should be a systematic search)
- the quality of the evidence reviewed
- the rigour of the processes used to assess/grade the evidence
- the people reviewing the evidence ('expert' panels are often used, but the structure and mix of panel members can vary)
- classification of what are deemed 'desirable' clinical outcomes (there is often debate about this even between experts within a particular field)

- the strength and quality of guideline recommendations
- the process and extent of obtaining feedback/pilot testing (if this process is conducted at all).

Three key processes that are essential for the development of a scientifically valid guideline have been described.[6,7] The first is that the panel that develops the guideline should contain representatives from all disciplines that the guideline is relevant to. Secondly, the scientific evidence should be synthesised in a systematic fashion, such as in a systematic review. The third process is that the recommendations should be explicitly linked to the evidence from which they were derived.

The steps involved in developing an *evidence-based* clinical guideline are more rigorous than the steps that are followed for other types of guidelines. The steps typically consist of:

1. Forming a development methods group—usually made up of published experts in the field who have experience in developing guidelines, as well as in judging levels of evidence, appraising the quality of evidence and appropriate statistical expertise
2. Searching systematically for evidence
3. Grading the evidence
4. Formulating a draft guideline
5. Forming an external multidisciplinary consensus panel to refine the draft guideline— the people in this group typically have similar expertise to the people in the methods group but are independent of the guideline development and can independently review the results of the draft guideline
6. Obtaining practitioner feedback and external review
7. Pilot testing the guideline
8. Disseminating (and implementing) the guideline
9. Scheduling a review of the guideline to ensure it remains based on the most current best available evidence—a timeframe of three years is often used

Can I trust the recommendations in a clinical guideline?

With such a large number of clinical guidelines available of varying quality, you may be left wondering which guidelines you should, or should not, use in your clinical practice. You need to ask yourself the same question that we asked when appraising various study designs in earlier chapters of this book—that is, are the results of this study valid? When appraising clinical guidelines, the 'results' are the recommendations, so you are trying to determine if you can trust the recommendations in a clinical guideline. As with the other types of evidence discussed in other chapters, it is important that you know how to appraise clinical guidelines and recognise the key features that discriminate high quality guidelines that can be used to guide practice from low quality clinical guidelines that should be used with caution. High quality guidelines can improve health care, but the adoption of low quality guidelines can lead to the use of ineffective interventions, the inefficient use of scarce resources and, most importantly, possible harm to clients.[8]

There are a number of instruments that can be used to help you appraise a guideline and establish the quality of its recommendations. However, just as guidelines themselves vary in quality, so too do the tools used to appraise them (see Box 13.1). One of the most comprehensive, easy-to-use and widely used tools to appraise guidelines is the AGREE instrument.[9] The Appraisal of Guidelines Research and Evaluation (AGREE) collaboration is an international group of researchers and policy makers. The instrument and instructions for its use can be downloaded for free from the collaboration website

A study that compared 24 different clinical guideline appraisal tools found considerable differences between the instruments.[10] These included the number of questions asked to assess the guidelines (from 3 to 52), whether a scoring system was used and whether it was validated. Overall, only four of the instruments had been subjected to a validation study. When all of the tools assessed in the study were rated on 10 dimensions (validity, reliability/reproducibility, clinical applicability, clinical flexibility, multidisciplinary process, clarity, scheduled review, dissemination, implementation and evaluation), the Cluzeau instrument was found to be the most comprehensive (covering all dimensions) and validated tool available. However, the AGREE instrument, which is based on the Cluzeau instrument, was reported as easier to use and more widely accepted.

(http://www.agreecollaboration.org/instrument/). The AGREE tool appraises guidelines based on how they score on 23 items, which are grouped into six major domains. Box 13.2 lists the domains and items of the AGREE instrument. Each item is rated on a 4-point scale (from 1 = strongly disagree to 4 = strongly agree), regarding the extent to which the item has been fulfilled by the guideline that is being appraised. For each domain, you are then able to sum the scores to obtain a domain score, which is then typically expressed as a percentage of the maximum total score that is possible for that domain.

The AGREE instrument and its accompanying user guide clearly explain how to assess a guideline according to the criteria that comprise the instrument. Most of the criteria are clearly explained in the user guide; however, it is worth elaborating a little about the domain that is concerned with evaluating the rigour of a guideline's development. In particular, we will consider/review item 10, which assesses whether the methods that were used for formulating the recommendations are clearly described. The process of formulating guideline recommendations is one of the most important, but difficult, steps when developing guidelines. Many guidelines grade the *strength of the recommendations* that they contain. It is important that this is done because the *strength of the evidence* behind recommendations can vary. Some guideline recommendations are based on high quality evidence, while others are based on lower quality evidence that is more susceptible to bias.[11] One difficulty that arises is that there is currently no commonly accepted method for grading the strength of the recommendations contained in a guideline. This lack of consensus on grading can make it confusing for readers, since the same recommendation could be graded as either 'strong evidence, strongly recommended', 'Level II-2, B evidence' or 'C+, 1 evidence', depending on which grading method/system was used.[12] The methods for grading the strength of recommendations continue to evolve—see, for example, the recommendations of the GRADE (Grading of Recommendations Assessment, Development, and Evaluation) working group[13] (http://www.gradeworkinggroup.org/index.htm).

We will briefly present the method that has been proposed by the NHMRC of Australia. At the time of writing this chapter, these NHMRC suggestions were contained in a draft document that was undergoing a stage of public consultation. We suggest you check the NHMRC website (http://www.nhmrc.gov.au) for the final document once it is published.

BOX 13.2 DOMAINS AND ITEMS CONTAINED IN THE AGREE INSTRUMENT

SCOPE AND PURPOSE

1. The overall objective(s) of the guideline is (are) specifically described.
2. The clinical question(s) covered by the guideline is (are) specifically described.
3. The clients to whom the guideline is meant to apply are specifically described.

STAKEHOLDER INVOLVEMENT

4. The guideline development group includes individuals from all the relevant professional groups.
5. The clients' views and preferences have been sought.
6. The target users of the guideline are clearly defined.
7. The guideline has been piloted among target users.

RIGOUR OF DEVELOPMENT

8. Systematic methods were used to search for evidence.
9. The criteria for selecting the evidence are clearly described.
10. The methods used for formulating the recommendations are clearly described.
11. The health benefits, side effects and risks have been considered in formulating the recommendations.
12. There is an explicit link between the recommendations and the supporting evidence.
13. The guideline has been externally reviewed by experts prior to its publication.
14. A procedure for updating the guideline is provided.

CLARITY AND PRESENTATION

15. The recommendations are specific and unambiguous.
16. The different options for management of the condition are clearly presented.
17. Key recommendations are easily identifiable.
18. The guideline is supported with tools for application.

APPLICABILITY

19. The potential organisational barriers in applying the recommendations have been discussed.
20. The potential cost implications of applying the recommendations have been considered.
21. The guideline presents key review criteria for monitoring and/or audit purposes.

EDITORIAL INDEPENDENCE

22. The guideline is editorially independent from the funding body.
23. Conflicts of interest of guideline development members have been recorded.

There is agreement that when grading the 'body of evidence' behind each recommendation, it is not sufficient to grade the strength of the recommendations only on the basis of the level of evidence (for example level I evidence—systematic review) that was available to develop the guideline. However, debate exists as to what components should be considered when grading the strength of recommendations. The NHMRC document suggests grading the evidence according to the following components:[14]

- the **evidence base**, in terms of the *number* of studies, *level* of evidence and the *quality* of studies (that is, their risk of bias)
- the **consistency** of the study results between studies

- the **potential clinical impact** of the proposed recommendation (for example, effect size, precision of the effect size estimate, clinical significance, balance of risks and benefits)
- the **generalisability** of the body of evidence to the target population for the guideline
- the **applicability** of the body of evidence to the Australian healthcare context.

For each 'body of evidence' that is being evaluated, each of these components should be given a rating of either A (excellent), B (good), C (satisfactory) or D (poor). Using this system, the developers of guidelines can then determine an overall grade, from A to D, for each of the recommendations that are contained in the guidelines,[14] where:

A = The body of evidence can be trusted to guide practice.

B = The body of evidence can be trusted to guide practice in most situations.

C = The body of evidence provides some support for recommendation(s) but care should be taken in its application.

D = The body of evidence is weak and the recommendations must be applied with caution.

How to use a guideline in practice

By now, it should be clear that there are many circumstances where you may wish to seek out a guideline to answer a clinical question. When searching for relevant guidelines, you should frame your clinical question of interest in a way that will help you to efficiently locate relevant information. The PICO method of formulating clinical questions, which was explained in Chapter 2, can also be used when searching for guidelines.

Once you have located and appraised a guideline and decided that it is valid, as with other types of evidence, you then need to assess its applicability. That is, is the guideline applicable to your client/clinical scenario? A key question that you need to ask is whether your client is similar to the clinical population to which the guidelines apply. For example, your client may have different risk factors to the clinical population which was targeted by the guidelines and, therefore, the guidelines cannot be applied to this client. You should also consider whether the setting of your clients is similar to the setting to which the guidelines apply. There are also organisational factors to bear in mind when considering implementing a guideline, such as whether the appropriate resources are available (for example, specialised equipment or staff with the necessary skills). Another issue to consider is whether the values that are associated with a guideline (either explicitly or implicitly) match the values of your client or your community.[11] Your client may have different values, preferences and beliefs to those that were assumed in the guideline.

A clinical guideline is not a mandate for practice. Regardless of the strength of the evidence on which the guideline recommendations are made, it is the responsibility of the individual health professional to interpret their application for each particular situation. Application involves taking account of client preferences as well as local circumstances.[15] For example, while two clients may have exactly the same risks for a particular health condition, we should not assume that they will react in the same way to a suggestion about commencing an intervention recommended in the guideline. As the two clients are likely to have different values, beliefs and preferences, one client may wish to proceed with the intervention that the guideline recommends, whereas another client may decide not to.

Do clinical guidelines change practice and improve care?

The use of clinical guidelines is not without some controversy. Despite the large amounts of human and financial resources that have been devoted to developing guidelines on a wide range of topics, there is no real clarity in the literature about whether the use of guidelines has led to an improvement in client outcomes. It is possible that the gap between what guidelines recommend and health professionals do is decreasing as health professionals increasingly become more familiar with guidelines and incorporate those recommendations into their practice. However, there is currently limited evidence that has investigated this issue.

The success of clinical guidelines at both changing practices and delivering better outcomes for clients is critically dependent on the methods used to develop, disseminate and implement those guidelines. While there is a substantial amount of literature about how to develop good quality guidelines, there is no consensus about which are the most effective methods for guideline dissemination and which implementation strategies are likely to be efficient under different circumstances.[16] When guidelines fail to improve outcomes, this could be due to failure at any one of these three stages. Clinical practice must change as new evidence becomes available. However, ensuring that there is a connection between the emergence of evidence, the development of clinical guidelines and subsequent changes in practice is not a simple process, with research showing that none of the many different approaches to changing practice are superior for all changes in all situations.[17] The process for implementing evidence into clinical practice, along with some of the barriers that may be encountered during the process and strategies for overcoming them, is discussed in Chapter 16.

Legal issues surrounding the use of clinical guidelines

We have seen that clinical guidelines are not a fool proof method of providing clinical care. Guidelines have, in the past, been criticised as being 'recipe book medicine' due to concerns that the rigid following of algorithms or care plans has the potential to de-skill health professionals. Certainly, if clinical guidelines are prescriptively applied, de-skilling may result. However, after reading this chapter, it should be clear that no matter how well clinical guidelines and their recommendations are linked to evidence, their interpretation and application should be guided by the health professional's clinical experience and judgement and the client's preferences and values. Clinical guidelines are a standardised approach to care that apply to general conditions (such as a person who has had a stroke) and not necessarily to the particular clinical situation at hand (for example, a 43-year-old woman who has had a cerebellar infarction and also has diabetes, osteoarthritis and a history of smoking). Therefore, health professionals should interpret the guidelines within the context of an individual client's circumstances.

The legal issues that surround the use of clinical guidelines can vary greatly between countries, because of different laws that exist in each country. Under common law in Australia, minimum acceptable standards of clinical care derive from responsible customary practice, not from guidelines. In England and Wales, the National Health Service Executive has stated that clinical guidelines cannot be used to mandate, authorise or outlaw treatment options.[18] While clinical guidelines may be used as evidence in court (either supporting or not supporting the actions of the health professional involved), they are unlikely to alter the usual evidentiary processes in litigation as, currently, the testimony of experts is used to help the courts to decide what is reasonable and accepted practice.[2] In other words, court decisions about whether a health professional provided reasonable care and skill are typically based on expert opinion rather than the contents of a clinical guideline. So, while guidelines may be introduced into courts by expert witnesses as evidence of accepted and customary standards of care, they cannot, as yet, be introduced as a substitute for expert testimony.

Although guidelines currently do not set legal standards for clinical care, they provide the courts with a benchmark by which to judge clinical conduct.[19] Because evidence-based clinical guidelines can set normative standards for practice, departure from them may require some explanation.[19] In clinical situations where there is a serious departure from guidelines, this will need to be well documented in the client's clinical records. The documentation should emphasise that the departure from the guidelines, and the possible consequences of this, have been thoroughly discussed and understood by the client and the relevant clinical, or other (for example, client choice), reasons for this departure provided.

Summary points of this chapter

- Clinical guidelines are systematically developed statements that are designed to help health professionals and their clients to make decisions about clients' health care. Guidelines aim to reduce unnecessary variations in care, encourage best practice and facilitate more informed and meaningful involvement of clients in making decisions about their health care.
- Clinical guidelines can be a useful tool for evidence-based practice. They translate evidence into actionable recommendations that can be applied to clinical situations. They do not take the place of informed clinical judgement and client choice in determining care, but can provide a useful adjunct to care.
- Clinical guidelines can be located using a variety of online resources, such as guideline-specific databases, bibliographic databases and the websites of disease-specific organisations.
- Clinical guidelines are typically developed by a range of stakeholders, including clinical experts, researchers and clients. Ideally, the development of guidelines should follow a rigorous process. However, the quality of guidelines varies according to the processes that occurred during their development.
- Because guidelines vary in quality, you should know how to appraise clinical guidelines and recognise the key features that discriminate high quality guidelines that can be used to guide practice from low quality clinical guidelines that should be dismissed. The AGREE instrument is a useful tool for appraising guidelines and helping you to determine if you can trust the recommendations that are in a clinical guideline.
- Medico-legal considerations in relation to guidelines need to be taken into account. If a considerable departure from guideline recommendations is agreed on by the client and the health professional, it is good practice to state the reason for this in the client's clinical records.

References
1. Institute of Medicine. Field M, Lohr K (eds). Guidelines for clinical practice: from development to use. Washington, DC: National Academy Press; 1992.
2. Dwyer P. Legal implications of clinical practice guidelines. Med J Aust 1998; 169:292–293.

3. Feder G, Eccles M, Grol R et al. Clinical guidelines: using clinical guidelines. BMJ 1999; 318: 728–730.
4. Craig J, Irwig L, Stockler M. Evidence-based medicine: useful tools for decision making. MJA 2001; 174:248–253.
5. Wilczynski N, Haynes RB, Lavis J et al. Optimal search strategies for detecting health services research studies in MEDLINE. CMAJ 2004; 171:1179–1185.
6. Grimshaw J, Russell I. Achieving health gain through clinical guidelines. Qual Health Care 1993; 2:243–248.
7. Grimshaw J, Eccles M, Russell I. Developing clinically valid practice guidelines. J Eval Clin Pract 1995; 1:37–48.
8. Graham I, Harrison M. Evaluation and adaptation of clinical practice guidelines. Evid Based Nurs 2005; 8:68–72.
9. The AGREE Collaboration. Development and validation of an international appraisal instrument for assessing the quality of clinical practice guidelines: the AGREE project. Qual Saf Health Care 2003; 12:18–23.
10. Vlayen J, Aertgeerts B, Hannes K et al. A systematic review of appraisal tools for clinical practice guidelines: multiple similarities and one common deficit. Int J Qual Health Care 2005; 17:235–242.
11. Straus S, Richardson W, Glasziou P et al. Evidence-based medicine: how to practice and teach EBM. 3rd edn. Edinburgh: Elsevier Churchill Livingstone; 2005.
12. GRADE working group. Online. 2008. Available: http://www.gradeworkinggroup.org/ (7 Sept 2008).
13. GRADE Working group. Grading quality of evidence and strength of recommendations. BMJ 2004; 328:1490–1497.
14. National Health and Medical Research Council (NHMRC). NHMRC additional levels of evidence and grades for recommendations for developers of guidelines. Online. 2008. Available: http://www.nhmrc.gov.au (23 Aug 2008).
15. Scalzitti D. Evidence-based guidelines: application to clinical practice. Phys Ther 2001; 81:1622–1628.
16. Grimshaw J, Eccles M, Thomas R et al. Toward evidence-based quality improvement. Evidence (and its limitations) of the effectiveness of guideline dissemination and implementation strategies 1966–1998. J Gen Intern Med 2006; 21:S14–S20.
17. Grol R, Grimshaw J. From best evidence to best practice: effective implementation of change in clients' care. Lancet 2003; 362:1225–1230.
18. Hurwitz B. Clinical guidelines: legal and political considerations of clinical practice guidelines. BMJ 1999; 318:661–664.
19. Hurwitz B. How does evidence based guidance influence determinations of medical negligence? BMJ 2004; 329:1024–1028.

CHAPTER **14**

Talking with clients about evidence

Tammy Hoffmann and Leigh Tooth

LEARNING OBJECTIVES

After reading this chapter, you should be able to:

- Describe why it is important that health professionals communicate effectively with their clients
- Understand what is meant by the term client-centred care
- Explain what is meant by shared decision making and discuss some of the challenges associated with it and the strategies that can be used to facilitate it
- List the key communication skills needed by health professionals when talking with clients about evidence
- Describe the various methods that can be used for communicating information to clients, the main considerations associated with each method and the major factors that should be considered when deciding which communication tool(s) to use with a client
- Explain how to effectively communicate statistical information to clients

At the heart of the definition of evidence-based practice that was provided in Chapter 1 lies the involvement of clients and the consideration of their values and preferences when making decisions regarding their health care. As part of the health care that they are receiving, clients often need to make decisions about aspects of their health care such as whether to proceed with a particular intervention. A health professional's ability to communicate effectively with clients and, often, also their family members is crucial to the successful involvement of clients in these decisions. For these decisions to be fully informed and ones with which the client is involved, clients need to know about the benefits, harms and risks associated with the various intervention options. Even when a decision about intervention is not needed, there are often many other aspects of their health care that clients can benefit from being knowledgeable about. Individualised education that is specific to the disease and the client is able to improve a client's self-efficacy to manage chronic conditions, assist with short-term behaviour change, improve quality of life and reduce morbidity and healthcare utilisation.[1] Effective communication can also help to build trust between clients and health professionals, make clinical practice more effective and reduce clinical mishaps and errors.[2]

Despite its importance, many health professionals are not specifically trained in how to effectively communicate with clients, and many clients do not know how to communicate with health professionals. Therefore, we have devoted a chapter of this book to this topic so that, when you are interacting with clients, you are aware of the importance of talking with your clients about evidence and are knowledgeable about the skills and resources that can assist you to do this successfully. In this chapter, we will discuss why effective communication is important, outline the steps to communicating effectively with clients and discuss some of the key communication skills that health professionals need, including sections on how to decide which communication method and tool(s) to use and how to communicate statistical information to clients. We will also outline the concept of client-centred care and one of the skills that is often central to achieving this, namely shared decision making.

Why is effective communication so important?

You may not think of communication as a particularly important or specialised skill for health professionals to have and often health professionals do not give it the emphasis that it needs. Health professionals often think of communication as secondary to their 'real' job of caring for clients. However, the success of an intervention is frequently dependent upon the health professional successfully providing the client with appropriate information. In addition, health professionals often do not realise that, as with many of the other interventions that they provide to clients, there are theories and principles that should be used to guide communication with clients.

Effective communication is central to a 'client-centred' approach by health professionals. The evolution and benefits of client-centred care are discussed in the following section.

Client-centred care

Client-centred care (also commonly referred to as patient-centred care or client-centred practice) is a broad umbrella term reflecting a particular approach to the health professional–client relationship that implies communication, partnerships and a focus beyond the specific clinical condition.[3] Client-centred practice by health professionals reflects their commitment to quality care by the way they respect clients' needs, goals, values, expectations and preferences and involve clients in the decision-making process.[4]

Central to client-centred care is treating clients with dignity, responding quickly and effectively to clients' needs and concerns[5] and providing clients with enough information to enable them to make informed choices about their health care.[6] Client-centred care has become the model that is advocated by health professionals and health professional associations. This model of care sits between the 'paternalistic' and 'informed patient or independent choice' models of care.[7,8] In the traditional 'paternalistic' model of care, the health professional is in control, discloses information as and when suitable and makes the decisions for the client who is expected to be passive, unquestioning and compliant. At the other end of the spectrum is the 'informed patient or independent choice' model in which health professionals present the facts and leave the decision making solely up to the client.[7]

There is emerging evidence of the benefits of client-centred care to health professionals and clients. Client-centred practice can increase client satisfaction and quality of life, reduce client anxiety and improve adherence to long-term medication use.[3,9] For health professionals, client-centred practice can contribute to more appropriate and cost-effective use of health services, such as reducing the number of diagnostic tests and unnecessary referrals.[3,9,10] Features of client-centred practice include shared decision making and tailoring communication and education to the needs, abilities and preferences of the client, each of which will be discussed in the following sections of this chapter.

Shared decision making

Shared decision making refers to clinical decision making as a partnership between the client and health professional, with communication focussed on achieving shared understanding of treatment goals and plans.[11] Shared decision making allows clients the opportunity to express their values. Client involvement in the decision-making process often extends beyond just choosing treatment options and can also involve:[7]

- recognition and clarification of the health issue
- identification of possible solutions
- appraisal of possible solutions
- implementation of the chosen solution
- evaluation of the solution.

Many leading health organisations now advocate client participation in clinical decision making. These include the National Health and Medical Research Council of Australia,[2] the USA Preventive Services Taskforce[7] and the General Medical Council of the UK.[12]

Shared decision making between clients and health professionals has been linked with improved client outcomes, for example improved control of hypertension,[13] better compliance,[14] greater family satisfaction with communication,[15] improved emotional status[16] and reduced visits to emergency departments and use of medications.[17] However, shared decision making is not possible in all clinical encounters, nor is it welcomed or desired by all clients. The next section presents some of the challenges that can be associated with shared decision making.

Shared decision making: the challenges

Challenges related to the availability of evidence

Sometimes shared decision making can be relatively straightforward, for example in common health problems where there is only one course of action or where the evidence is clear and most informed health professionals and clients would agree that the benefits outweigh the harms.[18] In other situations, shared decision making can be more difficult. For example, with some chronic conditions the research evidence that is provided by randomised controlled trials and systematic reviews often fails to endorse one intervention and instead highlights the benefits and harms of a number of interventions. While difficult, shared decision making can be particularly valuable in these situations, with health professionals helping clients to understand the risks, benefits and trade-offs of the various interventions.[14] Finally, for some medical conditions there may not be sufficient evidence about the benefits and harms of intervention options, in which case the health professional needs to assist the client to assess this uncertainty against the client's values and preferences.[18]

Clients' involvement in shared decision making

Shared decision making is not always possible, for example in medical emergencies or with clients who do not have the cognitive capacity to participate. Further, shared decision making is also not always welcomed or desired by clients. In a nationally representative sample of 2750 adults in the USA it was found that, while 96% of the participants wanted to be asked for their opinions and offered choices, half preferred to rely on their doctors for information and half wanted to leave the final decisions up to their doctors.[19] Clients' preferences for involvement in decision making were found to differ by health status and socio-demographic characteristics. For example, clients who were in poorer health, male, older than 45 years of age and with fewer years of education were less likely to want to participate in shared decision making.

Individual clients may also vary in the degree to which they want to participate in shared decision making depending upon the specific clinical situation.[2] This illustrates the need for you, as a health professional, to determine the role that each of your clients wishes to take in the management of their health. A simple question that you can ask to help establish this is 'How do you feel about being involved in making decisions about your treatment?'[20]

It is worth pointing out that shared decision making may also have unwanted effects. For example, once clients are fully informed about benefits, harms and risks, they may still decide not to undertake treatment for a health condition or to have a screening test because they are at low risk of developing future problems.[3] It has been suggested that this expression of 'fully informed choice may sometimes frustrate the health professional'[3] as it can lead to some clients choosing a path that results in harm or death. A clear example of this is when clients reject the need for blood transfusions due to religious beliefs.

Shared decision making also has legal implications, in particular concerning informed consent. Health professionals have been found legally liable for damages in instances where inadequate information has been provided to clients and harm has arisen following intervention.[21] In recent court cases, the High Court of Australia has referred to the importance of shared decision making, defining it as 'a shared exercise in which healthcare practitioners are obliged to take active steps to ensure that patients are empowered to make their own decisions about important procedures to be undertaken on their bodies'.[21]

The complexities of client and health professional involvement in shared decision making

Shared decision making is a complex process, which involves not only the client's values and preferences, but also their feelings and views about their relationship with the health professional and the degree of effort that both parties put into the decision making process and the communication between them.[7] Box 14.1 provides some examples of the complexities in health professional–client relationships that can influence shared decision making.[7]

BOX 14.1 EXAMPLES OF THE COMPLEXITIES IN THE HEALTH PROFESSIONAL–CLIENT RELATIONSHIP[7]

- Clients who believe that the health professional cares about them and is collaborating with them and making an effort on their behalf may be more likely to be encouraged to do their own bit in relation to their health care.
- Clients who doubt that their health professional likes them or doubt that their health professional is focussed on their best interests may be less confident about the recommended intervention options.
- Health professionals who have positive views of their clients as partners who are capable and able to be trusted are more likely to facilitate the involvement of clients in the decision-making process.
- Health professionals who are mentally disengaged from clients or the decision-making process may be less likely to facilitate other aspects of client involvement in the decision-making process.

Strategies to assist shared decision making

As a health professional, there are various strategies that you can use to facilitate effective shared decision making and these are presented in Box 14.2.[14–16,22–24] Central to successful shared decision making is effective communication, which involves communicating the evidence to clients and is informed by how clients prefer to receive information and their ability to understand it. These issues are described in more detail later in this chapter.

Assessment tools for health professionals to use in shared decision making

A number of scales have been developed to assess the involvement of clients and health professionals in shared decision making. The scales in these two areas will be discussed separately and one example of each will be described in detail. These scales can also assist

---

BOX 14.2 STRATEGIES TO FACILITATE SHARED DECISION MAKING

- Attend to the whole of clients' problems and take account of their expectations, feelings and ideas.
- Value clients' contributions, for example, the life experiences and values that clients bring to the decision-making process.
- Provide clear, honest and unbiased information.
- Assess the degree to which your clients understand the information that you have provided to them.
- Assess the degree to which your clients want to be involved in decision making.
- Provide a caring, respectful and empowering context in which clients can be enabled to participate in decision making.
- Be well informed about the most current evidence, particularly regarding issues such as diagnosis and intervention.
- Do not assume that your clients will make the same decisions as you just because the evidence has been provided to them in a manner that they can understand.

you by providing examples of questions that you can ask and competencies you can aim for in your own clinical practice.

Scales to measure health professionals' involvement in shared decision making
In a 2001 systematic review, eight instruments that assess various aspects of clinical decision making were described, but the authors of the review concluded that none of the eight instruments sufficiently captured the concept of whether the health professional encouraged client 'involvement' in the decision-making process.[24] The authors of the review subsequently developed and revised the 12-item OPTION (Observing Patient Involvement in Decision Making) scale to measure the extent that a health professional engages in shared decision making during client consultations.[25,26] Examples of the 12 'competencies' that are assessed in OPTION are:
- Item 1: The health professional draws attention to an identified problem as one that requires a decision-making process.
- Item 3: The health professional assesses the client's preferred approach to receiving information to assist decision making.
- Item 5: The health professional explains the pros and cons of options to the client (taking 'no action' is an option).
- Item 10: The health professional elicits the client's preferred level of involvement in decision making.

Each 'competency' is rated by observers on a scale that measures the order of magnitude to which the health professional demonstrates the skill. The scale is as follows:
- 0— 'The behaviour is not observed'
- 1— 'A minimal attempt is made to exhibit the behaviour'
- 2— 'The health professional asks the patient about their preferred way of receiving information to assist decision'
- 3— 'The behaviour is exhibited to a good standard'
- 4— 'The behaviour is observed and executed to a high standard'

Scales to measure clients' involvement in shared decision making
Questionnaires have been developed to assess clients' satisfaction with decision making,[27] degree of decisional conflict,[28] perceived involvement in care,[29] risk communication and confidence in decision making[20] and the extent of shared decision making.[30] One of these will now be further described.

The COMRADE (Combined Outcome Measure for Risk Communication and Treatment Decision Making Effectiveness) was developed by combining items from some existing shared decision-making scales and constructs identified by clients during focus groups.[20] It consists of 20 statements that represent two broad aspects of decision making—risk communication and confidence in the decision.

Each statement is scored on a five-point Likert scale from 1 (strongly agree) to 5 (strongly disagree). While the original scale statements use the term 'doctor', the COMRADE can be used by all health professionals. Examples of the 20 statements are as follows.

Statements about risk communication:
- The health professional gave me enough information about the treatment choices available.
- The health professional gave me the chance to express my opinions about the different treatments available.
- The health professional gave me the chance to decide which treatment I thought was best for me.

Statements about confidence in decision making:
- I am satisfied that I am adequately informed about the issues important to the decision.
- I am satisfied with the way the decision was made in the consultation.
- I am sure that the decision is the right one for me personally.

The COMRADE is intended to be used in conjunction with three other relevant instruments, the SF-12 measure of quality of life, the short-form anxiety instrument and the patient enablement instrument (see the reference that describes the COMRADE[20] for more details).

Key steps to communicating evidence to clients effectively

A five-step model for communicating evidence to clients in a way that facilitates shared decision making has been proposed[31] and is presented below. Although the model was developed as a guide for medical practitioners who are consulting with clients and helping them to make healthcare decisions, the key principles of the model can be used as a guide for any health professional who is communicating evidence to a client.

1. **Understand the client's (and family members') experiences and expectations.**

   You need to take the time and make the effort to understand the needs, fears, experiences, expectations and values of your client.

2. **Build partnerships.**

   Rather than just providing information to your client in an old-style paternalistic manner, you should try and gain your client's trust and build a partnership with them. Activities that may assist with this include: encouraging partnership (for example, 'This is a decision that we need to make together'), acknowledging the difficulty of the situation/decision that is being discussed, expressing empathy and expressing mutual understanding (for example, 'I think I understand …').[31]

3. **Discuss the evidence, including a balanced discussion about uncertainties.**

   In addition to answering your client's questions, you should also discuss issues that they may not have thought to ask or are reluctant to bring up. A discussion of the evidence needs to include a simple explanation of the uncertainties surrounding the evidence, but be aware that overemphasising the uncertainty can cause some clients to lose confidence.[31] Using an appropriate method to communicate statistical information can be beneficial at this stage and a discussion of the various methods for doing this are explained in a later section of this chapter.

4. **Present recommendations.**

   Obviously a healthcare decision does not need to be made every time that you communicate evidence to a client, particularly if it is evidence related to a prognostic or qualitative information need that you or your client had. However, when the clinical question is about the effect of an intervention, a decision may need to be made. This step should only occur after you have integrated the best quality clinical evidence that is available for the issue with your client's values and preferences. You should explain how your recommendation has been generated from both the evidence and your client's values.[31] In situations where the evidence is uncertain or contradictory and you do not have a specific recommendation, you should present each of the options neutrally.

5. **Check for understanding and agreement.**

   It is important to confirm that your client has understood the information that you have presented to them. You may wish to ask your client to briefly summarise their understanding of the information for you. You may need to repeat the information, explain it in a different way or provide more detailed information. There are various communication tools that can be used to share information with clients and, in some cases, help them to make decisions. These tools are discussed in a later section of this chapter.

Key communication skills needed by health professionals

In addition to the general communication and relationship-building skills that you should have as a health professional, some of the key skills that you need when talking with your clients about evidence are listed in Box 14.3.

BOX 14.3 KEY SKILLS NEEDED BY HEALTH PROFESSIONALS WHEN TALKING WITH THEIR CLIENTS ABOUT EVIDENCE

- Ability to communicate complex information using non-technical language
- Tailoring the amount and pace of information to the client's needs and preferences
- Drawing diagrams to aid comprehension
- Understanding the principles of shared decision making and how and when to implement this with clients
- Ability to determine how much involvement in decision making clients desire
- Considering the client's preferences and values and integrating this with the clinical evidence for the various treatment options
- Understanding the factors that can impede information exchange and shared decision making
- When a healthcare decision needs to be made, the ability to clearly explain the probability and risk for each option
- Facilitative skills to encourage client involvement
- Evaluation of internet information that clients might bring with them
- Creating an environment in which clients feel comfortable asking questions
- Giving clients time to take in the information
- Declaration of 'equipoise' when present—equipoise exists when there is uncertainty about which treatment option, including the option of no further treatment, will benefit a client the most
- Checking client understanding
- Negotiation skills

Adapted with permission from Ford S, Schofield T, Hope T. What are the ingredients for a successful evidence-based patient choice consultation? A qualitative study; published by Social Science and Medicine 2003.

Methods for communicating information

There are various formats that you can choose to use when providing clients with information, with the aim of increasing their knowledge and understanding of the evidence related to their situation. Using more than one method to provide the information can be a valuable way of increasing clients' retention of the information.[32]

Verbal information

Verbal education is the method that is most commonly used by health professionals for providing information. There are some general points that you should follow when providing clients with information verbally to improve the effectiveness of the information exchange[33] and these are listed in Box 14.4.

One of the major limitations of providing information verbally is that people often forget what they have been told. It has been estimated that most people remember less than a quarter of what they have been told.[34] For this reason, using written materials to supplement or reinforce information that has been presented verbally is recommended.[35]

Combination of verbal and written information

The combination of verbal and written information has the potential to maximise a client's knowledge.[36] A Cochrane systematic review that evaluated the effect of providing written summaries or recordings (such as an audiotape) of consultations found that between 83% and 96% of clients found the summaries to be valuable and that there was better recall of information and more satisfaction with information received by those who received summaries or recordings.[37] However, none of the studies in the systematic review found that the summaries had an effect on anxiety or depression.

Written information

Appropriate readability and design of written materials

There are many forms that written information can take, such as a pamphlet, booklet, printed information sheet or information from internet sites. Regardless of the form, for written information to be useful to clients, they need to notice, read, understand, believe

---

BOX 14.4 STRATEGIES FOR CLEARLY AND EFFECTIVELY PROVIDING INFORMATION VERBALLY TO CLIENTS

- Sit down with the client, maintain eye contact, remove any distractions and give the client your full attention.
- Use effective communication skills such as active listening, gesturing and responding to the client's nonverbal cues to facilitate communication.
- Do not speak too quickly.
- Use clear and simple language. Avoid jargon where possible. Explain any medical terminology that is used.
- Where possible, use the same terms consistently throughout the discussion rather than using a range of different terms that mean the same thing.
- Present the most important information first.
- Do not provide too much information at once. Present a few points and then pause to check the client understands.
- Observe for indicators that the client may not have understood, such as a look of confusion or a long pause before responding to a question.
- Have the client indicate their level of understanding. Having them repeat the main points of what you have said in their own words can often be more valuable than just asking 'Do you understand?'

and remember it. Many written materials that health professionals use with clients are written and designed in a way that can make it difficult for clients to understand the content that they contain. One of the most common problems is that many health education materials are written at a reading level that is too high for the majority of the clients who receive them.[38,39] A fifth to sixth grade reading level is recommended for written health information. There are various readability formulas that can be used to quickly and easily assess the readability of written information, including the SMOG[40] and the Flesch Reading Ease formula[41] (available in Microsoft Word).

In addition to readability, there are many other features of written health education materials that need to be given appropriate consideration in order to maximise the usefulness of the materials for clients. This includes features such as:
* the content in the material (for example, is it evidence-based?)
* the language used (for example, what types of words are used and how are sentences structured?)
* the organisation of content (for example, are bulleted lists used where possible?)
* the layout and typography throughout the material (for example, is an appropriate font size used throughout?)
* the illustrations within the material (for example, is each illustration appropriately labelled and explained in the text?)
* the incorporation of learning and motivation features into the content (for example, are there features in the material that actively engage the reader?)

It is beyond the scope of this chapter to discuss these features in detail. However, summaries of this information are readily available,[42] and there are a number of checklists that can be used to assess the quality of the written information that is used with clients.[42-44]

Assessing the quality of written information about treatment choices
In addition to having appropriate readability and design, it is important that written health information is evidence-based. DISCERN is a questionnaire designed to assess the quality of written information on treatment choices for a health problem. It consists of 16 items, each scored on a 5-point scale. Box 14.5 lists the main points that are covered in the DISCERN questionnaire.[45] The full questionnaire is available on the DISCERN website (http://www.discern.org.uk).

Computer-based information
In addition to accessing health information from the internet, there are other ways that computers can be used as a health information resource for clients. For example, providing clients with interactive information that is accessed by a touchscreen (see, for example, the study by Graham and colleagues[46]) or providing clients with tailored printed information (see, for example, the system described by Hoffmann and colleagues[47]). Computer-based materials can also be used to assist clients to make health-related decisions. More information about this is provided in the later section of this chapter about decision aids.

Internet-based health information
As much health information is obtained from the internet,[48] you should be prepared to evaluate health information from the internet that clients may bring with them and also to evaluate health information websites prior to recommending them to clients. There are various criteria that can be used to evaluate health information websites and these criteria relate to the content of the website, the credibility of the website's

---

BOX 14.5 MAIN ISSUES COVERED BY DISCERN—A QUESTIONNAIRE FOR ASSESSING THE QUALITY OF WRITTEN INFORMATION ON TREATMENT CHOICES FOR A HEALTH PROBLEM

- Is the publication reliable?
  - Are the aims clear?
  - Does it achieve its aims?
  - Is it relevant?
  - Is it clear what sources of information were used to compile the publication?
  - Is it clear when the information used or reported in the publication was produced?
  - Is it balanced and unbiased?
  - Does it provide details of additional sources of support and information?
  - Does it refer to areas of uncertainty?
- How good is the quality of the information on treatment choices?
  - Does it describe how each treatment works?
  - Does it describe the benefits of each treatment?
  - Does it describe the risks of each treatment?
  - Does it describe what would happen if no treatment was used?
  - Does it describe how the treatment choices affect overall quality of life?
  - Is it clear that there may be more than one possible treatment choice?
  - Does it provide support for shared decision making?
- Overall rating of the publication as a source of information about treatment choices

---

authors, disclosure on the website and the design and aesthetics of the website.[32] For internet sites that contain information about treatment options for a health problem, the DISCERN questionnaire (as shown in Box 14.5) can also be used to evaluate these sites.

As recommending health information websites to clients is now a common occurrence during health professional–client consultations, the following resources may be of use to you:

- The Cochrane Consumer Network (http://www.cochrane.org/reviews/en/)—is aimed at helping clients to make informed decisions and provides a plain language summary and abstracts of Cochrane reviews.
- MedlinePlus (http://www.nlm.nih.gov/medlineplus/)—is a free service provided by the USA National Library of Medicine that offers web links that meet pre-established quality criteria to health information on the internet. It is designed to help provide high quality health information to clients and their families. Health professionals can also use this site to obtain quick and easy access to images or videos to help when providing information to clients.
- Intute: Health and Life Sciences (http://www.intute.ac.uk/healthandlifesciences/)—is a free online service that allows users to access online resources that Intute staff have selected and evaluated according to agreed policies, priorities and criteria.
- Health on the Net (HON) Foundation (http://www.hon.ch)—is a foundation aimed at guiding internet users to reliable, understandable, accessible and trustworthy sources of health information. Using the HONcode (consists of eight criteria), the foundation evaluates websites and websites that meet the criteria become accredited websites and

can display the HON logo. On this site you can also access HONmedia, which contains a wide selection of medical illustrations that can be used when educating clients.
- HealthFinder (http://www.healthprovider.gov)—is a USA government gateway site to reliable health information resources that have been reviewed by HealthFinder staff.

Interactive computer-based information
Compared to standard methods of providing information (such as a booklet), interactive computer-based information has been found to increase clients' knowledge[46,49,50] and decrease clients' anxiety.[46] The use of computer programs to provide clients with interactive health information is generally well accepted by clients[49] and often preferred to reading a booklet or watching a videotape.[51]

Tailored print information
Tailored information is information which is customised according to an individual's characteristics or preferences. Although it is not essential to use a computer to provide clients with tailored information, doing so can make the process of tailoring information to individual clients' needs quick and easy. There is evidence that, compared to non-tailored information, tailored print information is better remembered, read and perceived as relevant and/or credible.[52] Tailored information is also more likely to influence changes in health behaviour[52] and result in greater client satisfaction with the information that is provided and better met informational needs.[53]

DVDs/videotapes and audiotapes
Use of media such as digital video discs (DVDs), videotapes and/or audiotapes can be a useful method for providing information to clients, particularly clients who have a low literacy level or English as a second language or for those who have an auditory (if audiotape) or visual (if DVD) learning style. There is some evidence that, compared with normal practice such as verbal information[54] or a leaflet,[55] using videotapes to provide clients with information can increase their knowledge, without increasing their anxiety levels.

Decision aids

What are decision aids?
For people who are facing decisions about the best way to manage their health, whether it is a decision about treatment or screening, decision aids are a communication tool that may be of some assistance for clients in certain situations. Decision aids are interventions designed to help clients make decisions by providing them with information about the options and the personal importance of possible benefits and harms and to encourage their active participation in the decision-making process.[56] Decision aids may be paper-based (such as a pamphlet) or involve a video (often with accompanying printed information). However, the majority of decision aids are internet-based.

What outcomes can decision aids have an effect on?
A Cochrane systematic review that evaluated the effectiveness of decision aids concluded that, compared to usual care, decision aids can result in clients having greater knowledge, more realistic expectations, lowered decisional conflict and improved agreement between values and choice.[56] Decision aids were also found to result in an increased proportion of clients who were active in decision making and, conversely, a reduced proportion of people who remained undecided following the intervention. However, compared to

comparison interventions, such as standard booklets, decision aids appeared to have no superior effect on satisfaction with decision making, anxiety or health outcomes.

Finding decision aids

Currently, the majority of decision aids that exist are on topics that are most appropriate for medical practitioners to discuss with their clients (for example, deciding between various treatments for cancer or deciding whether to receive hormone replacement therapy). However, other health professionals such as nurses and allied health professionals may find some of the decision aids that are currently available also useful in their clinical practice. For example, there are decision aids available on topics such as deciding about nursing home care for a family member who has dementia, options for managing back pain and options for managing carpal tunnel syndrome.

New decision aids are continually being developed so, when you have a client who needs to make a health care decision, it is worth searching on the internet to see if there is a relevant decision aid. A recommended resource is The Ottawa Health Research Institute (http://www.ohri.ca/decisionaid/), which maintains an inventory of decision aids. The Cochrane review on decision aids that was discussed earlier[56] also contains an extensive list of decision aids.

Using decision aids

As with other client education resources, if you are considering using a decision aid with a client, there are a number of factors that you need to take into account. These are detailed in the section below. If you choose to use a decision aid with a client, you need to ensure that it is of good quality. A set of criteria, known as the CREDIBLE criteria, has been developed for assessing the quality of decision aids and full details of the criteria are available in the Cochrane review on decision aids that was discussed earlier.[56,57] The main criteria are:

- C competently developed
- R recently updated
- E evidence-based
- DI devoid of conflicts of interest
- BL balanced presentation of options, benefits and harms
- E decision aid is efficacious at improving decision making.

Decision aids, particularly internet-based ones, are a relatively new tool that can be used for communicating evidence to clients and enabling them to participate in making decisions about their health care. However there are many gaps in the research related to decision aids, such as how they impact on health professional–client communication, factors that determine the successful use of decision aids in practice and what types of decision aids work best with different types of clients.[56]

Deciding which communication tool(s) to use with your clients

As discussed earlier in this chapter, there are various communication tools that you may choose to use when providing clients with information. Your choice will be influenced by a number of factors including:

- client's preference—this may also be influenced by your client's preferred learning style (for example, visual or auditory), cultural background, level of motivation, cultural background and primary language

- client's literacy level and education level—see below for more information
- client's cognitive ability and any impairments they have that may impact on their ability to communicate, understand or recall information or make decisions—see below for more information
- the educational resources/communication tools that are available to you
- time-related issues—see below for more information.

Literacy levels

If written (or printed or computer-based) health education materials are used to provide information or supplement information that is provided verbally, the literacy levels of the clients who are receiving the information need to be considered. Written materials will not benefit clients if they are unable to understand them. You should be aware of your client's literacy skills so that you can alter the educational intervention accordingly.[58] Be aware that people with poor literacy often use a range of strategies to hide literacy problems[58] and are often reluctant to ask questions so as not to appear ignorant.[59]

Although literacy levels can be influenced by education level, it has not been consistently found that reading skill is dependent on educational attainment.[60] Therefore, it is recommended that you assess clients' reading skills using one of the published tests that have been designed to do this, rather than relying only on their self-reported level of education.[59,60] Commonly used tests include: the Rapid Estimate of Adult Literacy in Medicine (REALM),[61] the Test of Functional Health Literacy in Adults (TOFHLA)[62] and the Medical Achievement Reading Test (MART).[63] All of these tests evaluate a client's ability to understand medical terminology and are quick and straightforward to administer and score.

Impairments which may impact on communication

Your client may have one or more impairments that can impact on how they are able to process information. This can include cognitive, hearing, visual or speech and language impairments. You need to consider how the presence of one or more of these impairments may result in the need for you to alter how you communicate with your client and which communication tool(s) you choose to use. There are various strategies that you can use to facilitate communication with clients who have one or more of these impairments; however, it is beyond the scope of this chapter to detail these. Further reading about strategies specific to different impairments is recommended; for example, refer to the client education book by McKenna and Tooth.[64]

Time-related issues

Time-related issues include both the amount of time that is available for communicating with your client and the timing of communicating with your client. Clients' needs vary at different times. For example, clients' informational needs during an initial consultation are different to their needs after a diagnosis or during follow-up consultations or treatment sessions. There may be various points in time (for example, after a diagnosis or when feeling acutely unwell) that clients are unable to process much information. You should be sensitive to when this may be the case and adapt your communication with the client accordingly. Providing only the most essential information may be sufficient initially. More detailed information can be provided to your client at a later, more appropriate time.

Various communication tools may also be indicated at different times. For example, verbal information is usually the main format that is used during initial consultations with clients, but in-between subsequent consultations, clients may be given written information or referred to recommended internet sites. This may be useful as a reinforcement of information already provided, to answer some of the client's questions and/or to generate more questions which can be discussed the next time that they see you.

Communicating statistical information to clients

Clients expect information about benefits and risks that is (as far as possible) accurate, unbiased, personally relevant to them and presented in a way that they can understand.[2]

Communicating statistical information, most notably information about probabilities and risks, in a manner that clients can understand is an area that health professionals need to be aware of. There are often differences between how health professionals and clients understand probability and risk. Health professionals have been trained to understand these as mathematical probabilities of an event happening within a whole population. Health professionals subsequently view these statistics as objective and impersonal. Conversely, clients' views and understanding of these concepts are commonly influenced by emotions, anxieties, concerns about the future, what they have seen and heard reported in the media and by the views of their social networks. Indeed, clients often personalise risk and are less interested in what happens to 'populations'.[2] Information about risks can also be hard for clients to understand when they do not have previous experience to compare the numbers to; for example, if the risk of an event is 20%, clients may not know whether this is relatively high or low.[2] Finally, for allied health professionals the responsibility for a good health professional–client information exchange process may be even greater in cases where clients have not had a prior referral from a medical practitioner and may have no understanding about the possible risks of treatments.[21]

There are different types of statistical information that health professionals need to communicate to clients. The next section describes the most frequently used statistics and how clients may misinterpret the meanings. Table 14.1 presents strategies that you can use to simplify how you present this information.

Types of data that health professionals use and how to present it to clients

Probability
Probability refers to the chance of an event occurring. Values for probability lie between 0 and 1 and are often presented as a percentage. For example, a probability of 0.5 may be expressed as 50%. Probability can occur as a single probability or as a conditional probability. Consider the situation where a client wants to know the likelihood of side effects that they might experience in relation to an intervention. An example of *single probability* is that there is a 20% chance that the client will have a particular side effect if they receive a certain intervention. The problem with this concept is that how it should be interpreted may be confusing. For example, a client may interpret this as meaning that 20% of clients will have the side effect or that all clients will have the side effect 20% of the time. The latter interpretation reflects the 'personal' as opposed to 'population' view that clients tend to have.[65] *Conditional probability* refers to the probability of an event, given that another event has occurred. An example of conditional probability is if a person has a disease, the probability that a screening test will be positive for the disease is 90%.

Risk of disease/side effect

Risk of disease/side effect refers to the probability of developing the disease/side effect in a stated time period. As we saw in Chapter 4, risk is often presented either as absolute risk or relative risk. When referring to the risk of a disease or a side effect, these concepts can be interpreted as follows:

- Absolute risk refers to the incidence (or natural frequency) of the disease or event in the population.
- Relative risk is the ratio of two risks (or, as we saw in Chapter 4, the flipside of the concept of relative risk is relative benefit): the risk in the population exposed to some factor (for example, having received a particular intervention), divided by the risk of those not exposed. Relative risk gives an indication of the degree of risk.
  - ‣ If the relative risk is *equal to 1*, the risk in the exposed population is *the same* as the unexposed population.
  - ‣ If the relative risk is *greater than 1*, the risk in the exposed population is *greater than* it is for those in the unexposed population.
  - ‣ If the relative risk is *less than 1*, the risk in the exposed population is *less than* it is for those in the unexposed population. Box 14.6 illustrates an example of *relative* risk.

Relative risk reductions (or increases) versus absolute risk reductions (or increases)

As was pointed out in Chapter 4, the use of relative risks alone when presenting information to clients can be misleading. As shown in the example in Box 14.6, while clients who take a medication may have a 50% higher risk of experiencing a side effect, in absolute terms, if a client's initial risk was only 22 in 1000 (or 2.2%), then taking the medication would increase this risk to only 34 in 1000 people (or 3.4%). An important factor to note is to avoid using descriptors, such as 'low', 'high', 'rare' and 'frequent', to quantify risk without clear explanation, as clients' and health professionals' perceptions of what such descriptors actually mean can vary dramatically.[31]

The importance of baseline risk was explained in Chapter 4. When explaining absolute and relative risk reduction (or increase) to clients, the baseline or starting level of risk to the client should also be presented to help the client interpret the risks appropriately.[66] For example, a 1995 warning by the Committee on Safety in the USA stated that third generation oral contraceptive drugs were associated with twice the risk compared with

---

BOX 14.6 **EXAMPLE OF RELATIVE RISK**

Incidence of a side effect among people exposed to medication A $\quad = \quad \dfrac{34}{1000} \quad = \quad 0.034$

Incidence of a side effect among people not exposed to medication A $\quad = \quad \dfrac{22}{1000} \quad = \quad 0.022$

$\text{Relative risk} = \dfrac{\text{Incidence in exposed}}{\text{Incidence in unexposed}} \quad = \quad \dfrac{0.034}{0.022} \quad = \quad 1.5$

Therefore, in people who have taken the medication, the risk of having the side effect is 1.5 times greater (or a relative risk increase of 50%) than in those people who have not taken the medication.

second generation contraceptives. This was reported by the media and it led to a dramatic reduction in the use of oral contraceptives and a subsequent increase in pregnancies and terminations. However, what the media did not inform people of was that the baseline risk was extremely low, at 15 cases per year per 100,000 users, and that the increased risk was still extremely low, at 25 cases per year.[66]

Number needed to treat

The concept of number needed to treat was explained in Chapter 4 and we saw that it can be a clinically useful concept for health professionals. Using number needed to treat (as a form of absolute risk) may be preferable to using relative risk values when communicating with clients during the decision-making process.[2] However, you should be aware that a recent randomised controlled trial found that the concept of number needed to treat was still difficult for clients to understand and may have limited use as a communication tool during shared decision making.[67]

Table 14.1 provides two examples of the issues surrounding the presentation of probability and risk to clients and shows how using natural frequencies or plain numbers (for example, '8 out of 100') can aid clients' understanding.

Factors for health professionals to consider when presenting statistical information to clients

Framing

Framing of information refers to whether the information is presented in a positive or negative manner. How information is framed has been found to influence clients' confidence in medical decision making. If information is positively framed it is

The clinical scenario	Expressed as a probability	How probabilities may be incorrectly understood	Expressed as natural frequencies (event rates)
Client needs to have a particular treatment but there is a 20% risk of a side effect	Single probability commonly expressed as 'There is a 20% chance that you will have a particular side effect if you follow the treatment'	That they will have the side effect 20% of the time	Of every 100 clients who have this treatment, 20 clients will experience this side effect
The clinical scenario	**Expressed as a relative risk**	**How relative risks may be incorrectly understood**	**Expressed in natural frequencies as an absolute risk**
By undergoing a particular screening test, the client's risk of dying from a disease may be reduced	For example, 'By having a screening test your risk of dying from the disease is reduced by 50%'	The large percentage may mislead the client into thinking that the reduction in the risk of their own possible death is large	The client's baseline risk of dying from the disease is 1 out of 1000. By undergoing the screening test, this is reduced by half, or to 0.5 in 1000

TABLE 14.1 The problem of probabilities and risk and how using natural frequencies can help when explaining this type of information

presented in terms of who will benefit. For example, out of 1000 clients who have this treatment, 800 (or 80%) will benefit. If information is negatively framed, it is presented in terms of who will not benefit (or possibly be harmed). For example, out of 1000 clients who have this treatment, 200 (or 20%) will experience an adverse side effect.

Positive framing has been linked with clients being more willing to undertake risky treatments.[65] Information can also be framed in terms of a gain or loss with respect to screening, for example gain or loss framing concerns the outcomes from having (gain) or not having (loss) a screening test. Loss framing, which outlines the possible adverse outcomes from not having the test, has been linked with a higher uptake by clients of screening tests than gain framing, which outlines the advantages of having the test.[65]

Current recommendations are that health professionals be unbiased and present clients with both the positive and negative aspects of an intervention by using the same statistical denominator: for example, telling a client that the risk of developing a disease is 34 in 1000 people who follow the treatment and that the risk of not developing the disease is 966 in 1000 people who follow the treatment. Gigerenzer and Edwards[65] describe an example of poor practice in an information brochure for clients about a particular screening test. In the brochure, health professionals presented information using relative risk statistics to make the benefits appear large, while they presented the risks of undertaking screening using absolute risk statistics (which were smaller).

Using graphs and pictures

Using graphs or pictures can assist clients to understand the information that you are presenting. For example, a pictograph of a population of 1000 people (represented by circles) which you can colour in to show how many will benefit (or be harmed) by a particular intervention is one way of showing data in an absolute manner. Figure 14.1 shows how a pictograph can be used, using a hypothetical example. Pictographs have been found to be more easily and accurately understood when the data are presented along the horizontal axis of the pictograph.[68] This presentation can assist clients to see the overall picture and help them put the information into perspective. For example, they can see the baseline level of risk and how much the level of risk changes following the intervention.

The pictograph in Figure 14.1 illustrates that:
- of 1000 people aged between 50 and 60 years, the chance of dying is 20 in 1000 if the medication is *not* taken (see second bottom row of the pictograph)

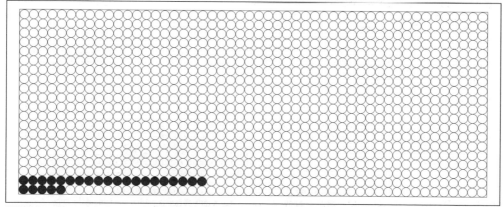

FIGURE 14.1 Pictograph of a population of 1000 people that can be used to illustrate the risk of a certain intervention

- of 1000 people aged between 50 and 60 years, the chance of dying is reduced to 5 in 1000 if the medication *is* taken (see bottom row of the pictograph).

Graphs representing benefit and harm can also be prepared. Figure 14.2 shows a hypothetical example of a graphical representation of risk for experiencing a side effect from taking a particular medication. The vertical (y) axis shows the number of clients per 1000 who experience this side effect. The horizontal (x) axis shows two groups. Group one is the general population (to represent baseline risk) and group two represents the clients who take the medication. The graph clearly shows the increased risk of experiencing the side effect for clients who take this particular medication, in comparison to the general population. Using this approach, graphs of benefits and harms can be presented side by side. However, if graphs of benefit and harm are presented side by side, the same y axis should be used in both graphs to ensure consistency.[65] There is some evidence that vertical bar graphs are better than horizontal bars, pie charts and systematic or random ovals in helping to explain differences in proportions to clients.[69] As we saw in Chapter 8, survival curves can sometimes be used to display prognostic information. A study that investigated using survival curves to inform clients found that survival curves were understood by clients if they were given more than one opportunity to see and discuss them.[69]

Consider time frames and social factors

You should be aware that how clients perceive probabilities and risks can differ according to their age. A lifetime risk may not mean much to a young person whereas a risk over the next 5 years may mean more to an older person.[2] There are also many social factors that can influence how clients interpret risk information. Clients can be influenced by the social context of the information, for example, the perceived relevance of it and the extent to which they trust the source. Health professionals need to understand that they are just one source of information about risk and may not be the source that clients trust the most.[70] In previous sections of this chapter we have described strategies that health professionals can use to help develop a relationship of trust with clients. These included: engaging in shared decision making; respecting the client's needs, views and preferences; and using effective communication techniques.

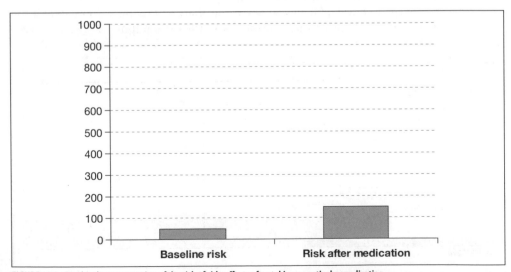

FIGURE 14.2 Graphical representation of the risk of side effects after taking a particular medication

The nature of the risk also influences how clients may react. For example, clients may be more sensitive to high consequence risks (such as being struck by lightning) than by the consequences of disease/disability from smoking.[70] These types of high consequence, but rare, risks often evoke a strong emotional reaction and a disproportionately large popular media coverage. To help clients put risk numbers into perspective, it can be useful to compare risk numbers with other more familiar risks, for example dying of any cause in the next year. Figure 14.3 provides an example of a perspective chart (based on one developed by Paling[71]) that can be used by health professionals when educating clients about the probability of developing melanoma. The chart provides the estimated risk of developing melanoma as well as the estimated risk of other events such as death by car accident, developing type 2 diabetes and being struck by lightning. The *British Medical Journal* also provides a website (http://bmj.bmjjournals.com/cgi/content/full/327/7417/694/DC1) that health professionals can use that provides general information about risks from numerous events, such as the annual risk of death from smoking cigarettes, dying from any cause in the next year and winning the lottery.

Box 14.7 summarises the strategies that health professionals can use to ensure that information about risks and probabilities is presented in the best possible way for clients to understand.

Summary points of this chapter

- It is important that health professionals communicate effectively with their clients for many reasons, such as obtaining fully informed consent, enabling clients to be involved in making decisions about their health care, building trust between the client and health professional and maximising the effectiveness of particular interventions.
- Client-centred care is an approach to the client–health professional relationship that can have benefits for both the client and the health professional. This approach involves forming a partnership with the client, engaging in shared decision making and responding effectively to the client's needs and concerns.

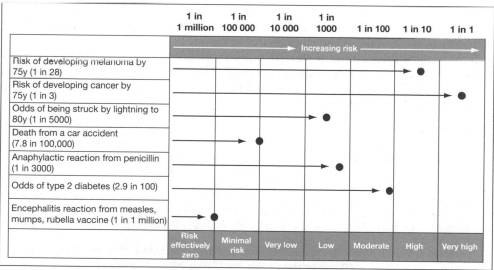

FIGURE 14.3 Presenting risk information in a way that gives perspective to the probability of an outcome
Based on: Risk Communication Format, © John Paling, 2000. (See www.riskcomm.com)

> **BOX 14.7 HOW TO PRESENT STATISTICAL INFORMATION TO CLIENTS**
>
> - Be open about uncertainties surrounding benefits and risks.
> - Give information in terms of both positive and negative outcomes to avoid bias.
> - Use the same denominator when presenting positive and negative outcomes.
> - Present natural frequencies (that is, plain numbers) rather than percentages or relative risks.
> - If you need to use relative statistics, supplement with absolute risks (natural frequencies) or benefits.
> - Use multiple formats: for example, verbal and written descriptions and, where possible, simple visual aids such as graphs.
> - Avoid using descriptors, for example 'high', 'low', 'rare' and 'frequent'.
> - Use visual aids such as graphs, pictures or perspective charts to aid in understanding where possible.

- In shared decision making, the client and health professional form a partnership to make decisions about the client's health care. Shared decision making is not always possible and sometimes there can be a number of challenges involved with achieving it. There are various strategies that health professionals can use to facilitate shared decision making. There are also tools that can be used to measure the extent of both client and health professional involvement in decision making.
- The steps involved in effectively communicating evidence to clients can include: understanding the client's experiences and expectations, building a partnership with them, discussing the evidence, presenting the recommendations and confirming the client's understanding and agreement.
- There is a range of formats that can be used when providing clients with information, including verbal information, written information, computer-based information, DVDs/videotapes and audiotapes and decision aids. Before using any of these formats with a client, there are issues that need to be considered, such as the quality, credibility and presentation of the information and the suitability of the format for that client and their needs, abilities and clinical circumstances.
- It can be difficult to communicate statistical information, such as risks and probabilities, to clients in a way that they will understand. There is a range of strategies, such as using natural frequencies, visual aids and framing information correctly, that can be used to aid clients' understanding.

References

1. Tooth L, Refshauge K. The effectiveness of client education: a review of the evidence and future challenges. In: McKenna K, Tooth L (eds). Client education: a partnership approach for health practitioners. Sydney: University of New South Wales Press; 2006:22–56.
2. National Health and Medical Research Council of Australia. Making decisions about tests and treatments: principles for better communication between healthcare consumers and healthcare professionals. Canberra: Australian Government Printer; 2006.
3. Bauman A, Fardy H, Harris P. Getting it right: why bother with patient centred care? MJA 2003; 179:253–256.
4. Bergeson S, Dean J. A systems approach to patient centred care. JAMA 2006; 296:2848–2851.
5. Coulter A. After Bristol: putting patients at the centre. BMJ 2002; 324:648–651.

6. McKenna T, Tooth L. Client education: a partnership approach for health practitioners. Sydney: University of New South Wales Press; 2006.
7. Entwistle V, Watt I. Patient involvement in treatment decision-making: the case for a broader conceptual framework. Patient Educ Couns 2006; 63:268–278.
8. Quill T, Brody H. Physician recommendations and patient autonomy: finding a balance between physician power and patient choice. Ann Intern Med 1996; 125:763–769.
9. Kahn K, Schneider E, Malin J et al. Patient centred experiences in breast cancer: predicting long-term adherence to Tamoxifen use. Med Care 2007; 45:431–439.
10. Coulter A. What do patients and the public want from primary care? BMJ 2005; 331:1199–1201.
11. Trevena L, Barratt A. Integrated decision making: definitions for a new discipline. Patient Educ Couns 2003; 50:265–268.
12. General Medical Council of the United Kingdom. Good medical practice: relationships with patients. Online. 2006. Available: http://www.gmc-uk.org/guidance/good_medical_practice/relationships_with_patients.asp (17 Sept 2008).
13. Naik A, Kallen M, Walder A et al. Improving hypertension control in diabetes mellitus: the effects of collaborative and proactive health communication. Circulation 2008; 117:1361–1368.
14. Frosch D, Kaplan R. Shared decision making in clinical medicine: past research and future directions. Am J Prev Med 1999; 17:285–294.
15. White D, Braddock C, Bereknyei S et al. Toward shared decision making at the end of life in intensive care units: opportunities for improvement. Arch Inter Med 2007; 167:461–467.
16. Stewart A. Effective physician-patient communications and health outcomes: a review. CMAJ 1995; 152:1423–1433.
17. McWilliams D, Jocobson R, Van Houten H et al. A program of anticipatory guidance for the prevention of emergency department visits for ear pain. Arch Pediatr Adolesc Med 2008; 162:151–156.
18. O'Connor A, Legare F, Stacey D. Risk communication in practice: the contribution of decision aids. BMJ 2003; 327:736–740.
19. Levinson W, Kao A, Kuby A et al. Not all patients want to participate in decision making: a national study of public preferences. J Gen Int Med 2005; 20:531–535.
20. Edwards A, Elwyn G, Hood K et al. The development of COMRADE: a patient-based outcome measure to evaluate the effectiveness of risk communication and treatment decision making in consultations. Patient Educ Couns 2003; 50:311–322.
21. Delany C. Cervical manipulation: how might informed consent be obtained before treatment? J Law Med 2002; 10:174–186.
22. Lockwood S. 'Evidence of me' in evidence based medicine? BMJ 2004; 329:1033–1035.
23. Ford S, Schofield T, Hope T. What are the ingredients for a successful evidence-based patient choice consultation? A qualitative study. Soc Sci Med 2003; 56:589–602.
24. Elwyn G, Edwards A, Mowle S et al. Measuring the involvement of patients in shared decision making. Patient Educ Couns 2001; 43:5–22.
25. Elwyn G, Edwards A, Wensing M. Shared decision making: developing the OPTION scale for measuring patient involvement. Qual Saf Health Care 2003; 12:93–99.
26. Elwyn G, Hutchings H, Edwards A et al. The OPTION scale: measuring the extent that health professionals involve patients in decision-making tasks. Health Expect 2005; 8:34–42.
27. Holmes-Rovner M, Kroll J, Schmitt N et al. Patient satisfaction with health care decisions: the satisfaction with decision scale. Med Decis Making 1996; 16:58–64.
28. O'Connor A. Validation of a decisional conflict scale. Med Decis Making 1995; 15:25–30.
29. Lerman C, Brody D, Caputo G et al. Patients' perceived involvement in care scale: relationship to attitudes about illness and medical care. J Gen Intern Med 1990; 5:29–33.
30. Simon D, Schorr G, Wirtz M et al. Development and first validation of the shared decision-making questionnaire (SDM-Q). Patient Educ Couns 2006; 63:319–327.
31. Epstein R, Alper B, Quill T. Communicating evidence for participatory decision making. JAMA 2004; 291:2359–2366.
32. McKenna K, Tooth L. Deciding the content and format of educational interventions. In: McKenna K, Tooth L (eds). Client education: a partnership approach for health practitioners. Sydney: University of New South Wales Press; 2006:128–158.

33. Tse S, Lloyd C, McKenna K. When clients are from diverse linguistic and cultural backgrounds. In: McKenna K, Tooth L (eds). Client education: a partnership approach for health practitioners. Sydney: University of New South Wales Press; 2006:307–326.

34. Boundouki G, Humphris G, Field A. Knowledge of oral cancer, distress and screening intentions: longer term effects of a patient information leaflet. Patient Educ Couns 2004; 53:71–77.

35. Hill J. A practical guide to patient education and information giving. Baillières Clin Rheumatol 1997; 11:109–127.

36. Raynor D. The influence of written information on patient knowledge and adherence to treatment. In: Myers L, Midence K (eds). Adherence to treatment in medical conditions. London: Harwood Academic; 1998:83–111.

37. Scott J, Harmsen M, Prictor M et al. Recordings or summaries of consultations for people with cancer. Cochrane Database Syst Rev 2003; 2: Art. No.: CD001539. DOI: 10.1002/14651858. CD001539.

38. Griffin J, McKenna K, Tooth L. Discrepancy between older clients' ability to read and comprehend and the reading level of written educational materials used by occupational therapists. Am J Occup Ther 2006; 60:70–80.

39. Hoffmann T, McKenna K. Analysis of stroke patients' and carers' reading ability and the content and design of written materials: recommendations for improving written stroke information. Patient Educ Couns 2006; 60:286–293.

40. McLaughlin H. SMOG grading: a new readability formula. J Reading 1969; 12:639–646.

41. Flesch R. A new readability yardstick. J Appl Psychol 1948; 32:221–233.

42. Hoffmann T, Worrall L. Designing effective written health education materials: considerations for health professionals. Disabil Rehabil 2004; 26:1166–1173.

43. Doak C, Doak L, Root J. Teaching patients with low literacy skills. 2nd edn. Philadelphia: J.B. Lippincott; 1996.

44. Paul C, Redman S, Sanson-Fisher R. The development of a checklist of content and design characteristics for printed health education materials. Health Promot J Austr 1997; 7:153–159.

45. Charnock D, Sheppard S, Needham G et al. DISCERN: an instrument for judging the quality of written consumer health information on treatment choices. J Epidemiol Commun Hlth 1999; 53:105–111.

46. Graham W, Smith P, Kamal A et al. Randomised controlled trial comparing effectiveness of touch screen system with leaflet for providing women with information on prenatal tests. BMJ 2000; 320:155–160.

47. Hoffmann T, Russell T, McKenna K. Producing computer-generated tailored written information for stroke patients and their carers: system development and preliminary evaluation. Int J Med Inform 2004; 73:751–758.

48. McMullan M. Patients using the Internet to obtain health information: how this affects the patient–health professional relationship. Patient Educ Couns 2006; 63:24–28.

49. Beranova E, Sykes C. A systematic review of computer-based softwares for educating patients with coronary heart disease. Patient Educ Couns 2007; 66:21–28.

50. Rostom A, O'Connor A, Tugwell P et al. A randomised trial of a computerised versus an audio-booklet decision aid for women considering post-menopausal hormone replacement therapy. Patient Educ Couns 2002; 46:67–74.

51. Stromberg A, Ahlen H, Fridlund, B. Interactive education on CD-ROM: a new tool in the education of heart failure patients. Patient Educ Couns 2002; 46:75–81.

52. Skinner C, Campbell M, Rimer B et al. How effective is tailored print communication? Ann Behaviour Med 1999; 21:290–298.

53. Hoffmann T, McKenna K, Worrall L et al. Randomised controlled trial of a computer-generated tailored written education package for patients following stroke. Age Ageing 2007; 36:280–286.

54. Agre P, Kurtz R, Krauss B. A randomised trial using videotape to present consent information for colonoscopy. Gastrointest Endosc 1994; 40:271–276.

55. Luck A, Pearson S, Maddern G et al. Effects of video information on precolonoscopy anxiety and knowledge: a randomised trial. Lancet 1999; 11:2032–2035.

56. O'Connor A, Stacey D, Entwistle V et al. Decision aids for people facing health treatment or screening decisions. Cochrane Database Syst Rev 2003; 1:Art. No.: CD001431. DOI: 10.1002/14651858.CD001341.

57. Stacey D, O'Connor A, Rovner D et al. Cochrane inventory and evaluation of patient decision aids. Med Decis Making 2001; 21:527.
58. Weiss B, Coyne C, Michielutte R et al. Communicating with patients who have limited literacy skills: report of the National Work Group on Literacy and Health. J Fam Pract 1998; 46:168–175.
59. Wilson F, McLemore R. Patient literacy levels: a consideration when designing patient education programs. Rehabil Nurs 1997; 22:311–317.
60. Weiss B, Reed R, Kligman E. Literacy skills and communication methods of low income older persons. Patient Educ Couns 1995; 25:109–119.
61. Murphy P, Davis T, Long S et al. REALM: a quick reading test for patients. J Reading 1993; 37:124–130.
62. Parker R, Baker D, Williams M et al. The Test of Functional Health Literacy in Adults: a new instrument for measuring patients' literacy skills. J Gen Intern Med 1995; 10:537–541.
63. Hanson-Divers E. Developing a medical achievement reading test to evaluate patient literacy skills: a preliminary study. J Health Care Poor Underserved 1997; 8:56–59.
64. McKenna K, Tooth L (eds). Client education: a partnership approach for health practitioners. Sydney: University of New South Wales Press; 2006.
65. Gigerenzer G, Edwards A. Simple tools for understanding risks: from innumeracy to insight. BMJ 2003; 327:741–744.
66. Berry D, Knapp P, Raynor T. Expressing medicine side effects: assessing the effectiveness of absolute risk, relative risk and number needed to harm and the provision of baseline risk information. Patient Educ Couns 2006; 63:89–96.
67. Halvorsen P, Kristiansen I. Decisions on drug therapies by numbers needed to treat: a randomised trial. Arch Int Med 2005; 165:1140–1146.
68. Price M, Cameron R, Butow P. Communicating risk information: the influence of graphical display format on quantitative information perception – accuracy, comprehension and preferences. Pat Educ Couns 2007; 69:121–128.
69. Trevena L, Davey H, Barratt A et al. A systematic review on communicating with patients about evidence. J Eval Clin Pract 2006; 12:13–23.
70. Alaszewski A, Horlick-Jones T. How can doctors communicate information about risk more effectively? BMJ 2003; 327:728–731.
71. Paling J. Strategies to help patients understand risks. BMJ 2003; 327:745–748.

CHAPTER 15

Clinical reasoning and evidence-based practice

Merrill Turpin and Joy Higgs

LEARNING OBJECTIVES

After reading this chapter, you should be able to:

- Describe some of the complexities and uncertainties of clinical practice
- Understand what is meant by the term clinical reasoning
- Be aware of the different perspectives about the concept of 'evidence'
- Understand the importance of clinical experience for evidence-based practice
- Understand what is meant by the term professional practice
- Explain how clinical reasoning can be used to integrate information from the different sources that are required for evidence-based practice
- Understand what is meant by critical reflection and how it might support evidence-based practice

Evidence-based practice aims to improve outcomes for clients.[1] This goal appears uncontentious and would generally be accepted by a range of stakeholders in health. Clients, health professionals, funding bodies and policy makers would all share in this aim. However, a range of issues make evidence-based practice problematic and the complexity of the problem becomes clearer when we question *how* best to achieve optimal health care.

Client outcomes are dependent on a range of factors, such as:

- the nature of the client's health problem
- the types of services that are available to and accessible by the client
- the practices of the health professionals working in those services
- the nature and quality of the interaction between the client and health professional
- the attitudes of the client towards the services offered
- the client's own conceptualisation of the health problem
- the ease with which any service recommendations that are made can be carried out by the client within the broader context of their life.

This list illustrates the complexity of the issue of improving client outcomes. If all of these issues interact together to impact upon the health outcomes for a particular client, where should planned improvements focus? Will a change in one factor be sufficient to obtain the desired result or do factors need to be considered in an integrated way? Health professionals face these kinds of questions on a daily basis, as well as the ever-present question, 'What can and should I do in this specific situation?'

Professional practice is complex and health professionals need to consider the range of factors that impact upon client outcomes when planning and delivering services. They are required to make decisions about what services they can and should offer, given the particular needs of and circumstances surrounding the individual client and the broader organisational and societal context. Making these kinds of decisions requires complex thinking processes as the 'problem' or situation about which decisions have to be made is often poorly defined and the desired outcomes are often unclear.[2] This thinking process is often referred to as clinical or professional reasoning, decision making and professional judgement.

Health professionals need to use their clinical reasoning to collect and interpret different types of information from a range of sources to make judgements and decisions regarding complex situations under conditions of uncertainty. In addition to the logical decisions that health professionals need to make, they also have to make ethical and pragmatic ones. They have to ask themselves questions like: 'What is the most effective thing I could do?', 'What is most likely to work in this situation?', 'What is the client most likely to accept and do?' and 'What should I do (ethically) in this situation?'

This chapter aims to explore the relationship between clinical reasoning and evidence-based practice. As you have seen throughout this book, evidence-based practice is a movement in health that aims to improve client outcomes by supporting health professionals to incorporate research evidence into their practice. Evidence-based practice also recognises that research evidence alone is not sufficient for addressing the complex nature of professional practice and that the ability to integrate different types of information from different sources is also required. Therefore, to practice in an evidence-based way, health professionals need to integrate research with their clinical experience, the preferences of their clients and the demands of the practice context. Clinical reasoning is the process by which health professionals integrate this information. In this chapter, we explore the notion of an evidence-based practice and the roles that a variety of types of information play in providing evidence for practice and highlight how the concept of practice should be viewed as being embedded within particular contexts.

We also explore the clinical reasoning processes that occur within practice and provide some brief suggestions for you to consider when critically reflecting on your own practice from the perspective of evidence-based practice.

What is an evidence-based practice?

The term evidence-based practice refers to a practice that is based on evidence. The assumption underpinning the perceived need for an evidence-based practice is that basing practice on rigorously produced information will lead to enhanced client outcomes. Given the complex range of factors that can affect client outcomes, how can we be sure that basing our practice on evidence will improve them and what kinds of information constitutes appropriate evidence? These are important questions for health professionals to ask.

The first question about whether basing practice on evidence does lead to better client outcomes has been examined widely in relation to specific interventions and specific outcomes. The broad assumption that basing practice on evidence leads to better client outcomes generally gives rise to the second question—what constitutes evidence? As much of the focus of evidence-based practice has been on the second question, 'What constitutes appropriate evidence?', the discussion of evidence-based practice in this chapter will consider that question. As we saw in Chapter 1, evidence-based practice evolved from its medical counterpart, evidence-based medicine and, as a consequence, many of the assumptions of medicine have been adopted by evidence-based practice. In the definition of evidence-based practice by Sackett and colleagues[3] that was examined in Chapter 1, the term 'current best evidence' was introduced as the criterion for evidence. Predictably, clarifying the nature of 'best' evidence has become the central concern of the evidence-based practice and evidence-based medicine movements. As the empirico–analytic paradigm is the dominant philosophy that underpins medicine, this also became the assumed perspective of the evidence-based practice movement.

The **empirico–analytic paradigm is** also known as the scientific paradigm or the empiricist model of knowledge creation. According to Higgs, Jones and Titchen[4] this paradigm 'relies on observation and experiment in the empirical world, resulting in generalisations about the content and events of the world which can be used to predict the future' (p 155). From the perspective of the empirico–analytic paradigm, the best form of evidence is evidence that is produced through rigorous scientific enquiry. It has been assumed that such rigour could be achieved best through the methods of research.[5] Therefore, information that has been generated from research became the concept of evidence that is used by the evidence-based practice movement. Many people take this assumption for granted and this is highlighted by the fact that some professions use the term 'research-based practice' rather than 'evidence-based practice'.

The position that scientific knowledge is the sole key to evidence has been questioned by a number of writers[5-7] who have argued that research evidence alone is not sufficient for addressing the complexities of professional practice and that the ability to generate and integrate different types of evidence from different sources is also required. However, this was the intent of early definitions of evidence-based medicine which emphasised that, to practise in an evidence-based way, professionals need to integrate research findings with the practical knowledge derived from their clinical experience and the preferences of their client.

In some ways, the assumption that 'evidence equals research' has been problematic for the evidence-based practice movement and has probably contributed to a strong division between those who align themselves with the evidence-based practice movement and those who oppose it. Critics of evidence-based practice argue that there are problems with the production, relevance and availability of research evidence and that it has limited capacity to address the problems of practice and enhance decision making in the context of complex practice situations.[8] Examples of criticisms include: that the research that is undertaken is often dependent on funding and, therefore, factors other than need and importance can influence what is researched; that the research undertaken can reflect what is easier to measure more than what is important to understand or most important to professional practice; and that, often, research findings are not presented in forms that are easily accessible to health professionals.

Perhaps the situation is summed up best by Naylor[9] who, in relation to evidence-based medicine (and his comments are just as relevant to evidence-based practice), stated that, 'A backlash is not surprising in view of the inflated expectations of outcomes-oriented and evidence-based medicine and the fears of some clinicians that these concepts threaten the art of patient care' (p 840). Exploring the assumptions about what is meant by the notion of 'evidence' can be a good start to examining what an evidence-based practice is and we will do this in the next section.

Evidence of what?

What is evidence? The Heinemann Australian Student Dictionary defines evidence as 'anything which provides a basis for belief'[10] and the Macquarie Dictionary defines it as 'grounds for belief'.[11] Thus, using this definition evidence might be considered by some as information that supports some sort of belief and an evidence-based practice would be a practice that is based on such information. But whose beliefs are referred to? Is it an individual health professional's beliefs, the beliefs of a particular health profession or the beliefs that underpin a particular health service or model of service delivery? Is it the beliefs of those receiving care from a particular service or those funding or providing the service? Are the beliefs of all of these stakeholders in health the same and of equal value?

Using this framework, these questions highlight that the types of information that could be appropriate to use as evidence for health practice can vary among different stakeholders. For example, if a service measures client outcomes in terms of reducing (or eliminating) impairments, then it is information about the effectiveness of interventions in reducing impairments that is used most often as evidence, regardless of the functional and practical implications of those changes. However, people using health services might use other criteria to measure outcomes. For example, they might value services that make an appreciable difference to their health experience, are accessible (physically and financially) and use interventions that are easy to implement within their own life context. Healthcare funding bodies might be most concerned with value-for-money and might seek information that substantiates the cost-effectiveness of interventions or services. That is, they might only look favourably on interventions and service provision models that have evidence to support their effectiveness in improving client outcomes as well as having an acceptable financial cost.

From the perspective of the empirico–analytic paradigm

As explained in the previous section, the evidence-based practice movement has so far taken its understanding of evidence from the empirico–analytic paradigm that underpins the assumptions of medicine. This perspective aims to develop a knowledge base generated from information about 'reality' or 'how the world is'. Therefore, the information that provides appropriate evidence about 'how the world is' tends to be observable (often with the assistance of technology), reliably generated and reproducible. To be dependable as evidence of how the world is, information needs to be free of bias when collected, the potential effects of the information collection process on the phenomena need to be minimised and any changes observed must be able to be reliably attributed to particular factors or variables.

To make the empirico–analytic concept of best evidence explicit, a number of hierarchies have been developed, based on the methodology that is used to generate the information. In Chapter 2 we explored the hierarchies and levels of evidence for questions about intervention, diagnosis and prognosis in detail. Developing levels of evidence was a strategy used to establish the degree to which information could be trusted as 'evidence'. For example, the top two levels of evidence in the hierarchy for intervention effectiveness are randomised controlled trials and their systematic reviews. As we saw in Chapter 4, randomised controlled trials (individual and systematically reviewed) generate knowledge that is considered to have a high degree of validity. By eliminating potential bias and controlling for variables that might influence the outcome, the confidence that any observed change can be attributed to one particular factor is very high. Therefore, in the empirico-analytic paradigm this study design represents the most trustworthy type of information to use as 'evidence' of how the world really is.

The accepted way that this kind of information is generated is through research that requires careful planning and, often, adequate funding. Therefore, it makes sense that, when considering the need for practice to be based on evidence, the evidence-based practice movement conceptualised 'best evidence' as information that is generated through research that is conducted within an empirico–analytic paradigm. This helps to explain the origins of the evidence-based practice movement's assumption of 'evidence equals research'. Further, as explained in Chapter 1, the use of the term 'evidence' in evidence-based practice serves the purpose of highlighting the use of research as an important source for decision making that had previously been undervalued. Hence, for the purpose of this book, the position taken is that 'evidence' means evidence from research, but it is considered to be only one of the many types of information that must be integrated for decision making. However, it is also important to consider other interpretations of the term 'evidence' that have been discussed in the literature.

From the perspective of technical rationality

A second approach that has influenced what is considered to be appropriate evidence for professional practice is technical rationality. The main aim of this approach to improving client outcomes is to regulate practice in order to enhance its efficiency and cost-effectiveness. Schon[12] claimed that, from the perspective of technical rationality, 'professional activity consists in instrumental problem solving made rigorous by the application of scientific theory and technique' (p 21). The major elements of this definition are problem solving and the rigorous use of scientific theory and technique. Whereas the empirico–analytic approach emphasises the trustworthiness of information in representing how things really are, this approach focuses on the problem solving of health professionals. Therefore, a major difference between these two approaches is that the former centres on the *quality* of the information whereas the latter targets the process of *using* the information.

From a technical rationalist perspective, human reasoning and judgement is understood in health care as problem solving, which requires the framing and definition of a problem and the search for a solution within a defined problem space. From this approach, efficiency and cost-effectiveness can be improved by providing tools that support the problem-solving process and minimise the likelihood of reasoning errors. As the technical rationalist approach values the rigorous use of the scientific method and technique, information that is generated using this method is incorporated into routines and procedures that aim to lessen the professional judgement required. The influence of technical rationality on health care is evident in the use of clinical pathways, protocols, decision trees and other tools that aim to systematise practice decisions. For example, the typical path to be taken by a health professional is clarified when a standard problem definition (often based on a medical diagnosis) can be used. Decision trees work in this way.

A major aim of using reasoning tools and research evidence is to reduce reasoning errors and the potentially biasing effects that can come from clinical opinions. An example of this type of bias is that health professionals can overemphasise the effectiveness of their own interventions because they might only see the short-term effects of the intervention. In addition, they might be overly influenced by situations and outcomes that they have access to, while potentially being unaware of or undervaluing other possibilities (such as interventions offered by other health professionals). In contrast, clinical protocols and research evidence are generated from information that is gathered from a broader range of sources. For example, protocols are often developed using information such as research evidence, broader trends in client outcomes or statistics about adverse incidents, epidemiological trends in population health and client opinions and experiences.

The technical rationalist approach shares a similar definition of evidence with the empirico–analytic approach. Both approaches value information that is generated using rigorous scientific methods and consider it to be appropriate evidence upon which to base clinical practice. While they share a concern for effectiveness, they often differ in relation to cost-effectiveness. In the empirico–analytic approach it might be argued that an intervention is essential, regardless of the cost. In all probability, the technical rationalist approach that incorporates the closest scrutiny of client outcomes and evidence would also include outcomes such as the reduction of health service costs and adverse incidents that occur during service delivery. However, a criticism of the technical rationalist approach is that it fails to give due attention to the complexity of professional practice and the individual nature of client experience.[13] This criticism is derived from the argument that the problems of professional practice are both specific and varied, which makes it impossible to develop protocols and procedures to cover the variety of situations that health professionals face.

What information helps health professionals to address the dilemmas of their practice?

A third approach to the question of what constitutes evidence is to consider the question, 'What information helps professionals to address the dilemmas of their practice?' Health professionals use judgement to deal with the complexity of professional practice,[14] which relies on their clinical or professional expertise. The concept of professional expertise is central to the evidence-based practice process. This is illustrated in Sackett and colleagues' 1996[3] definition of evidence-based medicine that was presented in Chapter 1. The beginning of Sackett and colleagues'[3] definition of evidence-based medicine, quoted earlier in the chapter, is well known. However, the section that follows has been quoted infrequently when definitions of evidence-based medicine (or practice) are presented. It reads (p 71):

The practice of evidence based medicine means integrating individual clinical expertise with the best available external clinical evidence from systematic research. By individual clinical expertise we mean the proficiency and judgement that individual clinicians acquire through clinical experiences and clinical practice. Increased expertise is reflected in many ways, but especially in more effective and efficient diagnosis and in the more thoughtful identification and compassionate use of individual patients' predicaments, rights, and preferences in making clinical decisions about their care.

As was pointed out in Chapter 1, this definition makes it clear that an evidence-based practice requires professional expertise, which includes thoughtfulness and compassion as well as effectiveness and efficiency.

Sociocultural theories of learning suggest that professional expertise is developed through interaction with communities of practice.[15,16] Health professionals learn the practices, activities and ways of thinking and knowing of their profession through participation in the community of practice. Expertise develops 'as an individual gains greater knowledge, understanding and mastery' (p 24)[16] in their practice area.

The work of Dreyfus and Dreyfus[17] has been widely used to understand the concept of professional expertise developing with experience. The different ways that professionals think as they gain experience have been characterised into five stages, namely: novice, advanced beginner, competent, proficient and expert. Essentially these five stages reflect a movement from a practice that is based on context-free information and generalised rules to a sophisticated and 'embodied' understanding of the specific context in which the practice occurs. While the earlier stages focus on the application of generalised knowledge, in the proficient and expert stages health professionals are able to recognise (often subtle) similarities between the current situation and previous ones and use their knowledge of the previous outcomes to make judgements about what might be best in the current situation.

Professional expertise is difficult to quantify as it is partly determined by the understandings that are shared by members of the community of practice. For example, Craik and Rappolt[1] selected health professionals who were 'deemed by their peers to be educationally influential practitioners' as a criterion for inclusion into their research study of 'elite' practitioners. In nursing, expertise has been associated with holistic practice, holistic knowledge, salience, knowing the client, moral agency and skilled know-how.[18] Fleming[19] reported that occupational therapists described videotapes of expert practitioners as appearing 'elegant and effortless' (p 27). Jensen and colleagues[20] developed a grounded theory of expert practice in physiotherapy and proposed that expertise in physiotherapy is a combination of multidimensional knowledge, clinical reasoning skills, skilled movement and virtue and that all four of these dimensions contribute to the therapist's philosophy of practice. It appears that members of a community of practice are able to recognise expertise, even thought it involves unstated and embodied knowledge, skills and attributes that can be difficult to quantify.

From this perspective, evidence could be conceptualised as including health professionals' memories of previous experiences and their specific outcomes. This is not to suggest that expert health professionals no longer use information that is generated from research. Professional communities of practice have codes of ethics that usually include the need to maintain up-to-date knowledge of the field and some professional bodies require members to undertake formal accreditation processes. Health professionals meet this ethical requirement through a range of activities such as attending conferences and workshops, reading professional journals, sharing this information with one another and discussing cases and experiences with one another. All of these activities can increase professional knowledge through exposure to findings from systematic research as well as expanding practice knowledge through vicarious learning. Thus, the use of knowledge that is generated from research as well as knowledge that is generated from practical experience is important, for health professionals are more able to undertake practice that is based on a rich evidence base.

Considering evidence from the client's perspective

A fourth approach is brought into focus when we ask the question, 'What is going to make the biggest difference to my client's life and health?' This question helps to turn our attention to the client's perspective. As we saw in Chapter 1, the definition of Sackett et al[3] of evidence-based medicine includes the 'thoughtful identification and compassionate use of individual patients' predicaments, rights, and preferences in making clinical decisions about their care' (p 71). Clients seek professional services because they need something that they cannot obtain in other ways. Professional services often come at substantial financial costs (and other costs such as time and effort) to clients. Attending to clients' predicaments, rights and preferences requires a developed ability to understand people, both as individuals and as members of groups within the overall population. Examples of understanding preferences and rights include giving an individual choice in relation to interventions and understanding and advocating for the rights of marginalised people to participate in social roles such as work. Understanding predicaments requires the ability to place clients within the context of their living situations and social roles. For example, a health professional might have to consider the need for support of a client's carer, the logistics of a client being able to follow an intervention recommendation when the client returns to their daily life context or the opportunities for social participation that a client has, given the attitudes of the society in which they live.

While clients expect health professionals to offer them services that will be effective, they also expect them to listen to their concerns and to validate their experiences of health. Therefore, clients might seek evidence of a health professional's interpersonal skills (for example, a professional's ability to listen to their concerns), the 'value for money' of the services that are being offered and the accessibility (physical and temporal) of the services as well as the effectiveness of the intervention that is being offered. Clients might seek this kind of information from sources such as the internet; friends, relatives and neighbours; and/or another trusted health professional. The importance of health professionals being able to communicate effectively with their clients was discussed in Chapter 14.

Evidence of what? A summary

In summary, asking the question 'Evidence of what?' can emphasise the fact that different stakeholders seek different types of information. People who work from an empirico–analytic paradigm are likely to seek information that is accepted as representing how things really are. Starting from this position, they are likely to value that kind of information over other types of information, as illustrated by the established hierarchies of evidence. People who work from a technical rationalist perspective are most likely to seek information that provides evidence of efficiency and cost-effectiveness and will aim to use this information to develop tools and strategies to standardise practice according to what is considered best practice. Health professionals are most likely to value and seek information that provides evidence to support the decisions that they need to make about what they, as a member of a specific health profession, should offer a particular client, given his or her life circumstances. Finally, clients are most likely to value and seek information that provides evidence of services and health professionals that offer effective, accessible, value-for-money interventions that they are likely to be able to incorporate into the context of their daily life.

All of these different perspectives are important when considering what an evidence-based practice might look like for health professionals as they highlight the complexity of professional practice. Health professionals are influenced by and need to consider all of the different types of information for their practice. In 2000, Sackett and colleagues[21] provided a more succinct definition of evidence-based medicine that emphasised the complexity of the task that faces health professionals in striving to create and sustain a practice that is evidence-based. The definition explicitly stated that the process of evidence-based medicine requires 'the integration of best research evidence with clinical expertise and patient values' (p 1). To understand this process of integration, it is important to contextualise professional practice as requiring art, science and ethics. In the following section, we will explore this process of integration.

Integrating information: the forgotten art?

Current conceptualisations of evidence-based practice define it as a process that requires the integration of information from different sources. However, an understanding of how such integration occurs is still in its infancy. Much of the early attention of the evidence-based practice movement centred on the nature of evidence that is appropriate for health practice (mainly research evidence) and little systematic investigation has been undertaken into how health professionals integrate information from different sources such as research, clinical expertise, client values and preferences and the practice context. Conceptualising evidence-based practice as a process of integration requires a focus on the activities of the health professional. This section of the chapter will explore the nature of professional practice.

Health professionals are required to provide services to their clients. They are required to think and act within particular contexts, which have been established to provide a particular type of service, and remain accountable to their funding bodies and clients. Health professionals also belong to particular professional groups or communities of practice. Therefore, professional practice needs to be understood within its social, organisational and professional contexts.

Professional practice has been described as a dynamic, creative and constructive phenomenon that flows constantly like a river that shapes and is shaped by the landscape over which it flows.[23] It is more than just a rational or routine practice. It requires the interaction between professions and clients and among professionals from different disciplines and ethical and professional behaviour. As Fish and Higgs[24] stated, 'As responsible members of a profession, [the health professional's] role is precisely to argue their moral position, utilise their abilities to wear an appropriate variety of hats on different occasions with proper transparency and integrity and exercise their clinical thinking and professional judgement in the service of differing individuals while making wise decisions about the relationship between the privacy of individuals and the common good' (p 21).

These descriptions illustrate the complexity of professional practice. It is not just a problem-solving exercise (as technical rationalists might argue), although it requires problem solving. It is not just a process of applying theories and other information to practice (as an empirico–analytic approach emphasises), although these are vital in guiding practice. It includes the fulfilment of role expectations and the delivery of services. As Coles[14] stated, 'professionals are asked to engage in complex and unpredictable tasks on society's behalf, and in doing so must exercise their discretion, making judgements' (p 3). Professional practice requires systematic thinking, social and contextual understanding, deep listening, good communication and the ability to deal creatively and ethically with uncertainty. Examples of the uncertainty of medical practice that have been described[25] include uncertainties about diagnosis, the accuracy of diagnostic tests, the natural history of a disease and the effects of interventions on groups and populations. Each health profession has its own complexity and areas of uncertainty.

Health professionals need to use their judgement to make decisions about the best course of action to take under conditions of uncertainty. Part of the complexity is dealing with different and often competing pieces of information from a variety of sources and considering the individual nature of client circumstances and preferences. Professional practice is an ethical and creative endeavour that requires the logical use of theory and research, good judgement and problem solving and the ability to implement protocols and procedures. Integrating information from research, clinical expertise, client values and preferences and information from the practice context requires judgement and artistry as well as science and logic.

The combining of science and art is embedded in the way that a variety of health professions think about their work. For example, in reference to occupational therapists, it has been stated that, 'When occupational therapists refer to the paired concepts of art and science, they express their moral dissatisfaction with being constrained by either. In isolation, art somehow seems too soft and unquantifiable and science too hard and unyielding' (p 482).[26] While science is generally associated with rigour, reliability and predictability, artistry is associated with judgement and being able to deal with unpredictability. In Sackett's 1996 definition of evidence-based medicine[3] that was referred to earlier, artistry is evident in the reference to 'thoughtful identification and compassionate use' of information that pertains to a particular client. While various health professions emphasise art and science to different degrees, they all appear to accept that a balance of some sort is required for professional practice.

Professional practice could be characterised as reasoned action, as it requires both knowing and doing. The concept of 'art and science' highlights that different types of knowledge are required for health professionals to undertake such reasoned action. Three types of knowledge that are required for practice have been identified:[27]

- **Propositional knowledge**, also known as theoretical knowledge, is an explicit and formal type of knowledge that is generated through research and scholarship and is associated with knowing 'what'. This type of knowledge is often thought of as 'scientific knowledge' and has been emphasised in the main conceptualisation of evidence-based practice to date.
- **Professional craft knowledge** refers to knowing 'how' to carry out the tasks of the profession. It is often associated with the idea of an 'art' of practice and includes the particular perspectives that characterise each profession.
- **Personal knowledge** refers to an individual health professional's knowledge about his or her self in relation to others. This type of knowledge is important for professional practice as the relationships that health professionals build with their clients are often central to that practice.

The last two types of knowledge 'may be tacit and embedded either in practice itself or in who the person is' (p 5)[23] and have been referred to collectively as 'non-propositional' knowledge.

Different types of knowledge can be gained from different sources. The definition of evidence-based practice that was explained in Chapter 1 and shown in Figure 1.1 included four sources: research, clinical expertise, the client's values and circumstances and the practice context. The practice context, which does not occur in any of Sackett's definitions[3,21] as an information source, provides important information about the local context.[5] This source draws attention to the context-specific nature of professional practice, to which insufficient attention has been paid when conceptualising a practice that is based on evidence. Health professionals need to know what and how things work in a particular context as well as with particular clients. Taken together, these four sources of information provide objective, experiential and contextual information from researchers, health professionals and clients.

The complexity of professional practice becomes evident if you consider that it requires the ability to obtain and use different types of information from a range of sources; to meet the demands of particular practice environments; to fulfil roles consistent with the perspectives of the professional communities of practice to which the health professional belongs; and to consider the predicaments, preferences and values of individual clients. Thus, the creation of a practice that is 'evidence-based', for the purpose of improving client outcomes, is equally complex. 'Evidence' and 'practice' are both important for understanding evidence-based practice. The study of clinical reasoning highlights one aspect of practice. As this investigation was initiated by medicine, the term *clinical reasoning* was used. However, as many of the settings within which various health professionals work are not considered 'clinical', the term *professional reasoning* has also been used.

Approaches to clinical reasoning

Higgs[28] defined clinical reasoning (or practice decision making) as (p 1):

> ... *a context-dependent way of thinking and decision making in professional practice to guide practice actions. It involves the construction of narratives to make sense of the multiple factors and interests pertaining to the current reasoning task. It occurs within a set of problem spaces informed by practitioners' unique frames of reference, workplace contexts and practice models, as well as by patients' or clients' contexts. It utilises core dimensions of practice knowledge, reasoning and meta-cognition and draws upon these capacities in others. Decision making within clinical reasoning occurs at micro-, macro- and meta-levels and may be individually or collaboratively conducted. It involves the meta-skills of critical conversation, knowledge generation, practice model authenticity, and reflexivity.*

Earlier approaches to the study of clinical reasoning were influenced by investigations into artificial intelligence and conceptualised clinical reasoning as a purely cognitive process. These emphasised the iterative process of obtaining cues or information about the clinical situation, forming hypotheses about possible explanations and courses of action, interpreting information in light of these hypotheses and testing them. This process is referred to as hypothetico–deductive reasoning. However, Higgs' definition[28] emphasises that clinical reasoning is a process that involves cognition, meta-cognition (that is, the process of reflective self-awareness) and interactive and narrative ways of thinking.

Higgs and Jones'[29] work presents a current approach to clinical reasoning. They broadly categorised approaches to clinical reasoning as cognitive and interactive. Table 15.1 outlines the main types of thinking that health professionals use. The wide range of clinical reasoning approaches presented in this table is related to the following factors.

1. **The inherently complex nature of clinical reasoning as a phenomenon.** Clinical reasoning models are essentially an interpretation or approximation of a very complex set of thinking processes at both cognitive and meta-cognitive levels. These processes use both domain-specific and generic knowledge. They operate in conjunction with other abilities such as communication and interpersonal interaction and are framed by the health professional's individual values, interests and practice model.

2. **The multiple, multi-dimensional ways of reasoning that evolve with growing expertise.** Health professionals, both within and across various health professions, do not reason in the same way. The assumption that there is one way of representing clinical reasoning expertise or a single correct way to solve a problem has been challenged.[30] The different ways that health professionals think as they gain expertise was explained earlier in this chapter.

3. **The embedding of clinical reasoning in decision–action cycles.** As discussed, professional practice requires action. Decisions and actions in professional practice influence each other. Decision making is a dynamic, reciprocal process of making decisions and implementing an optimal course of action.[31] These decision–action cycles form the basis for professional judgement.

4. **The influence of contextual factors.** It is important to remember that, in practice, health professionals are required to make decisions about particular actions that are going to be taken with particular clients in particular practice settings. The influence of context on clinical decision making has been examined and it was identified that the nature of the task (such as its difficulty, complexity and uncertainty), the characteristics of the decision maker (including frames of reference, individual capabilities and experience) and the external decision-making context (such as professional ethics, disciplinary norms and workplace policies) all influence the decision-making process.[32]

5. **The nature of collaborative decision making.** As you saw in Chapter 14, there is a growing trend, and indeed societal pressure, for clients and health professionals to adopt a collaborative approach to clinical reasoning which increases the client's role and power in decision making.[33] Shared decision making and being able to work together are important for creating and providing services that result in satisfactory outcomes for clients.

An interpretative model of clinical reasoning

These factors attest to the complexity and fluid nature of professional practice, which requires more than just cognitive processes. A model that views clinical reasoning as a contextualised interactive phenomenon has been developed by Higgs and Jones.[29] Figure 15.1 portrays the characteristics of this model, which include:

1. **Three core dimensions**
   a. **Discipline-specific knowledge**—propositional knowledge (derived from theory and research) and non-propositional knowledge (derived from professional and personal experience)
   b. **Cognition**—the thinking skills used to process clinical data against the health professional's existing discipline-specific and personal knowledge base in consideration of the client's needs and the clinical problem
   c. **Meta-cognition**—reflective self-awareness enables health professionals to identify limitations in the quality of information obtained, monitor errors and credibility in their reasoning and practice and recognise inadequacies in their knowledge and reasoning

2. **Interactive/contextual dimensions**
   a. **Mutual decision making**—the role of the client in the decision-making process
   b. **Contextual interaction**—the interactivity between the decision makers and the decision-making situation
   c. **Task impact**—the influence of the nature of the clinical problem or task on the reasoning process

3. **Four meta-skills**
   a. The ability to derive knowledge from reasoning and practice
   b. The capacity to locate reasoning within the health professional's chosen practice models
   c. The reflexive ability to promote clients' and health professionals' wellbeing and development
   d. The use of critical, creative conversations[28] to make clinical decisions

Model	Description
Hypothetico-deductive reasoning[34–36]	The generation of hypotheses based on clinical data and knowledge and testing of these hypotheses through further inquiry. It is used by novices and in problematic situations by experts.[37]
Pattern recognition[38]	Expert reasoning in non-problematic situations resembles pattern recognition or direct automatic retrieval of information from a well-structured knowledge base.[39] Through the use of inductive reasoning, pattern recognition/interpretation is a process characterised by speed and efficiency[40]
Forward reasoning; backward reasoning[40,41]	Forward reasoning describes inductive reasoning in which data analysis results in hypothesis generation or diagnosis, utilising a sound knowledge base. Forward reasoning is more likely to occur in familiar cases with experienced health professionals and backward reasoning with inexperienced health professionals or in atypical or difficult cases[41] Backward reasoning is the re-interpretation of data or the acquisition of new clarifying data invoked to test a hypothesis.
Knowledge reasoning integration[42,43]	Clinical reasoning requires domain-specific knowledge and an organised knowledge base. A stage theory which emphasises the parallel development of knowledge acquisition and clinical reasoning expertise has been proposed.[43] Clinical reasoning involves the integration of knowledge, reasoning and meta-cognition.[44]
Intuitive reasoning[45,46]	'Intuitive knowledge' is related to 'instance scripts' or past experience with specific cases which can be used unconsciously in inductive reasoning.
Multidisciplinary reasoning[47]	Occurs when members of a multidisciplinary team work together to make clinical decisions for the client, for example at case conferences and in multidisciplinary clinics.
Conditional reasoning[48–50]	Used by health professionals to estimate client's response to intervention and the likely outcomes of management and to help clients consider possibilities and reconstruct their lives following injury or the onset of disease.
Narrative reasoning[48,51,52]	The use of stories regarding past or present clients to further understand and manage a clinical situation. Telling the story of clients' illness or injury to help them make sense of the illness experience.
Interactive reasoning[48,49]	Interactive reasoning occurs between health professional and client to understand the client's perspective.
Collaborative reasoning[20,48,53,54]	The shared decision making that ideally occurs between health professionals and their clients. The client's opinions as well as information about the problem are actively sought and utilised.
Ethical reasoning[48,55–57]	Those less recognised, but frequently made decisions regarding moral, political and economic dilemmas which health professionals regularly confront, such as deciding how long to continue an intervention for.
Teaching as reasoning[48,58]	When health professionals consciously use advice, instruction and guidance for the purpose of promoting change in the client's understanding, feelings and behaviour.

TABLE 15.1 Summary of clinical reasoning approaches

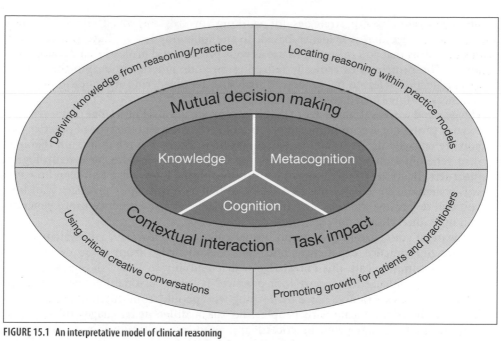

FIGURE 15.1 An interpretative model of clinical reasoning

Based on Higgs and Jones 2008.[29]

As this model demonstrates, health professionals use a range of cognitive, meta-cognitive and interactive skills to obtain and combine information from a range of sources when making clinical judgements. They need access to propositional knowledge that is appropriate to their professional discipline as well as knowledge about health and wellbeing more generally. This type of knowledge has been emphasised in conceptualisations of evidence-based practice to date. They also need access to non-propositional knowledge that is derived from professional and personal experience. They need the cognitive abilities to combine this information and the meta-cognitive skills to evaluate the trustworthiness and relevance of knowledge from these different sources and apply it to the practice decisions they have to make and to make changes to their practice accordingly. The capacity of a health professional to implement practice that aims to improve client outcomes through the use of 'evidence' to substantiate that practice must be developed over time as experience grows and through critical appraisal of one's practice.

How do I make my practice evidence-based?

In this chapter, we have presented professional practice as a complex and fluid process that is characterised by high levels of uncertainty that arise from the context-dependent nature of the tasks that are undertaken. Professional practice is difficult to describe specifically as it involves fulfilling particular professional roles with particular clients within particular contexts. Each of these factors contributes a unique aspect to the phenomenon, leading to a complex range of variations to what might be considered 'standard practice'. Therefore, there is no easy answer to the question, 'How do I make my practice evidence-based?' However, a number of principles and tools can provide health professionals with strategies for working towards improved client outcomes through a practice that is evidence-based. In the following list we have provided you with some ideas that you may wish to use as your practice and professional development requires. The principles of critically reflecting on your practice underpin these ideas. Critical reflection refers to the process of analysing, reconsidering and questioning your experiences within a broad context of issues.

- Have a good working knowledge of the current propositional knowledge that is relevant to your professional community of practice or profession and the type of practice that you are engaged in. For example, you might be working as a rehabilitation therapist in a rehabilitation ward where you primarily treat people who have neurological disorders. Be aware of the limits of your propositional knowledge and plan how you will systematically expand this knowledge to better inform your practice. Plan how you will determine the relevance of this knowledge to your practice more generally and individual clients more specifically.
- Be aware of your current non-propositional knowledge. How have you systematically tested your practice experiences and derived knowledge from these experiences? Can you communicate this knowledge with credibility to your colleagues and use it as sound evidence to support your practice? Is there personal knowledge derived from your life experiences (such as working with people from different cultures and learning to communicate with people who speak different languages to you) that you can use to enhance your practice? Planning to systematically enhance or expand this type of knowledge is an excellent way of drawing on your practice expertise and individualising the services that you provide to clients.
- Engage in empathic visioning and collaborative questioning with clients about their experiences, knowledge and values. Practice problem solving and mutual decision making with your clients to expand your collaboration skills and critically appraise your decision making.
- Reflect on how your actions are informed by research evidence, professional craft knowledge and an understanding of the practice context.
- Practice articulating your reasoning and your professional practice model.

As much of professional expertise becomes 'embodied' knowledge or practice wisdom, of which you might not be aware or able to articulate, raising awareness of those aspects of professional and personal thinking and action that have become taken-for-granted is vital for creating a practice that is evidence-based. This includes an ability to critically evaluate the types of knowledge that are available to health professionals, including the assumptions about knowledge that have become taken-for-granted. By engaging in critical reflection, you can become more systematic in your collection and use of the information upon which you base your practice. To conduct truly evidence-based practice, you need to be aware of the types of knowledge that you are using and the purpose of the use of that knowledge, ensuring that it constitutes appropriate evidence for the particular questions and problems about which you seek to be informed. You also need to be aware of the cognitive and meta-cognitive processes that you are using to combine information from different sources within the context of your discipline and practice context.

Summary points of this chapter
- Health professionals need to use clinical reasoning to collect and interpret different types of information from a range of sources to make judgements and decisions regarding complex situations under conditions of uncertainty.

- Clinical reasoning is a process that involves cognition, meta-cognition (that is, the process of reflective self-awareness) and interactive and narrative ways of thinking.
- Integrating information from research, clinical expertise, client values and preferences and information from the practice context requires judgement and artistry as well as science and logic.
- Critical reflection refers to the process of analysing, reconsidering and questioning your experiences within a broad context of issues. By engaging in critical reflection, you can become more systematic in your collection and use of the information upon which you base your practice.

References

1. Craik J, Rappolt S. Theory of research utilization enhancement: a model for occupational therapy. Can J Occup Ther 2003; 70:266–275.
2. Robertson L. Clinical reasoning part 1: the nature of problem solving, a literature review. Br J Occup Ther 1996; 59:178–182.
3. Sackett D, Rosenberg W, Gray J et al. Evidence based medicine: what it is and what it isn't: it's about integrating individual clinical expertise and the best external evidence. BMJ 1996; 312:71–72.
4. Higgs J, Jones M, Titchen A. Knowledge, reasoning and evidence for practice. In: Higgs J, Jones M, Loftus S et al (eds). Clinical reasoning in the health professions. 3rd edn. Edinburgh: Elsevier; 2008:151–161.
5. Rycroft-Malone J, Seers K, Titchen A et al. What counts as evidence in evidence-based practice? J Adv Nurs 2004; 47:81–90.
6. Higgs J, Andresen L, Fish D. Practice knowledge—its nature, sources and contexts. In: Higgs J, Richardson B, Abrandt Dahlgren M (eds). Developing practice knowledge for health professionals. Butterworth–Heinemann Oxford; 2004:51–69.
7. Jones M, Grimmer K, Edwards I et al. Challenges in applying best evidence to physiotherapy. The Internet Journal of Allied Health Sciences and Practice. Online. 2006;4. Available: http://ijahsp. nova.edu/ (7 Oct 2008).
8. Small N. Knowledge, not evidence, should determine primary care practice. Clinical Governance: An International Journal 2003; 8:191–199.
9. Naylor C. Grey zones of clinical practice: some limits to evidence-based medicine. Lancet 1995; 345:840–841.
10. Heinemann Australian Student's Dictionary. Melbourne: Reed Educational and Professional Publishing; 1992.
11. The Macquarie Concise Dictionary. 3rd edn Sydney: Macquarie Library; 1998.
12. Schon D. The reflective practitioner: how professionals think in action. New York: Basic Books; 1983.
13. Fish D, Coles C. Developing professional judgement in health care: learning through the critical appreciation of practice. Oxford: Butterworth–Heinemann; 1998.
14. Coles C. Developing professional judgement. J Contin Educ Health Prof 2002; 22:3–10.
15. Lave J, Wenger E. Situated learning: legitimate peripheral participation. Cambridge, UK: University Press; 1991.
16. Walker R. Social and cultural perspectives on professional knowledge and expertise. In: Higgs J, Titchen A (eds). Practice knowledge and expertise in the health professions. Oxford: Butterworth–Heinemann; 2001:22–28.
17. Dreyfus H, Dreyfus S. Mind over machine. New York: Free Press; 1986.
18. McCormack B, Titchen A. Patient-centred practice: an emerging focus for nursing expertise. In: Higgs J, Titchen A (eds). Practice knowledge and expertise in the health professions. Oxford: Butterworth–Heinemann; 2001:96–101.
19. Fleming M. The search for tacit knowledge. In: Mattingly C, Fleming M (eds). Clinical reasoning: forms of inquiry in a therapeutic practice. Philadelphia, PA: F A Davis; 1994:22–34.
20. Jensen G, Gwyer J, Hack L et al. Expertise in physical therapy practice. Boston: Butterworth–Heinemann; 1999.
21. Shepard K, Hack L, Gwyer J et al. Describing expert practice. Qual Health Res 1999; 9:746–758.
22. Sackett D, Straus S, Richardson W et al. Evidence-based medicine: how to practice and teach EBM. 2nd edn. Edinburgh: Elsevier Churchill Livingstone 2000.

23. Higgs J, Titchen A, Neville V. Professional practice and knowledge. In: Higgs J, Titchen A (eds). Practice knowledge and expertise in the health professions. Oxford: Butterworth–Heinemann; 2001:3–9.

24. Fish D, Higgs J. The context for clinical decision making in the 21st century. In: Higgs J, Jones M, Loftus S (eds). Clinical reasoning in the health professions. 3rd edn. Edinburgh: Elsevier; 2008: 19–30.

25. Hunink M, Glasziou P, Siegel J et al. Decision making in health and medicine: integrating evidence and values. New York: Cambridge University Press; 2001.

26. Turpin M. The issue is … recovery of our phenomenological knowledge in occupational therapy. Am J Occup Ther 2007; 61:481–485.

27. Higgs J, Titchen A. Propositional, professional and personal knowledge in clinical reasoning. In: Higgs J, Jones M (eds). Clinical reasoning in the health professions. Oxford: Butterworth–Heinemann; 1995:129–146.

28. Higgs J. The complexity of clinical reasoning: exploring the dimensions of clinical reasoning expertise as a situated, lived phenomenon. CPEA, Occasional Paper 6. Collaborations in Practice and Education Advancement. The University of Sydney, Australia; 2007.

29. Higgs J, Jones M. Clinical decision making and multiple problem spaces. In: Higgs J, Jones M, Loftus S (eds). Clinical reasoning in the health professions. 3rd edn. Edinburgh: Elsevier; 2008:3–17.

30. Norman G. Research in clinical reasoning: past history and current trends. Med Educ 2005; 39:418–427.

31. Smith M, Higgs J, Ellis E. Factors influencing clinical decision making. In: Higgs J, Jones M, Loftus S (eds). Clinical reasoning in the health professions. 3rd edn. Edinburgh: Elsevier; 2008: 89–100.

32. Smith M. Clinical decision making in acute care cardiopulmonary physiotherapy. Unpublished doctoral thesis, Sydney: The University of Sydney; 2006.

33. Trede F, Higgs J. Re-framing the clinician's role in collaborative clinical decision making: re-thinking practice knowledge and the notion of clinician–patient relationships. Learning in Health and Social Care 2003; 2:66–73.

34. Barrows H, Feightner J, Neufield V et al. An analysis of the clinical methods of medical students and physicians. Report to the Province of Ontario Department of Health McMaster University Hamilton, ONT; 1978.

35. Elstein A, Shulman S, Sprafka S. Medical problem solving: an analysis of clinical reasoning. Cambridge, Harvard University Press, MA; 1978.

36. Feltovich P, Johnson P, Moller J et al. LCS: The role and development of medical knowledge in diagnostic expertise. In: Clancey W, Shortliffe E (eds). Readings in medical artificial intelligence: the first decade. Reading, MA: Addison-Wesley; 1984:275–319.

37. Elstein A, Shulman L, Sprafka SA. Medical problem solving: a ten year retrospective. Eval Health Prof 1990; 13:5–36.

38. Barrows HS, Feltovich PJ. The clinical reasoning process. Med Educ 1987; 21:86–91.

39. Groen G, Patel V. Medical problem-solving: some questionable assumptions. Med Educ 1985; 19:95–100.

40. Arocha J, Patel V, Patel Y. Hypothesis generation and the coordination of theory and evidence in novice diagnostic reasoning. Med Decis Making 1993; 13:198–211.

41. Patel V, Groen G. Knowledge-based solution strategies in medical reasoning. Cogni Sci 1986; 10:91–116.

42. Schmidt H, Norman G, Boshuizen H. A cognitive perspective on medical expertise: theory and implications. Acad Med 1990; 65:611–621.

43. Boshuizen H, Schmidt H. On the role of biomedical knowledge in clinical reasoning by experts, intermediates and novices. Cogni Sci 1992; 16:153–184.

44. Higgs J, Jones M. Clinical reasoning. In: Higgs J, Jones M (eds). Clinical reasoning in the health professions. Butterworth–Heinemann: Oxford; 1995:3–23.

45. Agan R. Intuitive knowing as a dimension of nursing. Adv Nurs Sci 1987; 10:63–70.

46. Rew L. Intuition in critical care nursing practice. Dimens Crit Care Nurs 1990; 9:30–37.

47. Loftus S. Language in clinical reasoning: learning and using the language of collective clinical decision making. PhD Thesis, The University of Sydney, Australia; 2006. Available: http://ses.library.usyd.edu.au/handle/2123/1165.

48. Edwards I, Jones M, Carr J et al. Clinical reasoning in three different fields of physiotherapy – a qualitative study. In: Proceedings of the Fifth International Congress of the Australian Physiotherapy Association, Melbourne; 1998: 298–300.
49. Fleming M. The therapist with the three track mind. Am J Occup Ther 1991; 45:1007–1014.
50. Hagedorn R. Clinical decision making in familiar cases: a model of the process and implications for practice. Br J Occup Ther 1996; 59:217–222.
51. Benner P, Tanner C, Chesla C. From beginner to expert: gaining a differentiated clinical world in critical care nursing. Adv Nurs Sci 1992; 14:13–28.
52. Mattingly C, Fleming MH. Clinical reasoning: forms of inquiry in a therapeutic practice. Philadelphia: F A Davis; 1994.
53. Coulter A. Shared decision-making: the debate continues. Health Expect 2005; 8:95–96.
54. Beeston S, Simons H. Physiotherapy practice: practitioners' perspectives. Physiother Theory Pract 1996; 12:231–242.
55. Barnitt R, Partridge C. Ethical reasoning in physical therapy and occupational therapy. Physiother Res Int 1997; 2:178–194.
56. Gordon M, Murphy C, Candee D et al. Clinical judgement: an integrated model. Adv Nurs Sci 1994; 16:55–70.
57. Neuhaus B. Ethical considerations in clinical reasoning: the impact of technology and cost containment. Am J Occup Ther 1988; 42:288–294.
58. Sluijs EM. Patient education in physiotherapy: towards a planned approach. Physiotherapy 1991; 77:503–508.

CHAPTER **16**

Implementing evidence into practice

Annie McCluskey

LEARNING OBJECTIVES

After reading this chapter, you should be able to:

- Describe the process of transferring evidence into practice
- Explain what is meant by an evidence–practice gap and describe methods that can be used to demonstrate an evidence-based gap
- Explain various types of barriers to successfully implementing evidence and how barriers and enablers can be identified
- Describe strategies and interventions that can be used to facilitate the implementation of evidence
- Describe theories which can inform the development of implementation strategies and help explain behaviour change as it relates to the implementation of evidence

As we have seen throughout this book, searching for and appraising research articles are key components of evidence-based practice. However, while they are worthy activities, on their own they do not change client outcomes. To improve outcomes, health professionals need to do more than read the evidence. Transferring the evidence into practice is also required. Professionals need to translate research that has proven value, for example evidence from evidence-based clinical guidelines, systematic reviews and high quality randomised controlled trials. Findings from research projects which have involved years of hard work, many participants and often substantial costs should not remain hidden in journals. Translating or implementing evidence into practice is the final step in the process of evidence-based practice, but it is often the most challenging step.

Implementation is a complex but active process which involves individuals, teams, systems and organisations. Translating evidence into practice requires careful forward planning.[1] While some planning usually does occur, the process is often intuitive.[2] There may be little consideration of potential problems and barriers. As a consequence, the results may be disappointing. To help increase the likelihood of success when implementing evidence, this chapter provides a checklist for individuals and teams to use when planning the implementation of evidence.

In this chapter, definitions of implementation jargon are provided, followed by examples of evidence that different disciplines have applied in practice. A description is provided of the steps that health professionals follow when translating evidence into practice. Steps include collecting and analysing local data (gap analysis) and identifying possible barriers and enablers to change. Barriers might include negative attitudes, limited skills and knowledge or limited access to medical records and equipment. A menu of implementation strategies is presented, along with a review of the evidence for the effectiveness of these strategies. Finally, theories which can help us predict and explain individual and group behaviour change are considered.

Implementation terminology

A number of confusing terms appear in the implementation literature. Different terms may mean the same thing in different countries. To help you navigate this new terminology, definitions relevant to this chapter are provided in Box 16.1.

Implementation case studies

To help you understand the process of implementation, we will now consider three case studies. The first case study involves reducing referrals for a test procedure (X-rays) by general practitioners for people who present with acute low back pain.[7] This case example involves the overuse of X-rays. The other two case studies involve increasing the uptake of two underused interventions: cognitive behavioural therapy for adolescents with depression[8] and community travel and mobility training for people with stroke.[9,10]

Case study 1: Reducing the use of X-rays by general practitioners for people with acute low back pain

Low back pain is one of the most common musculoskeletal conditions seen by general practitioners,[11] but also by allied health practitioners such as physiotherapists, chiropractors and osteopaths. Clinical guidelines recommend that people presenting with an episode of acute non-specific low back pain should *not* be sent for an X-ray because of the limited diagnostic value of this test for this condition.[12] In Australia,

BOX 16.1 DEFINITIONS OF IMPLEMENTATION TERMINOLOGY

Implementation of evidence—A planned and active process of using published research in practice; for example, delivering an effective therapy from a randomised controlled trial to clients in a local setting.

Implementation science—The science of applying ideas, innovations and practices within the constraints of real healthcare settings. Implementation scientists typically use theories (for example, behaviour theory) to help explain why some ideas fail and others succeed and which professionals or teams are more likely to adopt an evidence-based intervention than others. Implementation also involves a systematic (and scientific) approach, with careful planning and preparation.[3]

Diffusion of innovations—The process of spreading new ideas, behaviours or routines across a population. The adoption of new ideas typically starts with a slow initial phase, followed by a period of acceleration as more people adopt the behaviours of the innovators, then a corresponding period of deceleration with adoption by the last few individuals.[4] Examples of health 'innovations' include the introduction of a new outcome measure, screening procedure or intervention.

Translational (or implementation) research—The scientific study of methods to promote the translation (or uptake) of research knowledge into practice. The aim is to ensure that new interventions or practices reach intended client groups and are implemented routinely. This type of research typically involves studying the process of behaviour change, barriers to change and the place of reminders and decision-support tools.[5]

Knowledge transfer (or translation)—A process of synthesising and exchanging knowledge between researchers and users (professionals, clients and policy makers). A primary aim of knowledge transfer is to accelerate the use of research by professionals, in order to improve health outcomes.[6] Multiple disciplines, such as health informatics, health education and organisational theory are involved in the knowledge translation process, to help close evidence–practice gaps.

Evidence–practice gaps—Areas of practice where routines or behaviour differ from clinical guideline recommendations or known best practice; areas of practice where quality improvement is required. For example, clients may be referred for an unnecessary and costly test procedure, while others may not be receiving an intervention that could improve their health.

Practice behaviour—A routine used by health professionals which can be observed. Practice behaviours include the ordering of diagnostic tests, use of assessments and outcome measures, clinical note writing and the delivery of interventions to clients and carers.

about 28% of people who visit their local general practitioner with acute low back pain are X-rayed,[13] with even higher estimates in the USA and Europe.[7] Put simply, X-rays are over-prescribed and costly. Instead of recommending an X-ray, rest and passive treatments, general practitioners should advise people with acute low back pain to remain active.[12]

In this instance, the evidence–practice gap is the overuse of a costly diagnostic test which can delay recovery. Recommendations about the management of acute low back pain, including the use of X-rays, have been made through national clinical guidelines.[12] A program to change practice, in line with guideline recommendations, is the focus of one implementation study in Australia[7] and will be discussed further throughout this chapter.

Case study 2: Increasing the delivery of cognitive behavioural therapy to adolescents with depression by community mental health professionals

Cognitive behavioural therapy has been identified as an effective intervention for adolescents with depression, a condition that is on the increase in developed countries.[14] Outcomes from cognitive behavioural therapy that is provided in the community are superior to usual care for this population.[15] Clinical guidelines recommend that young people who are affected by depression should receive a series of cognitive behavioural therapy sessions. However, a survey of one group of health professionals in North America found that two-thirds had no formal training in cognitive behavioural therapy and no prior experience using a treatment manual for cognitive behavioural therapy.[8] In other words, they were unlikely to deliver cognitive behavioural therapy if they did not know much about it. Furthermore, almost half of the participants in that study reported that they never or rarely used evidence-based treatments for youths with depression, and a quarter of the group had no plans to use evidence-based treatment in the following six months. Subsequently, that group of mental health professionals was targeted with an implementation program to increase the uptake of the underused cognitive behavioural therapy. The randomised controlled trial that describes this implementation program[8] and the evidence–practice gap (underuse of cognitive behavioural therapy) will also be discussed throughout this chapter.

Case study 3: Increasing the delivery of travel and mobility training by community rehabilitation therapists to people who have had a stroke

People who have had a stroke typically have difficulty accessing their local community. Many experience social isolation. Up to two-thirds of people who have had a stroke do not return to driving[16,17] and up to 50% experience a fall at home in the first six months.[18] Australian clinical guidelines recommend that community-dwelling people with stroke should receive a series of escorted visits and transport information from a rehabilitation therapist, to help increase outdoor journeys.[19] Although that recommendation is based on a single randomised controlled trial,[20] the size of the treatment effect was large. The intervention doubled the proportion of people with stroke who reported getting out as often as they wanted and doubled the number of monthly outdoor journeys, compared to participants in the control group.[20]

In order to see whether people with stroke were receiving this intervention from community-based rehabilitation teams in a region of Sydney, local therapists and the author of this chapter (AMC) conducted a retrospective medical record audit. The audit revealed that therapists were documenting very little about outdoor journeys and transport after stroke. Documented information about the number of weekly outings was present in only 14% of medical records (see Table 16.1). Furthermore, only 17% of people with stroke were receiving six or more sessions of intervention that targeted outdoor journeys, which was the 'dose' of intervention provided in the original trial by Logan and colleagues.[20,21] The audit data highlighted an evidence–practice gap, specifically, the underuse of an evidence-based intervention. This example will be used as the third case study throughout the chapter, to illustrate the process of implementation.

	N	%
Screening for outdoor mobility and travel		
Driving status documented (pre-stroke or current)	37	48
Preferred mode of travel documents	27	35
Reasons for limited outdoor journeys documented	26	34
Number of weekly outdoor journeys documented	11	14
Outdoor journey intervention		
At least 1 session provided	44	57
2 sessions or more provided	27	35
6 sessions or more provided	13	17

*Intervention to help increase outdoor journeys as described by Logan and colleagues.[20, 21]

TABLE 16.1 Summary of baseline file audits (n=77) involving five community rehabilitation teams describing screening and provision of an evidence-based intervention* for people with stroke

The process of implementation

The following sections summarise two models that may help you better understand the steps and factors involved in implementing evidence.

Model 1: The evidence-to-practice pipeline

The 'evidence pipeline' described by Glazsiou and Haynes[22] and shown in Figure 16.1 provides a helpful illustration of steps in the implementation process. This metaphoric pipeline highlights how leakage can occur, drip by drip, along the way from awareness of evidence to the point of delivery to clients. First, there is an ever-expanding pool of published research to read, both original and synthesised research. This large volume of information causes busy professionals to miss important, valid evidence (*awareness*). Then, assuming they have heard of the benefits of a successful intervention (or the overuse of a test procedure), professionals may need persuasion to change their practice (*acceptance*). They may be more inclined to provide a familiar intervention with which they are confident and which clients expect and value. Hidden social pressure from clients and other team members can make practice changes less likely to occur. Busy professionals also need to recognise appropriate clients who should receive the intervention (or not receive a test procedure). Professionals then need to apply this knowledge in the course of a working day (*applicability*).

Some test procedures and interventions will require new skills and knowledge. For example, the delivery of cognitive behavioural therapy to adolescents with depression involves special training, instruction manuals, extra study and supervision. A lack of skills and knowledge may be a barrier to practice change for professionals who need to deliver the intervention (*able*). A further challenge is that, while we may be aware of an intervention, accept the need to provide it and are able to deliver it, we may not act on the evidence all of the time (*acted on*). We may forget—or more likely—we may find it difficult to change well-established habits. For example, general practitioners who have been referring people with acute back pain for an X-ray for many years may find this practice difficult to stop.

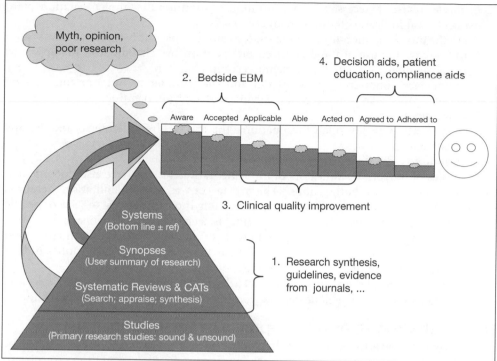

FIGURE 16.1 The research-to-practice pipeline

Reproduced from: Glasziou P and Haynes B, The paths from research to improved health outcomes, 10, 4–7, 2005, with permission from BMJ Publishing Group Ltd[22]

The evidence-to-practice pipeline illustrates the steps involved in maximising the acceptance and uptake of research findings. The final two steps rely on clients agreeing to a different test procedure than they expect (*agree*) and changing their behaviour to comply with an intervention. For example, people with low back pain will need to stay active within the level of comfort permitted by their low back pain (*adherence*). Any intervention that involves a major change in behaviour, for example exercise or the use of cognitive behavioural therapy principles, is likely to be difficult for many people to adopt and maintain.

Model 2: Plan and prepare model

A different process of implementation has been proposed by Grol and Wensing.[3] Their bottom line is 'plan and prepare'. While intended for the implementation of clinical guidelines, the principles apply equally well to the implementation of test ordering, outcome measurement or interventions and for procedures that are either under- or overused. The 'plan and prepare' model involves five key steps:

1. *Write* a proposal for change with clear aims and target groups.
2. *Analyse* the target groups and setting for barriers, problems, enablers and other factors that may hinder or help the change process.
3. *Decide* on implementation strategies to help professionals learn about, adopt and sustain the practice change.
4. *Execute* the implementation plan, documenting a list of activities, tasks and a timeline.

5. *Evaluate,* revise if necessary and continuously monitor the implementation plan, using clinical indicators to measure ongoing success.

Using the travel and mobility training study as an example, the two primary aims were:
- to increase the use of the underused intervention by rehabilitation therapists, as recommended by a national guideline recommendation
- to increase community participation and the number of outdoor journeys by people with stroke who received the evidence-based intervention.

The two target groups were:
- rehabilitation professionals (occupational therapists, physiotherapists and therapy assistants)
- community-dwelling people with stroke.

Examples of 'targets' or indicators of implementation success were also documented early in this project, for both groups.[9] The first target was that rehabilitation therapists would deliver an outdoor mobility and travel training intervention[20,21] to 75% of people with stroke who were referred to the service (that is, a change in professional behaviour). The second target was that 75% of people with stroke who received the intervention would report getting out of the house as often as they wanted and take more outdoor journeys per month compared to pre-intervention.

Other steps in the 'plan and prepare' model (identifying barriers and enablers, selecting implementation strategies) will be discussed, using examples, in the following sections.

Demonstrating an evidence–practice gap (gap analysis)

A common first step is to identify and clarify the evidence–practice gap which needs to be bridged. Most health professionals who seek funding for an implementation project, and post-graduate students who write research proposals, will demonstrate their evidence–practice gap using simple data collection methods. Surveys and medical record audits are the most popular methods.

Surveys for gap analysis

A survey can be developed and used, with health professionals or clients, to explore attitudes, knowledge and current practices. If a large proportion of health professionals admit to knowing little about, or rarely using, an evidence-based intervention, this information represents the evidence–practice gap. In the cognitive behavioural therapy example discussed earlier,[8] a local survey was used to explore attitudes to, knowledge and use of cognitive behavioural therapy by community mental health professionals.

The process of developing a survey to explore attitudes and behavioural intentions has been well documented in a manual by Jill Francis and colleagues.[23] The manual is intended for use by health service researchers who want to predict and understand behaviour and measures constructs associated with the Theory of Planned Behaviour. Behavioural theories will be discussed in a later section of this chapter. If you intend to develop your own local survey or questionnaire, whether the survey is for gap analysis or barrier analysis, it is recommended that you consult this excellent resource. Sample questions include: 'Do you intend to do (intervention X) with all of your clients?' and 'Do you believe that you will be able to do X with your clients?'

Audits for gap analysis

Audit is another method which can be used to demonstrate an evidence–practice gap. A small medical record audit can be conducted using local data (for example, 10 medical records may be selected, reflecting consecutive admissions over three months). The audit can be used to determine how many people with a health condition received a test or an evidence-based intervention. For example, we could determine the proportion of people with acute back pain for whom an X-ray had been ordered in a general practice over the previous three months. We could also count how frequently (or rarely) an intervention was used.

In the travel and mobility training study, it was possible to determine the proportion of people with stroke who had received one or more sessions from an occupational therapist or physiotherapist to help increase outdoor journeys.[9] Baseline medical record audits of 77 consecutive referrals across five services in the previous year revealed that 44/77 (57%) people with stroke had received at least one session targeting outdoor journeys, but 22/77 (35%) had received two or more sessions, and only 13/77 (17%) had received six or more sessions. In the original randomised controlled trial that evaluated this intervention,[20, 21] a median of six sessions targeting outdoor journeys had been provided by therapists. This number of sessions was considered the optimal 'dose' (or target) of intervention.

It has been recommended that more than one method should be used to collect data on current practice, as part of a gap analysis (for example, an audit and a survey).[2] Collecting information from a small but representative sample of health professionals or clients, using both qualitative and quantitative methods, can be useful.[2]

In Australia, examples of evidence–practice gaps in health care are summarised annually by the National Institute of Clinical Studies (NICS).[24] This organisation highlights gaps between what is known and what is practised. For example, recent reports have described evidence–practice gaps in the following areas: underuse of smoking cessation programs by pregnant mothers, suboptimal management of acute pain and cancer pain in hospitalised patients and underuse of preventative interventions for venous thromboembolism in hospitalised patients.[25]

After collating quantitative and qualitative information from a representative sample of health professionals and/or clients in a facility, the next step is to identify potential barriers and enablers to implementation.

Identifying barriers and enablers to implementation (barrier analysis)

Barriers are factors or conditions that may prevent successful implementation of evidence. Conversely, enablers are factors that increase the likelihood of success. Barriers and enablers can be attributed to individuals (for example, attitudes or knowledge), groups and teams (for example, professional roles) or clients (for example, expectations about treatment). When barriers and enablers have been identified, a tailored program of strategies can be developed.

Attitudinal barriers are easy to recognise. Most health professionals will know someone in their team or organisation that resists change. Perhaps they have been exposed to too much change and innovation. Knowledge, skill and systems barriers are often less obvious (for example: Do team members know how to deliver cognitive behavioural therapy? Do they have access to manuals, video-recorders or vehicles for community visits?). Experienced health professionals may be reluctant to acknowledge a lack of skills, knowledge or confidence. Qualitative methods such as interviews can be useful for investigating what people know, how confident they feel and what they think about local policies, procedures and systems. Social influences can also be a barrier (or an enabler), but may be invisible. For example, clients may expect and place pressure on health professionals to order tests or deliver particular interventions.

Methods for identifying barriers are similar to those used for identifying evidence–practice gaps: surveys, individual and group interviews (or informal chats) and observation of practice.[26,27] Sometimes it may be helpful to use two or more methods. The choice of method will be guided by time and resources, as well as local circumstances and the number of health professionals involved.

The travel and mobility training study involved community occupational therapists, physiotherapists and therapy assistants from two different teams. Individual interviews were conducted with these health professionals. Interviews were tape-recorded with their consent (ethics approval was obtained), and the content was transcribed and analysed. The decision to conduct individual interviews was based on a desire to find out what different disciplines knew and thought about the planned intervention and about professional roles and responsibilities. Rich and informative data were obtained;[10] however, this method produced a large quantity of information which was time-consuming to collect, transcribe and analyse. A survey or focus group would be more efficient for busy health professionals to use in practice. Examples of quotes from the interviews and four types of barriers from this study are presented in Figure 16.2.

Examples of questions to ask during interviews or in a survey, and potential barriers and enablers to consider, are listed in Box 16.2. The list has been adapted from a publication by Michie and colleagues.[28]

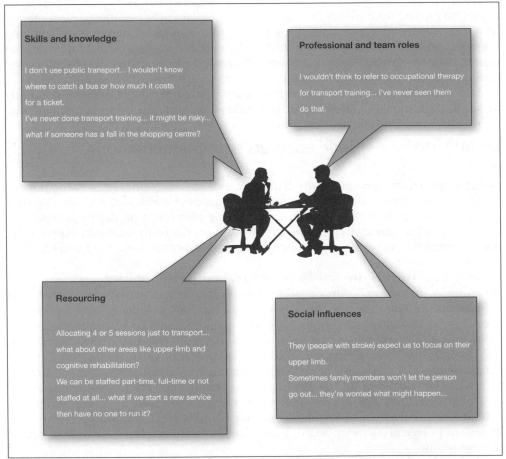

FIGURE 16.2 Barriers to the delivery of a communication-based outdoor journey intervention for people with stroke, identified through qualitative interviews with allied health professionals (n=13)

> ## BOX 16.2 **EXAMPLES OF QUESTIONS TO ASK DURING AN INTERVIEW OR IN A SURVEY WHEN IDENTIFYING POTENTIAL BARRIERS AND ENABLERS**
>
> - Do health professionals know about, accept and believe the evidence? **(knowledge, attitudes, values)**
> - Does the original research describe what to do and how to do it in sufficient detail? Is there a protocol for the intervention? Do health professionals know what to do? **(knowledge, skills, abilities)**
> - Are health professionals confident that they can provide the intervention? **(attitudes, capabilities, confidence)**
> - Do health professionals want to provide the intervention? **(motivation)**
> - Do health professionals intend to provide the intervention? **(intention)**
> - Is there an expectation from other team members or clients that the intervention will be provided? **(social influence)**
> - Do health professionals have the necessary equipment, space, manuals and staff to provide the intervention routinely? **(resources and staffing)**

While client expectations of intervention can be sought, this step often appears to be omitted during barrier analysis. A systematic review of treatment expectations confirmed that most people with acute low back pain who consult their general practitioner expect additional diagnostic tests to be ordered and a referral to be made to specialists.[29] General practitioners in another study also reported a tendency to 'give in' to client demands for an X-ray and referral to a physiotherapist.[30] McKenzie and colleagues[7] targeted this lack of confidence as part of their implementation strategy. To help practitioners refer fewer clients for an X-ray, workshops were conducted to model, rehearse and practise persuasive communication techniques during client consultations. Such strategies targeted the skills, knowledge and confidence of health professionals, who had to overcome pressure and social influence from clients.

Resources which can be used to identify barriers and enablers include those produced by the National Institute for Health and Clinical Excellence (NICE) in the UK[26] and the National Institute of Clinical Studies (NICS) in Australia.[27] An important next step is selecting evidence-based strategies to target identified barriers.

Implementation strategies and interventions

A range of strategies and interventions have been used to target barriers, help health professionals change their behaviour and get evidence into practice. The list is extensive. Frequently used strategies are listed below:

- Educational materials[31,32]
- Educational meetings[33]
- Educational outreach visits[34,35] including academic detailing
- The use of external facilitators[36]
- The use of opinion leaders
- Reminders[37,38] including client-mediated and computer-aided interventions
- Audit and feedback[39,40]
- Team building/practice development
- Tailored (targeted) interventions to overcome identified local barriers[41]
- Multifaceted interventions, including several of the above strategies[42]

Only some of these strategies have been evaluated for effectiveness and summarised in systematic reviews or 'overviews' of reviews.[43,44] Some of the commonly used strategies, and findings from more recent systematic reviews, are discussed next.

Educational materials

This strategy includes the distribution of published or printed materials such as clinical guideline summaries and guideline recommendations. Some authors also include audiovisual materials and electronic publications in their definition of educational materials. Content may be delivered personally or through mass mailouts. Materials may or may not target known knowledge and skill barriers. Such materials are relatively low cost and feasible to provide, but are unlikely to be effective if they do not target local knowledge barriers.

In Chapter 13, you learnt about the potential value of evidence-based clinical guidelines. In an attempt to get health professionals to use clinical guidelines, they are typically printed and mailed out to them. On its own, mailed dissemination of guidelines is known to have little or no effect on behaviour. Consequently, this process of mailing out guidelines to professionals is often used with control groups, in cluster randomised controlled trials. For example, in the study by McKenzie and colleagues,[7] doctors in the control group of practices received guideline recommendations about the management of acute low back pain. These guidelines were not expected to change doctors' X-ray ordering behaviour.

A recent Cochrane review on the effect of printed educational materials located and appraised 23 studies.[31] When randomised controlled trials were analysed alone (n=6), the median effect was a 4% absolute improvement, with an interquartile range of −8% to 10% for categorical outcomes such as X-ray requests and smoking cessation. The relative risk difference for continuous process outcomes such as medication change and X-ray requests per practice was greater (median change 14%, interquartile range −5% to 27%) based on four randomised controlled trials. However, there was no positive effect on clients' outcomes. Indeed, a negative effect or deterioration in client outcomes was reported when data were analysed. The median effect was −4% (interquartile range −1% to −5%) for categorical outcomes such as return to work, screening for a health condition or smoking cessation. The authors concluded that, when compared to no intervention, printed educational materials may positively influence practitioner behaviour, but they do not improve client outcomes. An earlier review of studies up to 1998, which included five randomised controlled trials, reported a median effect of 8% (interquartile range 4% to 17%) improvement in practitioner performance, but did not report on client outcomes.[32]

The overall effect of educational materials probably lies somewhere between 4% and 8%, but certainly less than 10% improvement. As will be shown in this chapter, few interventions to change practitioner behaviour result in changes greater than 10%.

Educational meetings

This strategy includes workshops, conferences, meetings and in-services, which are intended to increase awareness, impart knowledge and develop skills. Meetings can be interactive or didactic. The former may target skills, attitudes and knowledge, whereas didactic sessions mainly target knowledge barriers. Ideally, these sessions target identified skills or knowledge barriers. If practitioners indicate lack of confidence with a new practice, such as cognitive behavioural therapy in the study by Kramer and Burns,[8] educational meetings can help to address the need. In response to therapists' preferences, Kramer and Burns provided a one-day training session which prepared therapists to deliver motivational interviewing and cognitive behavioural therapy, educate adolescents about depression, promote medication adherence and assess ongoing suicide risk.

In the travel and mobility training study, occupational therapists and physiotherapists indicated a lack of awareness about the published evidence, as well as a need for information about local transport systems (for example, local bus routes and ticketing systems) and risk management strategies when escorting a person with stroke across roads, to local shops and on public transport.[10] They also indicated a preference for a half-day workshop, which was provided.

Two reviews have examined the effect of educational meetings and both were published in 2001.[33,44] Thompson O'Brien and colleagues reported on 32 studies which evaluated the effect of educational materials.[44] Appraisal of these studies revealed much variation in the complexity of behaviours targeted, characteristics of interventions used and results. Mixed effects were reported for didactic sessions alone, with no statistically significant differences in the majority of studies. Didactic sessions used as part of a workshop, and involving some interaction, resulted in small to moderate effects, with 11 of 12 comparisons being statistically significant. Moderate to moderately large effects, which were statistically significant, were reported for interactive workshops, in six of ten comparisons.

A second review of systematic reviews examined the effect of professional educational interventions, including continuing medical education meetings, on quality of care.[44] Grimshaw and colleagues found 41 reviews published up to July 1998, with 15 focussing on broad strategies including continuing education. However, none of the tabled results comment specifically on the effect of educational interventions such as workshops and conferences.

The effect of educational meetings was also reported in 1998, in another review of systematic reviews.[43] In total, 18 reviews were located and appraised. Consistent with the findings of Thompson O'Brien and colleagues,[33] these reviewers found that interactive educational meetings which included discussion or practice of skills seemed to consistently improve professional behaviour. On the contrary, didactic educational meetings such as lectures had little or no effect on professional behaviour.

Educational outreach visits

An educational outreach visit is defined as a face-to-face visit by a trained person to the practice setting of health professionals, with the intent of improving practice.[32,35] This strategy is also known as educational or academic detailing and educational visiting.[35] The aim may be to decrease prescribing or test-ordering behaviours and/or increase screening practices and/or the routine delivery of an evidence-based intervention. This strategy is derived from social marketing and uses social persuasion methods to target individual knowledge and attitudes. Sessions aim to transmit a small number of messages (two or three) in 15 to 20 minutes, using an approach tailored to individual professionals or practices. Typically, the focus is on simple behaviours such as medication prescribing habits.

An example of the use of outreach visits to change practice is where a trained pharmacist visited general practitioners to discuss childhood asthma management, while also leaving educational materials about best practice. The effect of the educational outreach visits was tested using a cluster randomised controlled trial design and involved multiple general practices in a township near Cape Town, South Africa.[34] Parents of children provided survey data on asthma severity and symptom frequency. Asthma symptom scores declined by 0.84 points more (on a 9-point scale, $p = 0.03$) in children whose doctors had received outreach visits compared to the control group of children.

For every child with asthma seen in a practice which received outreach visits, the authors report that one extra child will experience substantially reduced symptoms.

A systematic review of studies published up until 1998 examined the effect of outreach visits on professional practice.[32,38] This review located and analysed 13 cluster randomised controlled trials and five controlled before and after studies, with most evaluating outreach visits as part of a multifaceted intervention. When outreach visits were provided as part of a multifaceted intervention, they improved practice by a median of 6% (interquartile range –4% to 17%). The reviewers suggested that organisations should carefully consider the resources and cost involved in providing outreach visits for this modest (6%) change in behaviour. More recently, a Cochrane review on the effect of educational outreach visits was updated.[35] This review appraised 69 studies published up until March 2007, involving more than 15,000 health professionals; 28 studies contributed to the median effect size. The reviewers reported a median (adjusted risk) difference in practice of 6% (interquartile range 3% to 9%). Many of the studies evaluated the effect of outreach visits on prescribing practice. The median effect was more varied when other types of professional practice were examined (median 6%, interquartile range 4% to 16%). The effect of outreach visits was slightly superior to audit and feedback when the two strategies were compared (in eight trials). When individual visits were compared to group visits (three trials), the results were mixed.

Reminders

Reminders aim to prompt a health professional to recall information, such as performing or avoiding some action, to improve individual client care. These strategies include client-mediated information, encounter-specific information and computer-aided decision support.

Encounter-specific information refers to the use of reminders that are delivered to a health professional and are associated with particular encounters, such as breast screening or dental reviews, or a particular test result. In one example, educational messages about diabetes care were delivered to general practitioners with blood test results to help improve the quality of diabetes care.[37] Two examples of messages attached to HbA_{1c} (haemoglobin/blood test) reports were: 'If HbA_{1c} <6.5% = within target for type 2 diabetes'; and 'If HbA_{1c} 6.5–7.0% = for type 2 diabetes, consider increasing oral therapy'. Reminders might also prompt health professionals to conduct a foot examination or discuss smoking cessation with at-risk people with diabetes.

Client-mediated information involves giving the person with the health condition information which helps to drive health professionals' practice. One example is the use of a 'diabetes passport'[45]—a client-held record. A client takes the passport to appointments, to help prompt monitoring by health professionals of blood pressure and foot health care, among other health indicators. After introducing the passports to clients and embedding the passport into general practices in the Netherlands, the effect on client health outcomes was evaluated using a randomised controlled trial design.[46] Diabetes passports were issued to 87% of eligible clients. After 15 months, 76% of clients reported that the passport was being used, and referred to, during clinic visits.

In the travel and mobility training study, fluorescent pink stickers were provided as a reminder to therapists, containing the messages 'Screened for outdoor journeys' and 'Intervention provided targeting outdoor journeys'. These stickers were placed on the desks of occupational therapists and physiotherapists. The first sticker reminded therapists to ask a series of screening questions about driving status and community outings, complete a screening form and place the form in the client's file, accompanied by the sticker and a file entry. The second sticker prompted therapists to deliver an outdoor journey intervention to people with stroke who were not getting out as often as they wanted, then document the content of sessions in the client's file, accompanied by the sticker.

Evidence for the effectiveness of reminders is higher than for most other implementation strategies. In a review of 14 trials that had been published up until 1998, it was found that the median effect of reminders was 14% (interquartile range, −1% to 34%).[38] While 14% may seem a small effect size for an intervention, the amount of change from implementation strategies is typically lower than 10%. A change of 14% in behaviour is considered a good outcome for a first 'round' of implementation. Behaviour can be expected to improve further with continuous monitoring and feedback, or when combined with other strategies.

Audit and feedback

Audit refers to any summary of clinical performance over a specified period of time. Feedback about audit findings may be written or oral, and the summary may or may not include details of compliance with audit criteria and recommendations for action. Audit information can be obtained from medical records, computerised databases or by observing clients and professionals. Implementation literature describes audit and feedback together because there is limited value in conducting an audit if the target professionals do not receive feedback about the findings. Thus, some form of feedback about audit findings is needed.

One aim of audit and feedback is to create some urgency in the health professionals about the need for change. Without objective data from audits, health professionals are likely to perceive that their practice is within acceptable levels. However, it has been demonstrated that self-reports of behaviour are likely to overestimate performance by up to 27%.[47]

Audits are the mainstay of quality improvement activities, yet surprisingly few health professionals have conducted a medical record audit. If they have, the audit has typically focussed on compliance with note writing and record keeping (for example, whether or not notes were initialled, dated and profession-specific stickers were used). Rarely do medical record audits focus on the content of the interventions. Even fewer audits seem to focus on evidence-based interventions. Audits conducted as part of an implementation process focus on evidence-based processes; for example, 'Of 50 medical records audited, what proportion of clients were asked screening questions, as recommended in a clinical guideline?' or 'What proportion of clients were given written educational materials, as recommended in a clinical guideline?'

A recent Cochrane review of randomised trials investigated the effect of clinical audits, with or without feedback.[40] It was found that feedback does improve practice, but the effects are small to moderate. Comparison of dichotomous outcome data from 118 trials, involving 13,500 health professionals, resulted in a median-adjusted risk difference in compliance with desired practice of 5% (interquartile range, 3% to 11%). Thus, the probability of compliance with desired practice due to audit and feedback was approximately 5% greater, compared to other interventions or no intervention. For continuous outcomes, the median-adjusted risk percentage change in practice compared to controls was 16% (interquartile range 5% to 37%). Larger effects were seen if baseline adherence to recommended practice was low and feedback intensity was high. Audit and feedback should therefore be viewed as a helpful quality improvement strategy, but cannot yet be recommended as part of 'evidence-based' implementation to effect change because of the costs associated with data extraction and analysis.

In summary, the effects of several implementation strategies have been evaluated in systematic reviews. Most strategies lead to a small change in practice (no greater than

10%). Larger changes can be expected if compliance with practice at baseline is low. Health professionals and service managers who evaluate change due to implementation should not be surprised by small changes of this magnitude. A process of continuous quality improvement is the best way to improve practice in line with the evidence. For updates on the effectiveness of these and other strategies to change behaviour, visit the website of the Cochrane Effective Practice and Organisation of Care (EPOC) review group (http://www.epoc.cochrane.org/en/index. html).

The use of theory to support evidence implementation

Implementation of evidence is a complex process involving change in attitudes, systems and behaviour. Theories and frameworks are helpful for explaining complex processes. Thus it is helpful to theorise about why a person, organisation or profession succeeded or had difficulty with change such as delivering an intervention or ceasing to use a test procedure. Theories can also be used for planning. We can anticipate potential problems, such as a change in professionals' (or client) roles, and target these in advance.

The use of a theory or theoretical framework is now recommended to help identify and address factors that influence the adoption of a new practice behaviour.[48,49] Change theories can help us predict who might change, who might be resistant to change, how change might be experienced and the stages of change that most people will move through. Theories can also help inform the development of survey instruments[23,50] and interview questions about barriers to evidence uptake.[28] Researchers seeking funding and postgraduate students investigating the implementation of innovations are now expected to use theories to guide their research.

Grol and colleagues[49] have proposed a taxonomy of theories which aim to explain or predict 1) individual behaviour change (for example, attitudes, routines, motivation), 2) the effect of social context on change (for example, social/peer pressure, opinion leaders, role models) and 3) organisational or team behaviour change (for example, culture, systems, resources). The authors note that most theories overlap, sometimes to a large extent. Grol and colleagues summarised each 'type' of theory. Behaviour theories aim to explain behaviour. Cognitive theories aim to explain thought processes, attitudes and values. Social theories aim to explain how social groups or systems operate. Problems can occur at any level. For more in-depth information about this, you may wish to read their summary.[49]

Theories which explain behaviour change

Some theories explain how change is experienced and factors which promote change. Examples include the **transtheoretical stages of change theory** by Prochaska and DiClemente and the diffusions of innovation theory by Rogers.[51] The stages of change theory has been used to guide many implementation studies, particularly those targeting public health behaviours such as cigarette smoking and alcohol consumption.[52] Individuals at each of the stages (for example, pre-contemplation, contemplation, preparation and action) are typically targeted with different behaviour change strategies. However, a systematic review which examined the body of research on interventions based on the stages of change theory found no difference in outcomes (amount of behaviour change) in studies using this theory, compared to studies that were not based on this theory.[53]

Another use of the stages of change theory has been for the development of an instrument to measure attitudes and readiness to change (Clinician Readiness to Measure Outcomes Scale (CReMOS)).[50] The aim of the CReMOS is to measure health professionals' attitudes to outcome measurement and self-reported changes in attitude and practice, as a result of learning about standardised outcome measures. Sample statements from the 26-item CReMOS questionnaire, associated with the five stages of change, include:

- I know my interventions work. I do not need to measure them. *(Precontemplation)*
- Measuring outcomes would be good if it did not mean spending time doing extra paperwork. *(Contemplation)*
- I have had someone teach me how to search electronic databases to locate relevant outcome measures for my clients. *(Preparation)*
- I have trialled some outcome measures with my clients. *(Action)*
- I have been measuring outcomes with my clients for at least 6 months. *(Maintenance)*

The highly influential **theory of diffusion of innovations** has been used to help spread many innovations in health services and has been comprehensively reviewed by Greenhalgh and colleagues.[4,54] Diffusion is a passive process of social influence, whereas dissemination and implementation are active, planned processes that aim to encourage the adoption of an innovation. The original theory proposed that the spread or diffusion of ideas about a new practice could be achieved by harnessing the influence of opinion leaders and change agents. The social networks of targeted individuals could be mapped and targeted during the diffusion process (who knows whom, and who copies whom). Some individuals lead the adoption (innovators), while others become champions and opinion leaders (the early adopters). A large proportion of individuals adopt the change in practice when change becomes inevitable (the early majority) and can be used to encourage and persuade others (the late majority). And finally, there are always non-adopters who will only change when forced to do so by policy or performance review (the laggards).

Studies and organisations which talk about using 'opinion leaders' and 'champions' are using ideas from the diffusion of innovations theory. One such study in occupational therapy[55] involved using a local opinion leader to teach therapists about evidence-based practice, when the phenomenon was new and considered an 'innovation'. Funding was obtained to train 100 occupational therapists how to search for, and critically appraise, research evidence. The local opinion leader delivered a two-day workshop and encouraged therapists to become 'champions' of evidence-based practice in their organisation. To help spread the innovation, therapists provided in-services at work for other staff and established journal clubs.[56]

Theories which predict behaviour change

Theories which can help us to anticipate or predict behaviour change include Ajzen's theory of planned behaviour[57] and a psychological theory of behaviour change developed by Michie and colleagues.[28] When planning to implement evidence, we are often interested in theories which help predict who will, and will not, adopt new practice behaviours. Questions and topics derived from these theories have been used in surveys and interviews and to map results.

The **Theory of Planned Behaviour**[23,57] is one of the most frequently used theoretical frameworks. This theory proposes that intention and perceived control over behaviour are proxy predictors of behaviour and, while these constructs cannot be directly observed, they can be inferred from questionnaire or survey responses.[23] To predict whether a person intends to do something, we need to know whether that person is in favour of doing it ('attitude'), how much the person feels social pressure to do it ('subjective norm') and whether they feel in control of the action in question ('perceived behavioural control'). The Theory of Planned Behaviour proposes that these three constructs—attitudes, subjective norms and perceived behavioural control—predict the intention to perform a behaviour. A recent systematic review reported that there is, indeed, a predictable relationship between the intentions of a health professional and their subsequent behaviour.[58] Surveys and questionnaires based on the theory have been developed and used to investigate attitudes to and beliefs about the uptake of evidence.[23]

The **Psychological Theory of Behaviour Change**[28] is a more recent addition to the list of theories and also aims to help professionals and researchers anticipate and predict behaviour change. The authors of this theory have proposed 12 domains which can be used to inform the implementation of evidence, in particular for identifying barriers and strategies to target known barriers. The domains are shown in Table 16.2.

Focus/domain of question	Theory of planned behaviour[23]	Psychological theory of behaviour change[28]
Knowledge		Do you know about the evidence/guideline? Do you know you should be doing X?
Skills		Do you know how to deliver X? How easy or difficult do you find performing X? How confident are you about being able to perform X to the required standard in the required context?
Intentions, motivations and goals	Do you intend to do X with all of your clients? Of the next 10 clients you see with a diagnosis of Y, for how many would you expect to do X?	How much do you want to do X? How much do you feel a need to do X? Are there other things you want to do or achieve that might interfere with X? Does the evidence/guideline conflict with other interventions you want to deliver? Are there incentives to do X?
Attitudes and emotions	Are there any issues that come to mind when you think about doing X? Overall do you think that doing X is harmful/pleasant; the right thing to do; the wrong thing to do; good practice?	Does doing X evoke an emotional response? To what extent do emotional factors facilitate or hinder X?
Professional/ social roles	Is it expected that you will do X?	Do you think guidelines or evidence should determine your behaviour? Is doing X compatible or in conflict with your professional role/standards/identity? Would this be true for all professional groups involved?

TABLE 16.2 Examples of questions to ask about barriers to implementation based on two theories of behaviour change— (Cont'd)

Focus/domain of question	Theory of planned behaviour[23]	Psychological theory of behaviour change[28]
Beliefs about capabilities	Do you believe that you will be able to do X with the client?	How easy or difficult is it for you to do X? How confident are you that you can do X in spite of the difficulties? What would help you do X? How capable are you of maintaining X? How well equipped/comfortable do you feel about doing X?
Beliefs about consequences		What do you think will happen (to yourself, clients, colleagues and the organisation—positive and negative, short- and long-term consequences) if you do X? What are the costs of X? What do you think will happen if you do not do X? Do the benefits of doing X outweigh the costs? Does the evidence suggest that doing X is a good thing?
Memory, attention and decision processes		Is X something you usually do? Will you think or remember to do X? How much attention will you have to pay to doing X? Might you decide not to do X? Why?
Environmental context and resources		To what extent do physical or resource factors facilitate or hinder X? Are there competing tasks and time constraints? Are the necessary resources (staff, equipment etc) available to you and others who are expected to do X?
Social influence or pressure	Are there any individuals or groups who would approve or disapprove of you doing X? Do you feel under any social pressure to do X with your clients? Do your clients expect or want X?	To what extent do social influences (for example peers, managers, other professional groups, clients, clients' relatives) facilitate or hinder X? Do you observe others performing X? (i.e. Do you have role models?)
Behavioural regulation		What preparatory steps (individual or organisational) are needed to do X? Are there procedures or ways of working that encourage you to do X?
Nature of the behaviours		What is the proposed behaviour? Who needs to do what differently, when, where, how, how often and with whom? What do you currently do? Is this a new behaviour or an existing behaviour that needs to become a habit? Are there systems for maintaining longer term change?

TABLE 16.2 Examples of questions to ask about barriers to implementation based on two theories of behaviour change

As an example, in the travel and mobility training study involving occupational therapists and physiotherapists,[10] interview questions probed for therapists' attitudes, skills and knowledge, as well as role expectations about an outdoor journey intervention for people with stroke. The Psychological Theory of Behaviour Change provided a structure during interviews and, later, during analysis. Some brief examples of comments from therapists are presented in Figure 16.2. The majority of comments made during the 13 interviews could be mapped to two domains: beliefs about capabilities and social influences.

- **Beliefs about capabilities:**

  It is quite a time-consuming intervention, in terms of the number of clients you can see, and the number of hours. I think it would be hard to get to the six [sessions of the outdoor journey intervention].

  The whole scooter thing is still something they [occupational therapists] are nervous about. How do we know the person's appropriate for a scooter? How do you assess a person … ? and stuff around insurance and all that sort of thing … ? A lot of therapists don't get much exposure (to motorised scooters). I have never done a scooter prescription.

  Asking about driving, when someone is so unwell, can be an area that you don't want to go to. It can be the last thing on their mind, and the carers' mind. 'Oh no! He won't get back to driving!' These sorts of things could be a bit difficult to initiate in conversation.

- **Social influence (from clients and carers):**

  Sometimes they (people with stroke) are completely focussed on their mobility, and tend to think of it (an outdoor journey intervention) as more of a physio thing. Maybe they won't bring it up with us (the occupational therapists). Others are more focussed on getting their arm to work again. Trying to identify goals different from that can be hard. Usually they have been told 'We're referring you for upper limb therapy' and they become very focussed on that. They don't want to look at getting out and about.

  We could only achieve the goals he wanted to (work on) and would agree to.

  His wife isn't confident that he can do it. She says, 'No, he won't be able to do it'. Last week they had the opportunity to catch the train into the therapy session here, but the wife called the son to tell him to take the day off work to bring him in. So we've planned a visit to the coffee shop that he went to. It means catching a train, getting him to buy the tickets and so on. It's cognitive as well as language. But his wife isn't confident he can do it ….

Summary points of this chapter

- Implementation is a planned and active process of using published research in practice. Another term for implementation is knowledge transfer. Both processes aim to help close evidence–practice gaps.
- The process of implementation involves a series of steps which include demonstrating an evidence–practice gap; identifying barriers and enablers to implementation; deciding on the best strategies and interventions to help health professionals learn about, adopt and sustain behaviour change; and then executing and evaluating the implementation plan.

- Surveys and medical record audits are popular methods for identifying an evidence–practice gap. These methods explore and measure attitudes, knowledge and practice behaviours. More than one method should be used to collect data on current practice for a gap analysis, from a small but representative sample of health professionals and/or clients, preferably using both qualitative and quantitative methods.
- Common barriers to evidence implementation include: attitudes, beliefs, skills and knowledge of professionals; role expectations (professional and social); influences of other professionals, clients and family members; systems; and policies. Barriers are unique to local teams and organisations and time should be spent identifying local barriers. These can then be targeted with tailored implementation strategies.
- Strategies for implementing evidence in practice include, but are not limited to: educational materials, meetings and outreach visits, external facilitators, local opinion leaders, reminders and audit and feedback.
- None of these implementation strategies is likely to change practice by more than 10% at any one time. Behaviours with low baseline compliance are likely to change the most.
- Surveys and questionnaires, as well as focus groups and interviews, should be informed by theoretical constructs from behaviour, cognitive or social theories. This means that questions should ask about intentions, beliefs, attitudes, values, expectations, social systems and networks.

References

1. Grol R. Implementation of changes in practice. In: Grol R, Wensing M, Eccles M (eds). Improving patient care: the implementation of change in clinical practice. Edinburgh: Elsevier Butterworth–Heinemann; 2005:6–15.
2. van Bokhoven M, Kok G, Weijden V. Designing a quality improvement intervention: A systematic approach. Qual Saf Health Care 2003; 12:215–220.
3. Grol R, Wensing M. Effective implementation: a model. In: Grol R, Wensing M, Eccles M (eds). Improving patient care: the implementation of change in clinical practice. Edinburgh: Elsevier Butterworth–Heinemann; 2005:41–57.
4. Greenhalgh T, Robert G, Bate P et al. Diffusions of innovations in health service organisations: a systematic review. Oxford, UK: BMJ Books; 2005.
5. Woolf SH. The meaning of translational research and why it matters. JAMA 2008; 299:211–213.
6. Davis DA, Evans M, Jadad AR et al. The case for knowledge translation: shortening the journey from evidence to effect. BMJ 2003; 327:33–35.
7. McKenzie J, French S, O'Connor D et al. IMPLEmenting a clinical practice guideline for acute low back pain evidence-based manageMENT in general practice (IMPLEMENT): cluster randomised controlled trial study protocol. Implement Sci 2008; 3:11.
8. Kramer T, Burns B. Implementing cognitive behavioural therapy in the real world: a case study of two mental health centres. Implement Sci 2008; 3:14.
9. McCluskey A, Middleton S. Feasibility of implementing an evidence-based outdoor journey intervention in community stroke rehabilitation: changes in team behaviour and patient outcomes. Unpublished data.
10. McCluskey A, Middleton S. Delivering an evidence-based outdoor journey intervention to people with stroke: barriers and enablers experienced by community rehabilitation teams. Under review.
11. Britt H, Miller G, Charles J et al. General practice activity in Australia 2005–06. General Practice Series No 19 AIHW Cat No GEP 19. Canberra: Australian Institute of Health and Welfare; 2007.
12. Australian Acute Musculoskeletal Pain Guidelines Group (AAMPGG). Evidence-based management of acute musculoskeletal pain. Brisbane: Australian Academic Press; 2003.
13. McGuirk B, King W, Govind J et al. Safety, efficacy and cost effectiveness of evidence-based guidelines for the management of acute low back pain in primary care. Spine 2001; 26:2615–2622.
14. Klein J, Jacobs R, Reinecke M. Cognitive-behavioural therapy for adolescent depression: a meta-analytic investigation of changes in effect-size estimates. J Am Acad Child Adolesc Psychiatry 2007; 46:1403–1413.

15. Weersing V, Weisz J. Community clinic treatment of depressed youth: benchmarking usual care against CBT clinical trials. J Consult Clin Psychol 2002; 70:299–310.
16. Turnbull M. Return to driving following stroke: prevalence and associated factors [Unpublished masters thesis]. Faculty of Health Sciences. Sydney: The University of Sydney, 2007.
17. Fisk G, Owsley C, Pulley L. Driving after stroke: driving exposure, advice and evaluations. Arch Phys Med Rehabil 1997; 78:1338–1345.
18. Mackintosh S, Goldie P, Hill K. Falls incidence and factors associated with falling in older, community-dwelling, chronic stroke survivors (> 1 year after stroke) and matched controls. Aging Clin Exp Res 2005; 17:74–81.
19. National Stroke Foundation. Clinical guidelines for stroke rehabilitation and recovery. Melbourne, Australia: National Stroke Foundation; 2005.
20. Logan P, Gladman J, Avery A et al. Randomised controlled trial of an occupational therapy intervention to increase outdoor mobility after stroke. BMJ 2004; 329:1372–1377.
21. Logan P, Walker MF, Gladman, J. Description of an occupational therapy intervention aimed at improving outdoor mobility. Br J Occ Ther 2006; 69:2–6.
22. Glasziou P, Haynes B. The paths from research to improved health outcomes. Evid Based Med 2005; 10:4–7.
23. Francis JJ, Eccles MP, Johnstone M et al. Constructing questionnaires based on the theory of planned behaviour: a manual for health services researchers. Newcastle upon Tyne, UK: Centre for Health Services Research, University of Newcastle; 2004.
24. National Institute of Clinical Studies. Evidence–practice gaps report (volumes 1 and 2). Melbourne, Australia: National Institute of Clinical Studies; 2005.
25. National Institute of Clinical Studies. Evidence–practice gaps report, volume 1: a review of developments 2004–2007. Melbourne: National Institute of Clinical Studies; 2008.
26. National Institute for Health and Clinical Excellence. How to change practice: understand, identify and overcome barriers to change. London: National Institute for Health and Clinical Excellence; 2007.
27. National Institute of Clinical Studies. Identifying barriers to evidence uptake. Melbourne, Australia: National Institute of Clinical Studies; 2006.
28. Michie S, Johnston M, Abraham C et al. Making psychological theory useful for implementing evidence based practice: a consensus approach. Qual Saf Health Care 2005; 14:26–33.
29. Verbeek J, Sengers M, Riemens L et al. Patient expectations of treatment for back pain: a systematic review of qualitative and quantitative studies. Spine 2004; 29:2309–2318.
30. Schers H, Wensing M, Huijsmans Z et al. Implementation barriers for general practice guidelines on low back pain: a qualitative study. Spine 2001; 26:E348–E353.
31. Farmer A, Legare F, Turcot K et al. Printed educational materials: effects on professional practice and health care outcomes. Cochrane Database Syst Rev 2008; 3: Art. No.: CD004398. DOI: 10.1002/14651858.CD004398.pub2.
32. Grimshaw J, Eccles M, Thomas R et al. Toward evidence-based quality improvement: evidence (and its limitations) of the effectiveness of guideline dissemination and implementation strategies 1966–1998. J Gen Intern Med 2006; 21:S14–S20.
33. Thompson O'Brien M, Freemantle N, Oxman A et al. Continuing education meetings and workshops: effects on professional practice and health care outcomes. Cochrane Database Syst Rev 2001; 1: Art.No.: CD003030. DOI: 10.1002/14651858.CD003030.
34. Zwarenstein M, Bheekie A, Lombard C et al. Educational outreach to general practitioners reduces children's asthma symptoms: a cluster randomised controlled trial. Implement Sci 2007; 2:30.
35. O'Brien M, Rogers S, Jamtvedt G et al. Educational outreach visits: effects on professional practice and health care outcomes. Cochrane Database Syst Rev 2007; 4: Art. No.: CD000409. DOI: 10.1002/14651858. CD000409.pub2.
36. Stetler C, Legro M, Rycroft-Malone J et al. Role of 'external facilitation' in implementation of research findings: a qualitative evaluation of facilitation experiences in the Veterans Health Administration. Implement Sci 2006; 1:23.
37. Foy R, Hawthorne G, Gibb I et al. A cluster randomised controlled trial of educational prompts in diabetes care: Study protocol. Implement Sci 2007; 2:22.
38. Grimshaw J, Eccles M, Matowe L et al. Effectiveness and efficiency of guideline dissemination and implementation strategies. Health Technol Assess 2004; 8:1–72.

39. Jamtvedt G, Young J, Kristoffersen D et al. Audit and feedback: effects on professional practice and health care outcomes. Cochrane Database Syst Rev 2006; 2: Art. No.: CD000259. DOI: 10.1002/14651858. CD000259.pub2.
40. Jamtvedt G, Young J, Kristoffersen D et al. Does telling people what they have been doing change what they do? A systematic review of the effects of audit and feedback. Qual Saf Health Care 2006; 15:433–436.
41. Shaw B, Cheater F, Baker R et al. Tailored interventions to overcome identified barriers to change: effects on professional practice and health care outcomes. Cochrane Database Syst Rev 2005; 3: Art. No CD005470. DOI: 10.1002/14651858. CD005470. pub2.
42. Wright J, Bibby J, Eastham J et al. Multifaceted implementation of stroke prevention guidelines in primary care: cluster-randomised evaluation of clinical and cost effectiveness. Qual Saf Health Care 2007; 16:51–59.
43. Bero L, Grilli R, Grimshaw J et al. Closing the gap between research and practice: an overview of systematic reviews of interventions to promote the implementation of research findings. BMJ 1998; 317:465–468.
44. Grimshaw J, Shirran L, Thomas R et al. Changing provider behaviour: an overview of systematic reviews of interventions. Med Care 2001; 39:II2–45.
45. Dijkstra R, Braspenning J, Huijsmans Z et al. Introduction of diabetes passports involving both patients and professionals to improve hospital outpatient diabetes care. Diabetes Res Clin Pract 2005; 68:126–134.
46. Dijkstra R, Braspenning J, Grol R. Implementing diabetes passports to focus practice reorganisation on improving diabetes care. Int J Qual Health Care 2008; 20:72–77.
47. Adams AS. Evidence of self-report bias in assessing adherence to guidelines. Int J Qual Health Care 1999; 11:187–192.
48. Ceccato N, Ferris L, Manuel D et al. Adopting health behaviour change theory through the clinical practice guideline process. J Contin Educ Health Prof 2007; 27:201–207.
49. Grol R, Wensing M, Hulscher M et al. Theories of implementation of change in healthcare. In: Grol R, Wensing M, Eccles M (eds). Improving patient care: the implementation of change in clinical practice. Edinburgh: Elsevier Butterworth–Heinemann; 2005:15–40.
50. Bowman J, Lannin N, Cook C et al. Development and psychometric testing of the Clinician Readiness for Measuring Outcomes Scale (CReMOS). J Eval Clin Pract. 2009; 15:76–84.
51. Rogers EM. Diffusion of innovations. 4th edn. New York: Free Press; 1995.
52. Prochaska JO, DiClemente CC. In search of how people change: applications to addictive behaviours. Am Psychol 1992; 47:1102–1114.
53. Reisma RP, Pattenden J, Bridle C et al. A systematic review of the effectiveness of interventions based on a stages of change approach to promote individual behaviour change. Health Technol Assess 2002; 6:1–243.
54. Greenhalgh T, Robert G, Macfarlane F et al. Diffusion of innovations in service organisations: systematic review and recommendations. Milbank Q 2004; 82:581–629.
55. McCluskey A, Lovarini M. Providing education on evidence-based practice improved knowledge but did not change behaviour: a before and after study. BMC Med Educ 2005; 5:40.
56. McCluskey A, Home S, Thompson L. Becoming an evidence-based practitioner. In: Law M, MacDermid J (eds). Evidence-based rehabilitation: a guide to practice. 2nd edn. Thorofare, NJ: Slack; 2008:35–60.
57. Ajzen I. The theory of planned behaviour. Organ Behav Hum Decis Process 1991; 50:179–211.
58. Eccles M, Hrisos S, Francis J et al. Do self-reported intentions predict clinicians' behaviour: a systematic review. Implement Sci 2006; 1:28.

Index

➡

Note: Page numbers followed by b, f, and t indicate boxes, figures, and tables, respectively.